INTRODUCTION

Welcome to the world of the most demanding puzzles.

This book is full of the challenging, mind-bending mazes for all the hard puzzle lovers. You can push your maze skills to the limits by confronting yourself to some of the most advanced labyrinths out there. This awesome book has been created for all the ladies that want to test their maze solving abilities.

You will find here various kinds and shapes of puzzles, some of them accompanied by little funny drawings. The cell sizes and difficulty increase as you progress in the book

Note: There is no solution key to the mazes in this book. You will either solve them or give up.
Starting point are mostly on the top and bottom sides, sometimes they are marked, sometimes no. Just keep your eye out.

The mazes are appropriate for all the girls and women that love puzzle challenges
There are 6 levels of difficulty starting from intermediate to expert.
Your persistence and brilliance will be put to the ultimate test. Do you feel you have what it takes to become a master maze puzzler? Believe me, if you can solve all these mazes you are a puzzle champion.

If you like the book please type a short review. We would do appreciate that.

We would be grateful if you see our other products including cute notebooks, journals, planners and more, on Amazon, typing **Orex Publishing Group** in the search bar. You are very welcome to visit as on Instagram, Pinterest on Facebook.

Thank you for your purchase.

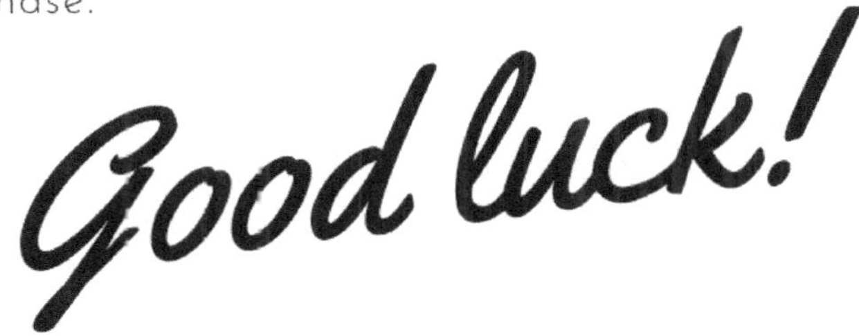

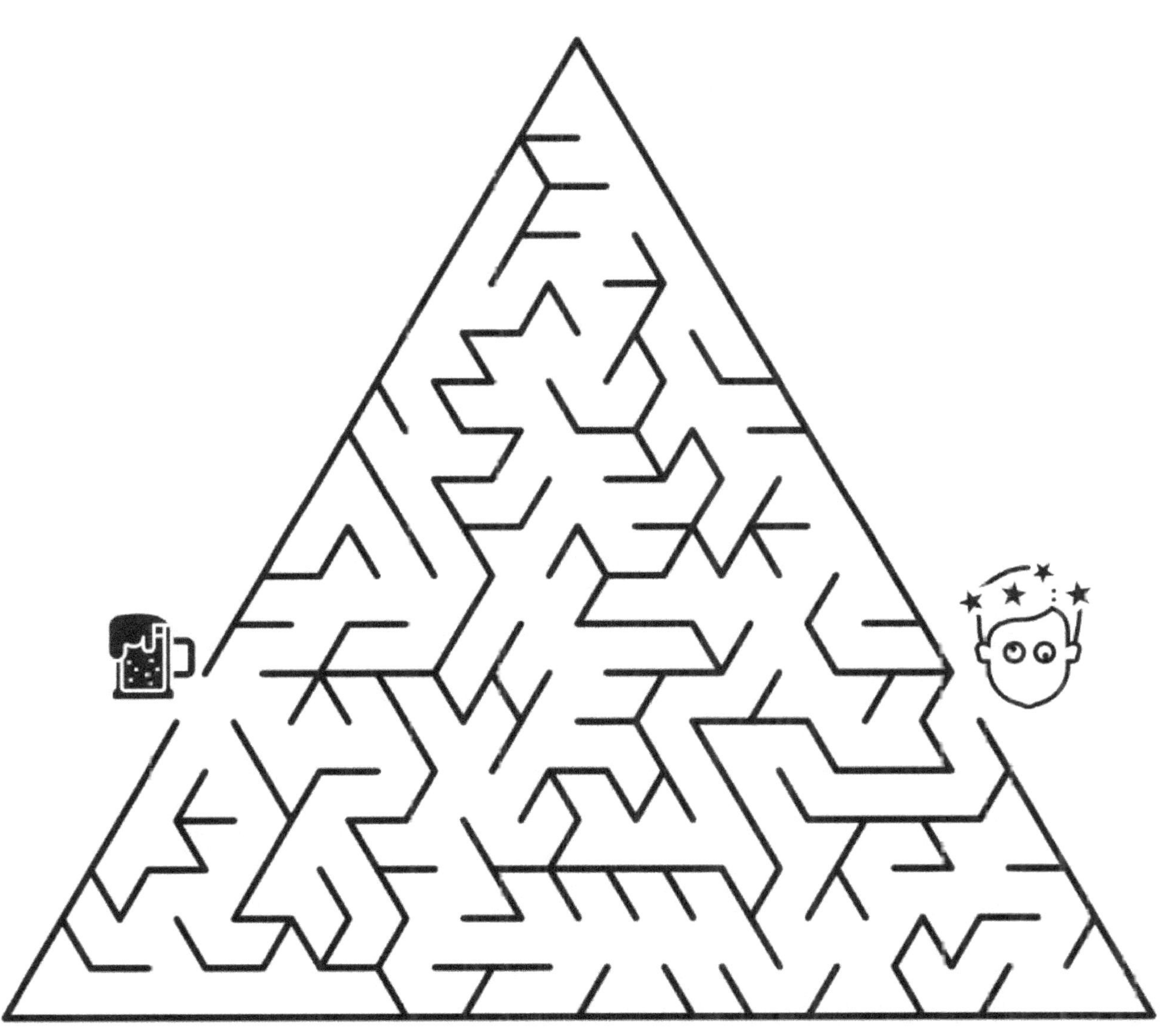

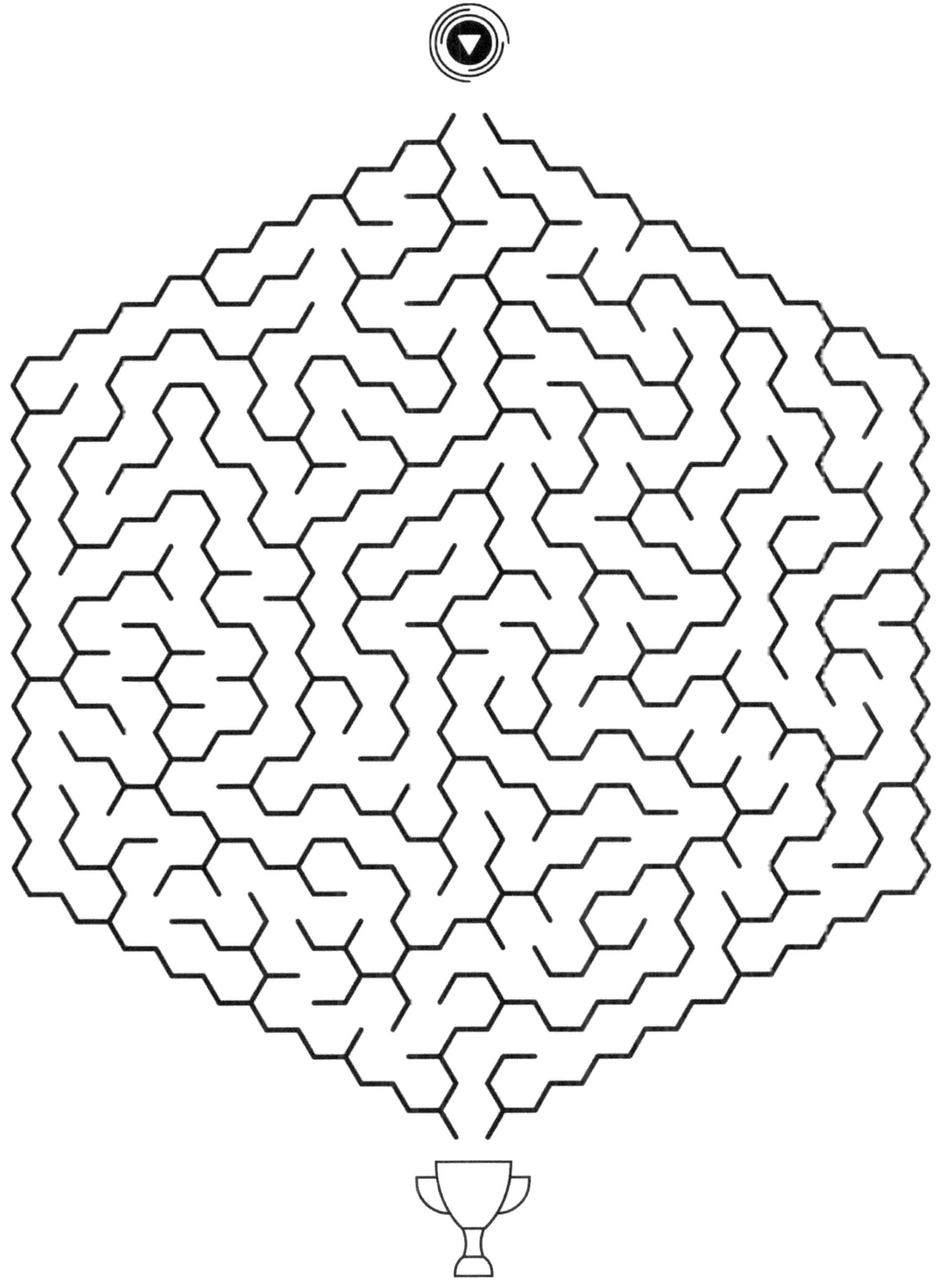

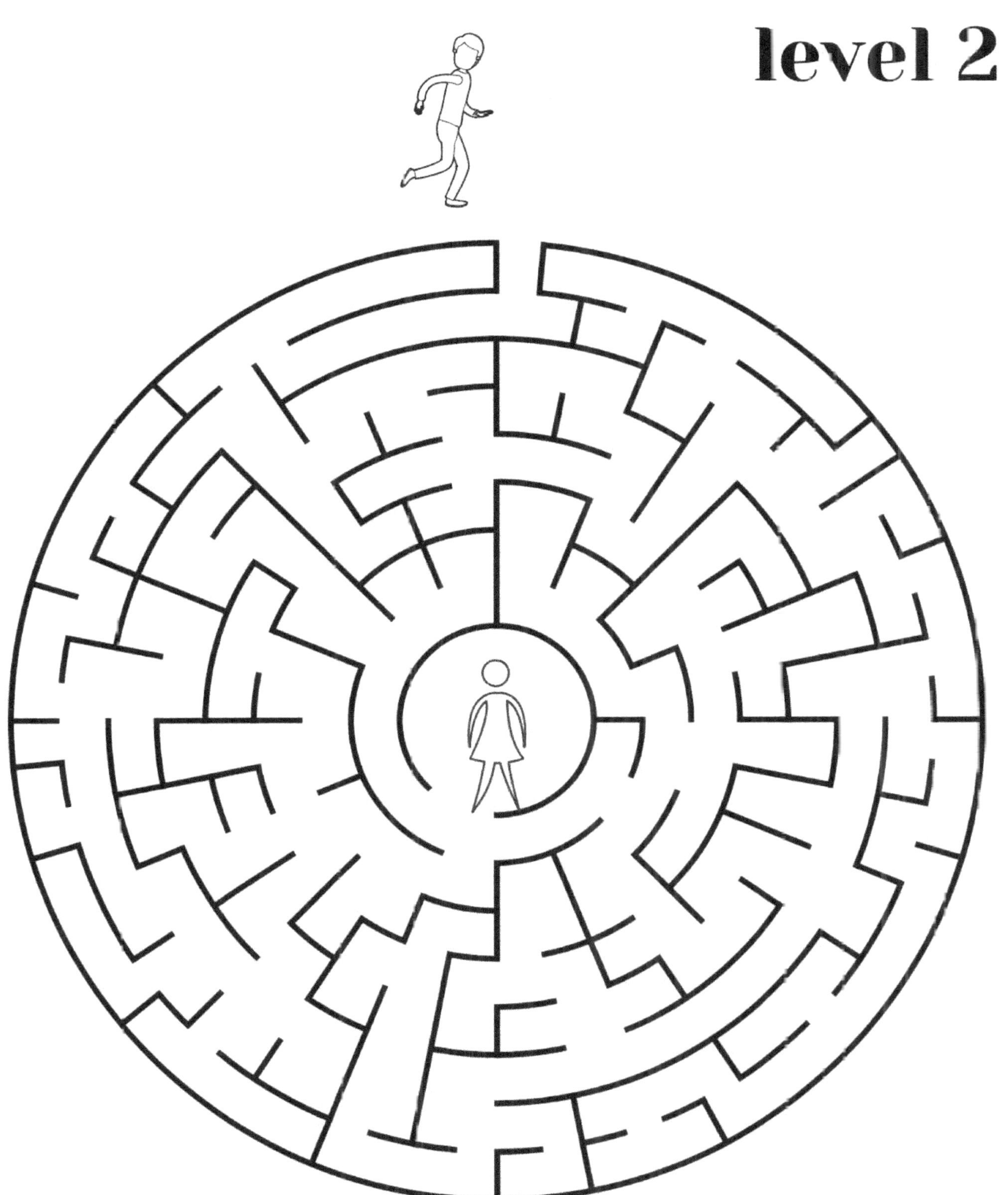

level 2

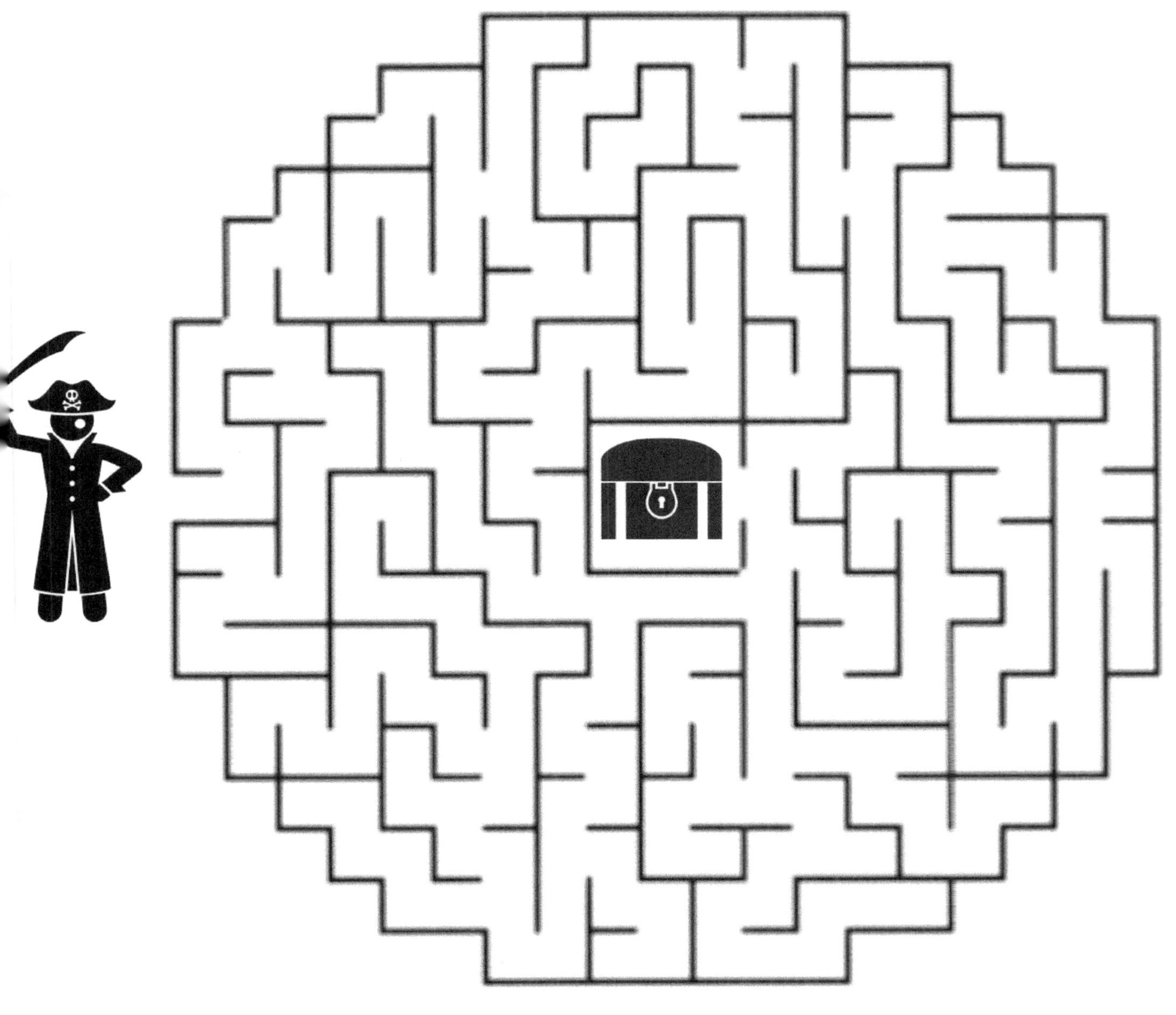

level 2

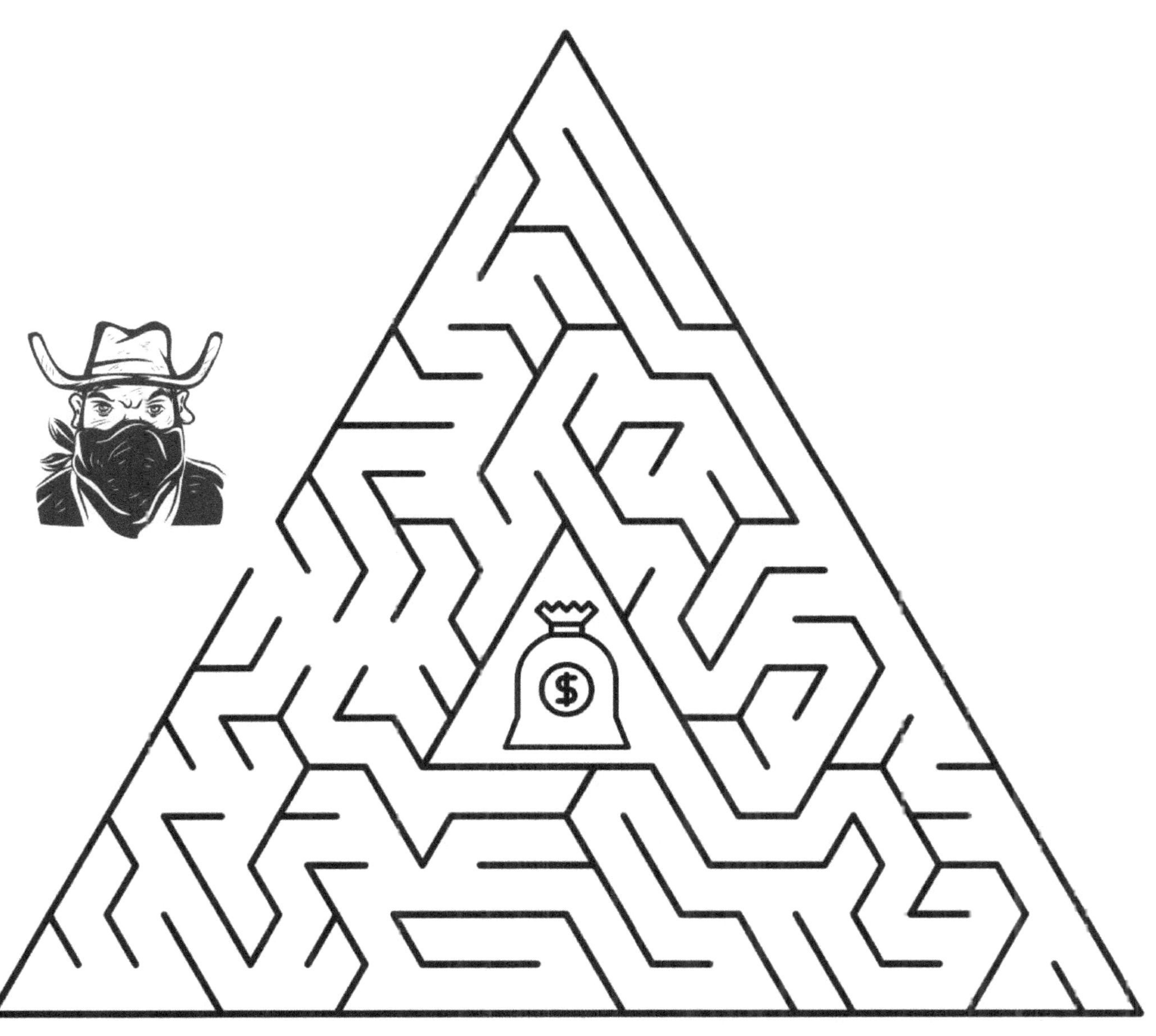

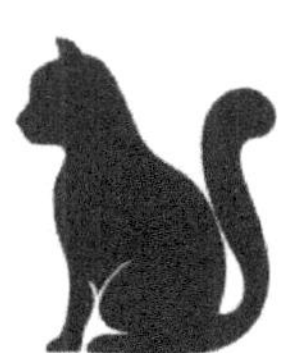

level 3

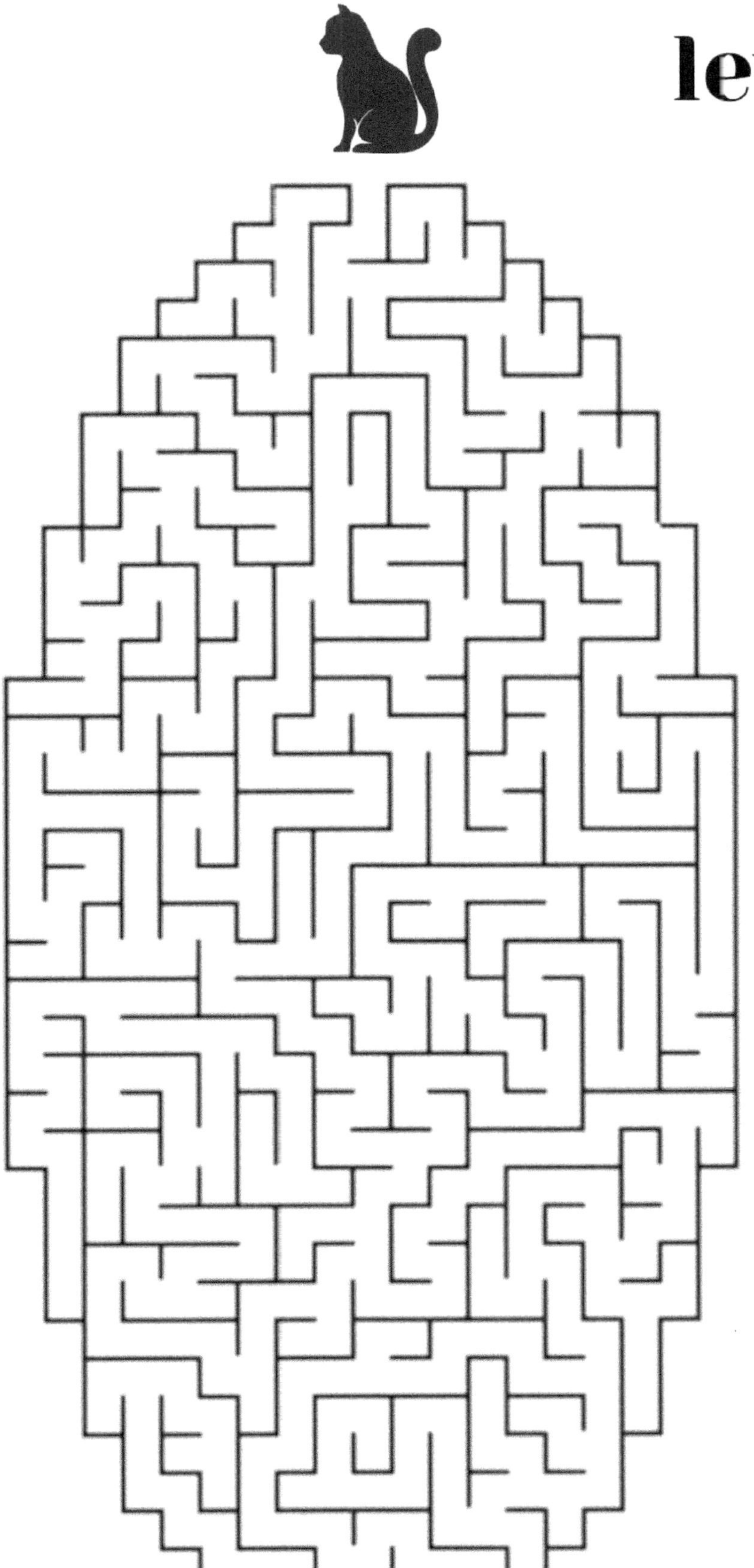

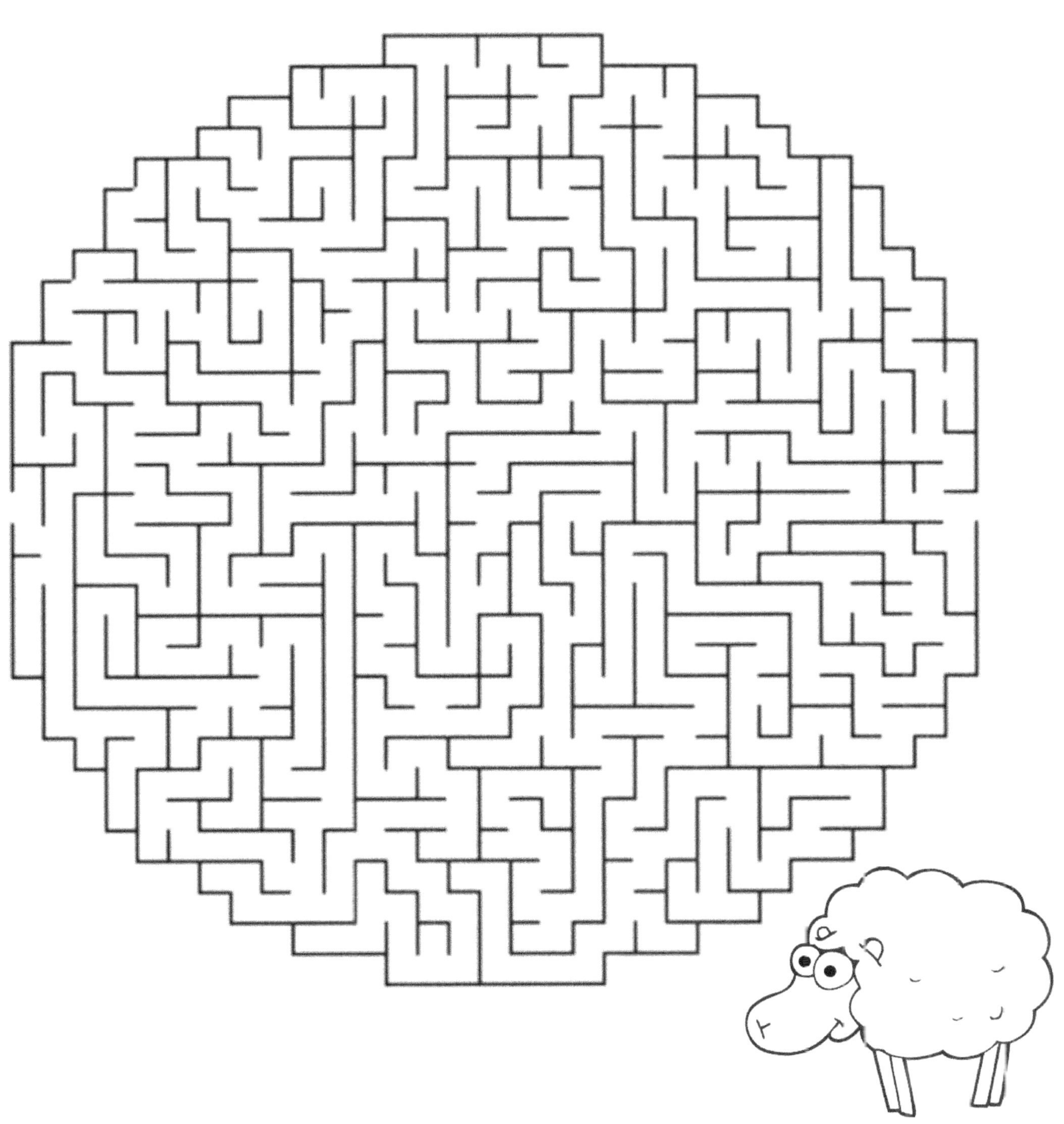

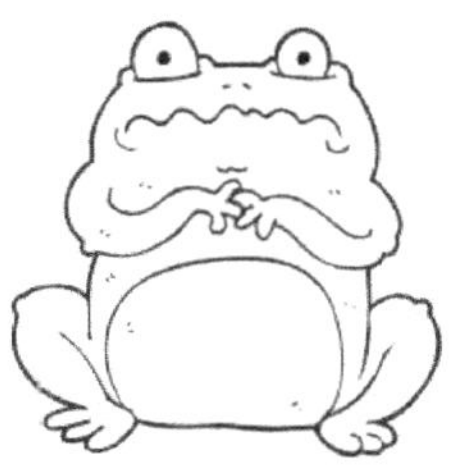

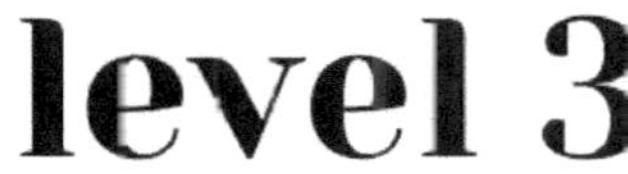

level 3

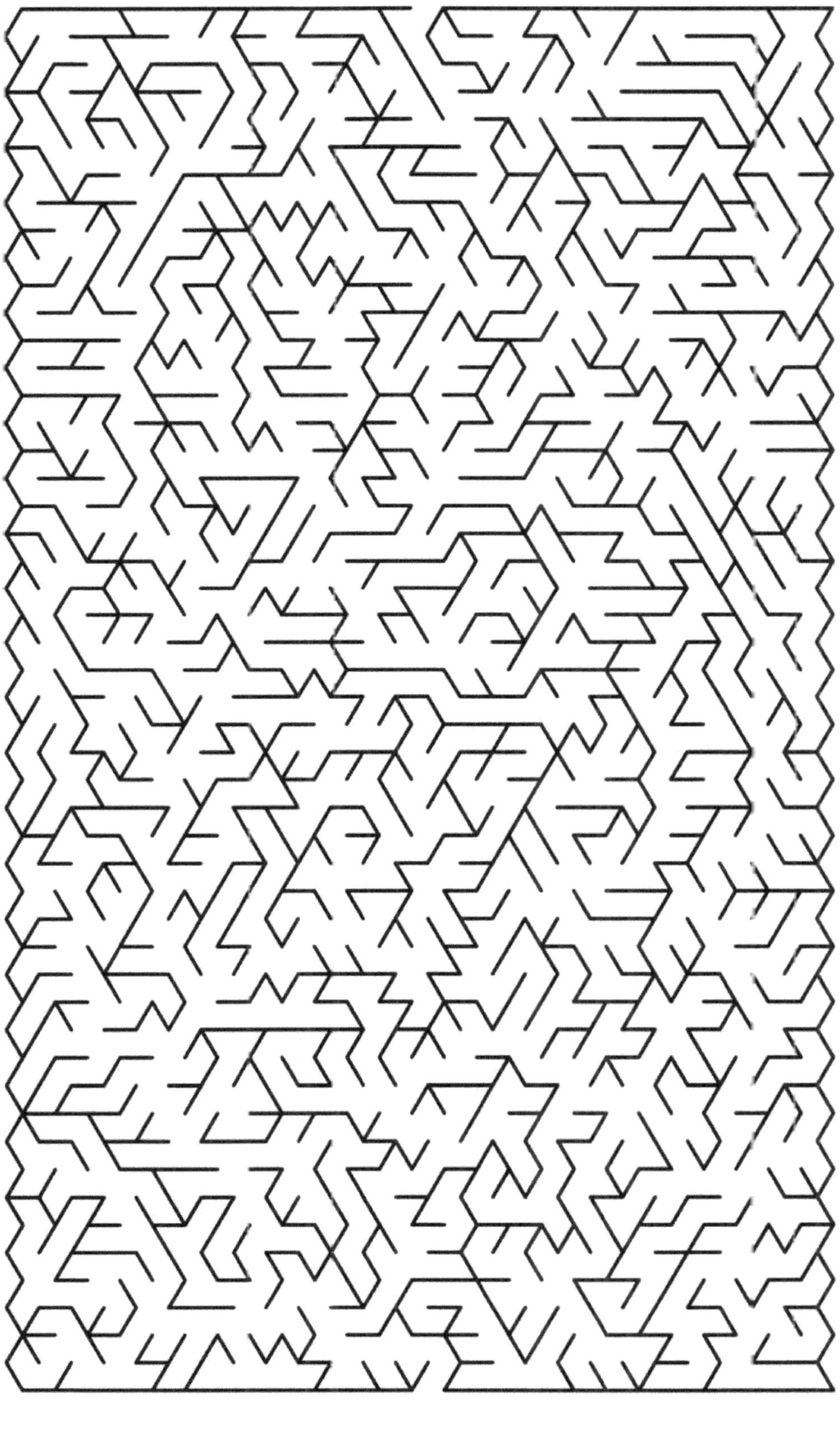

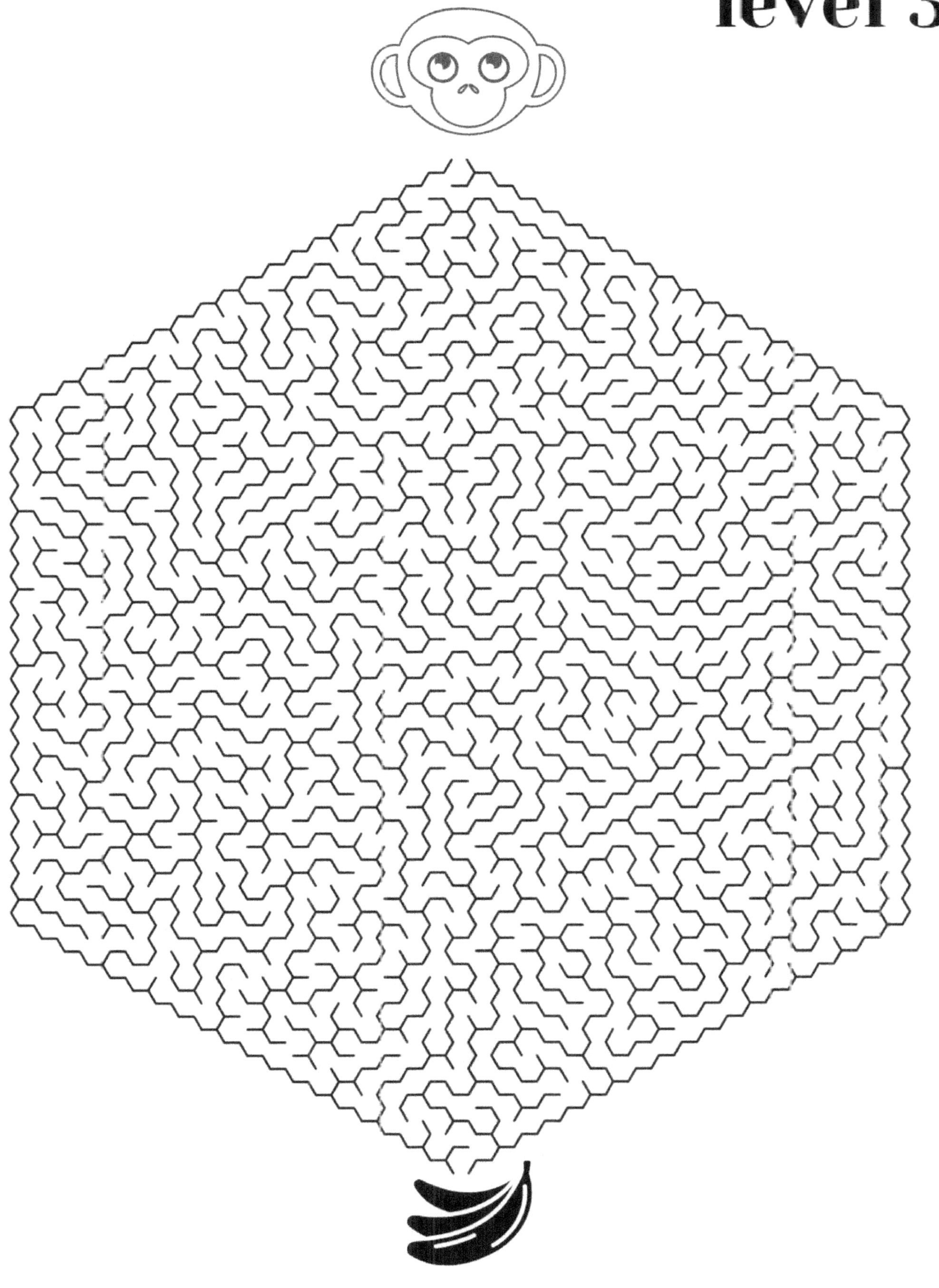

level 3

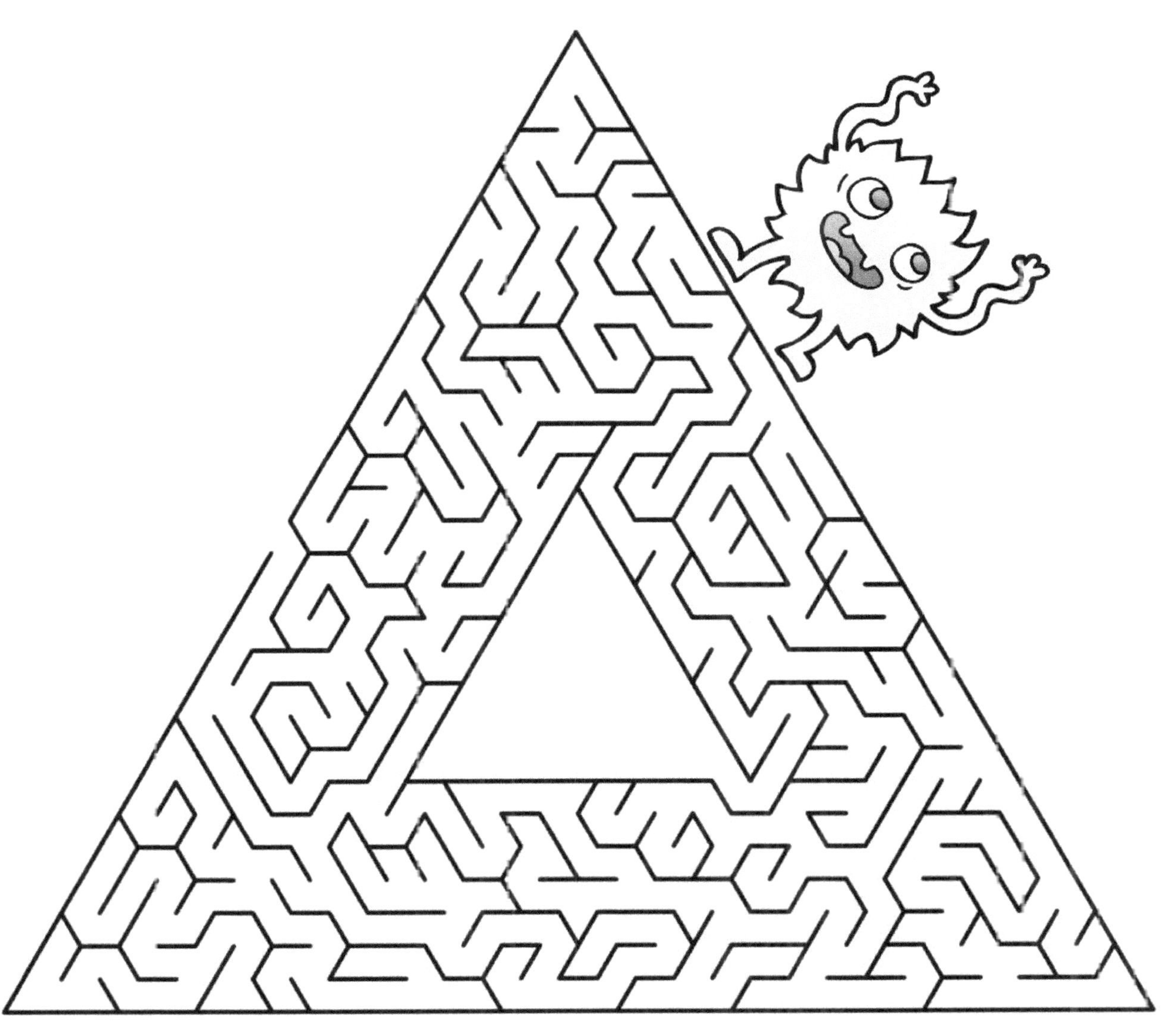

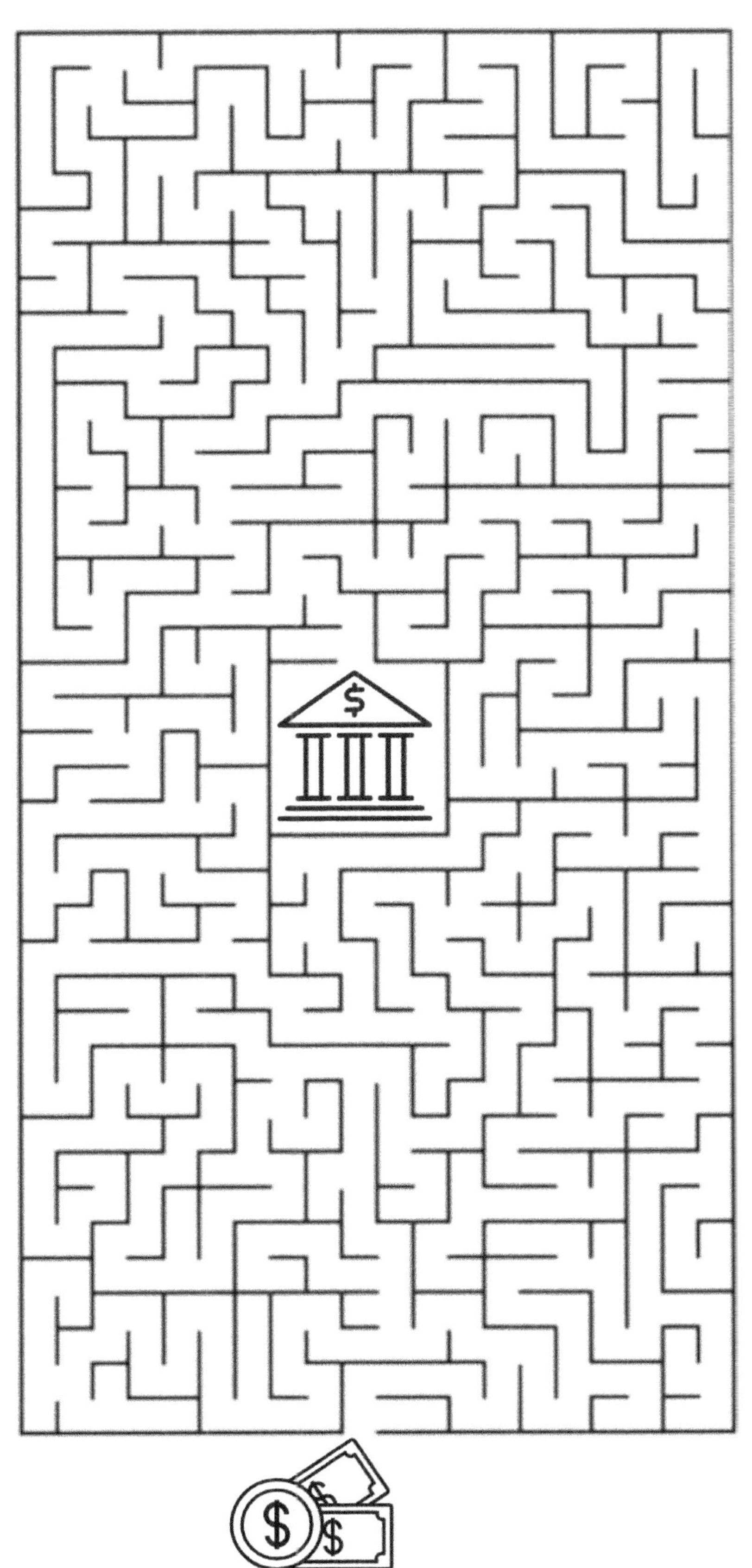

level 3

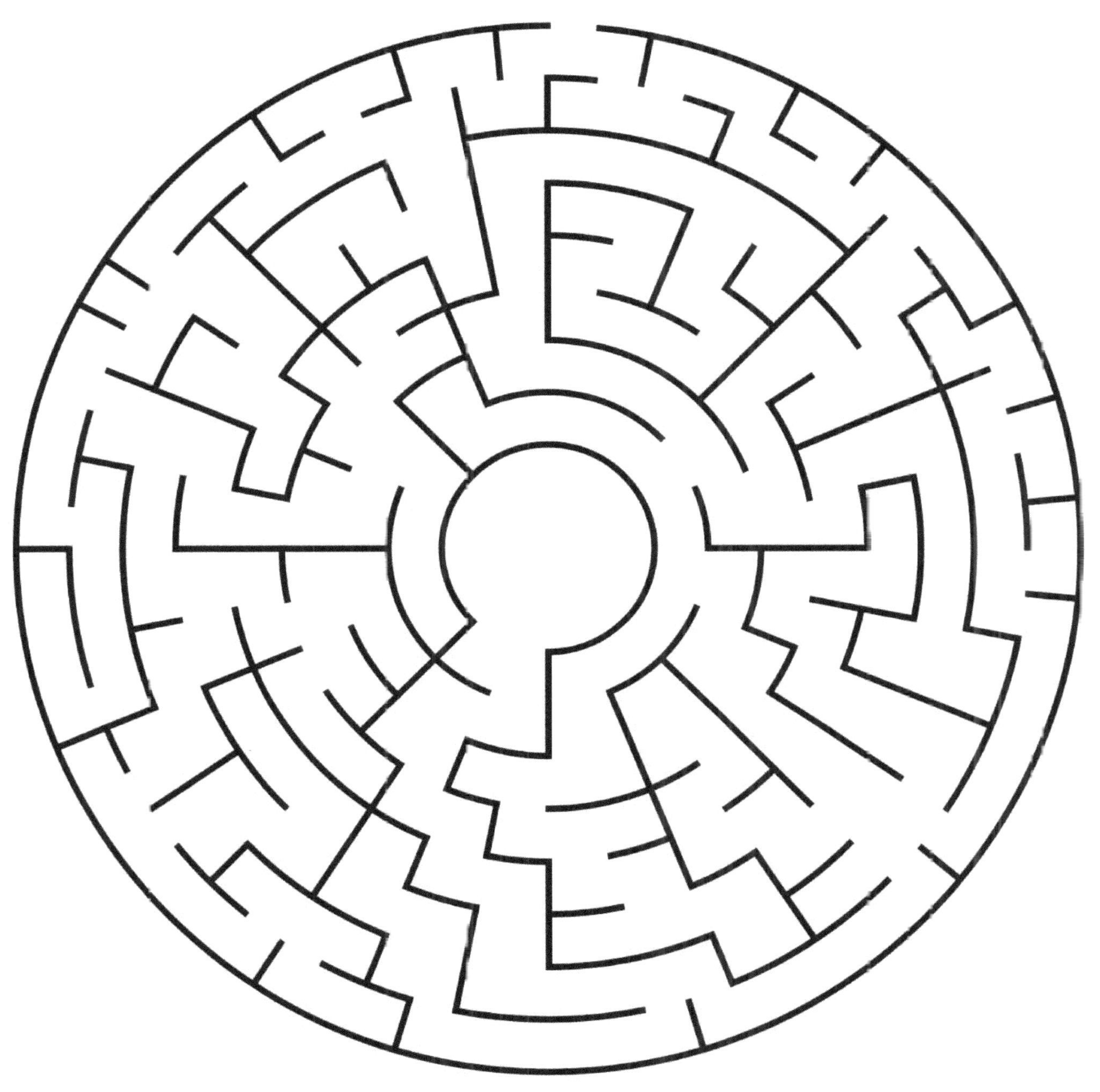

YOUR MIND IS A MAZE OF POSSIBILITIES.
DON'T GET LOST

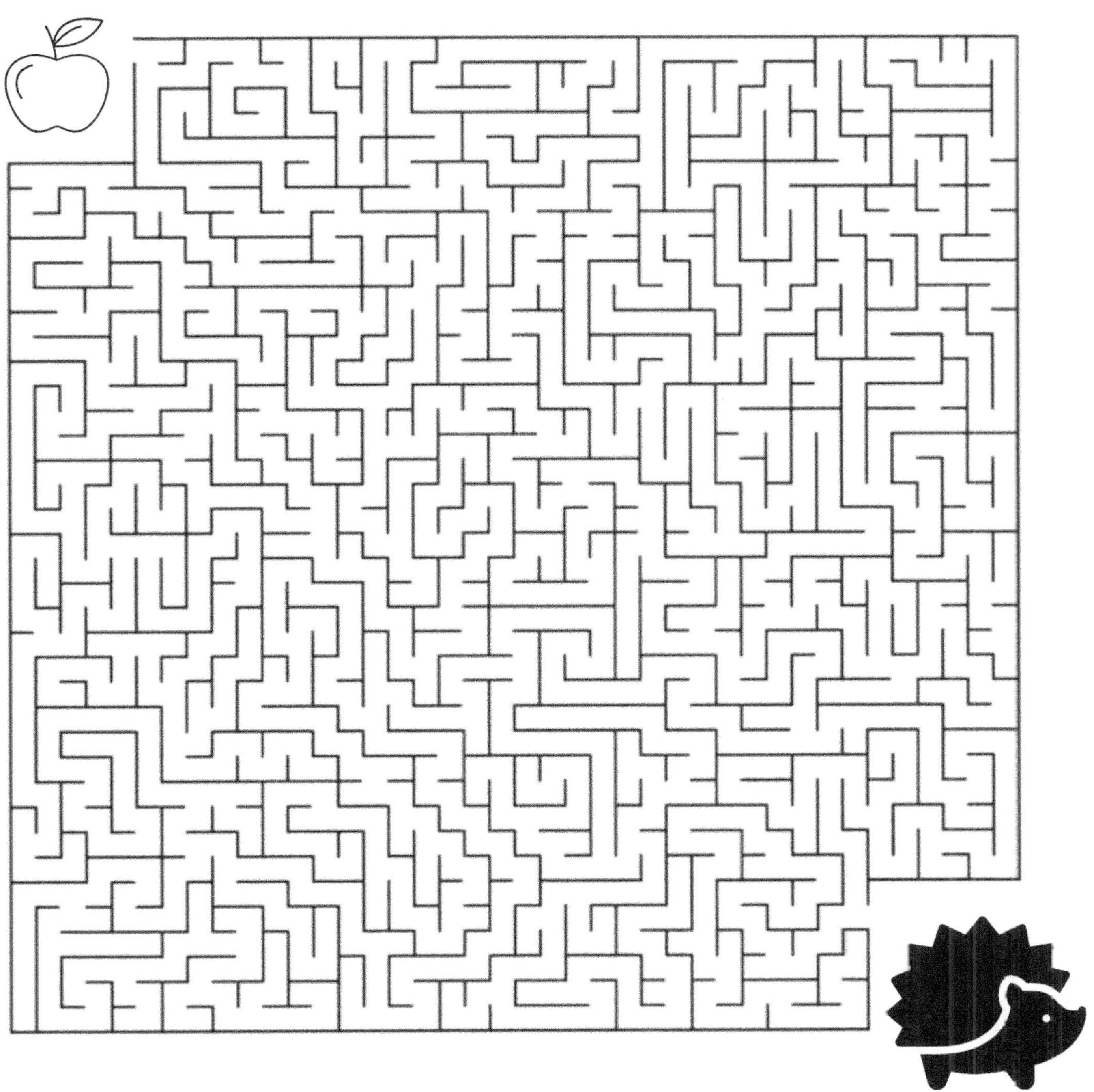

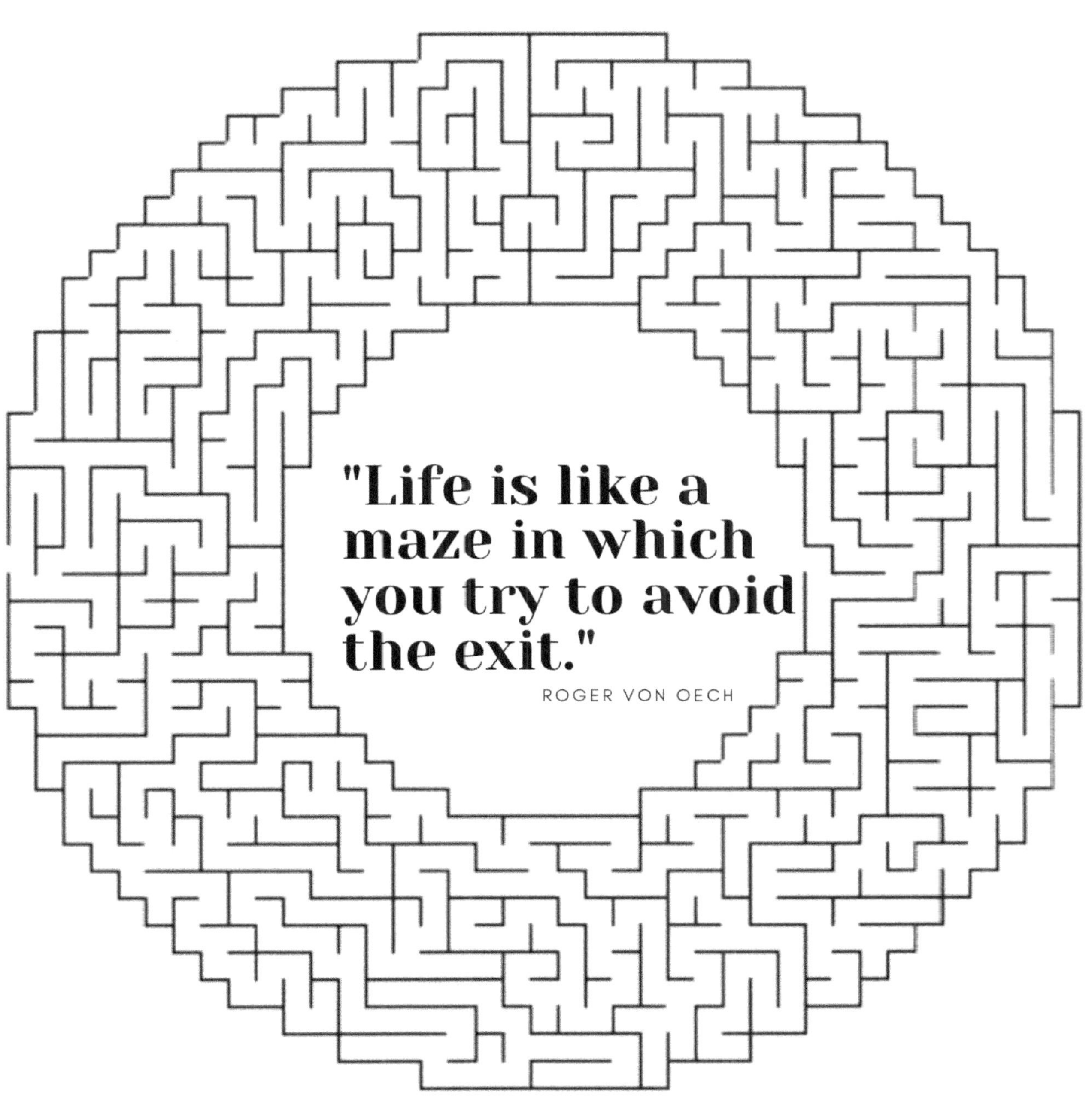
"Life is like a
maze in which
you try to avoid
the exit."
ROGER VON OECH

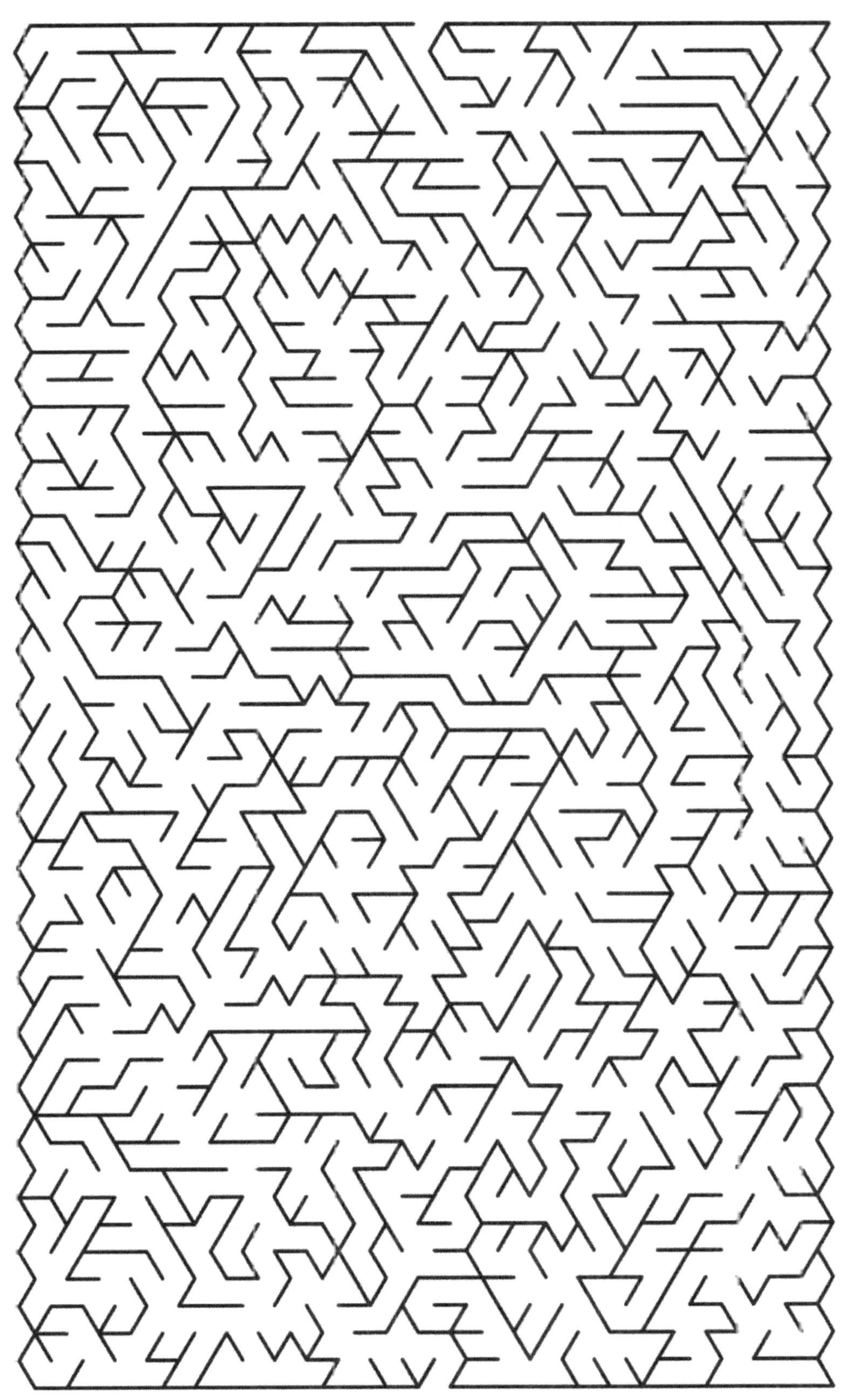

level 4

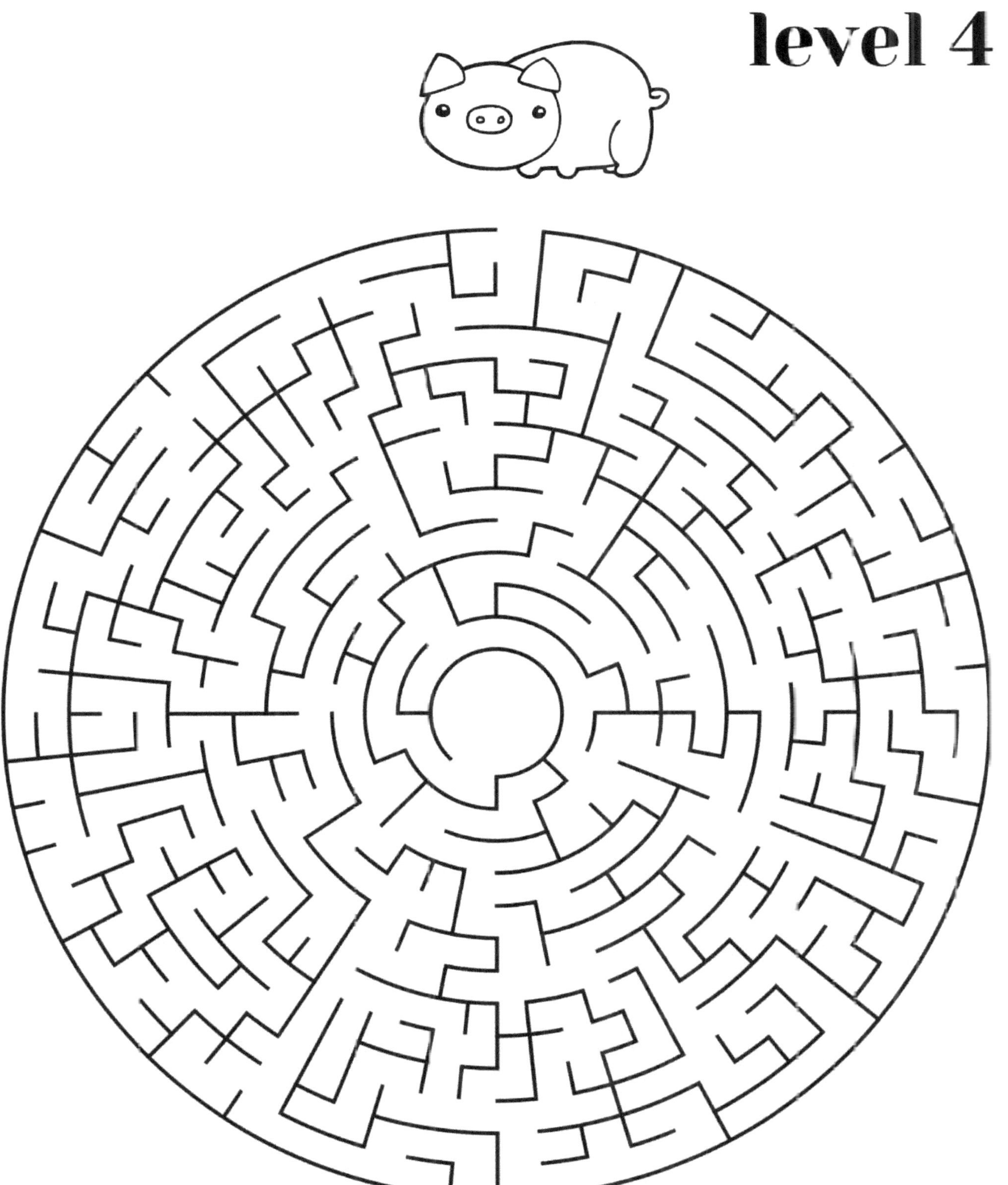

level 4

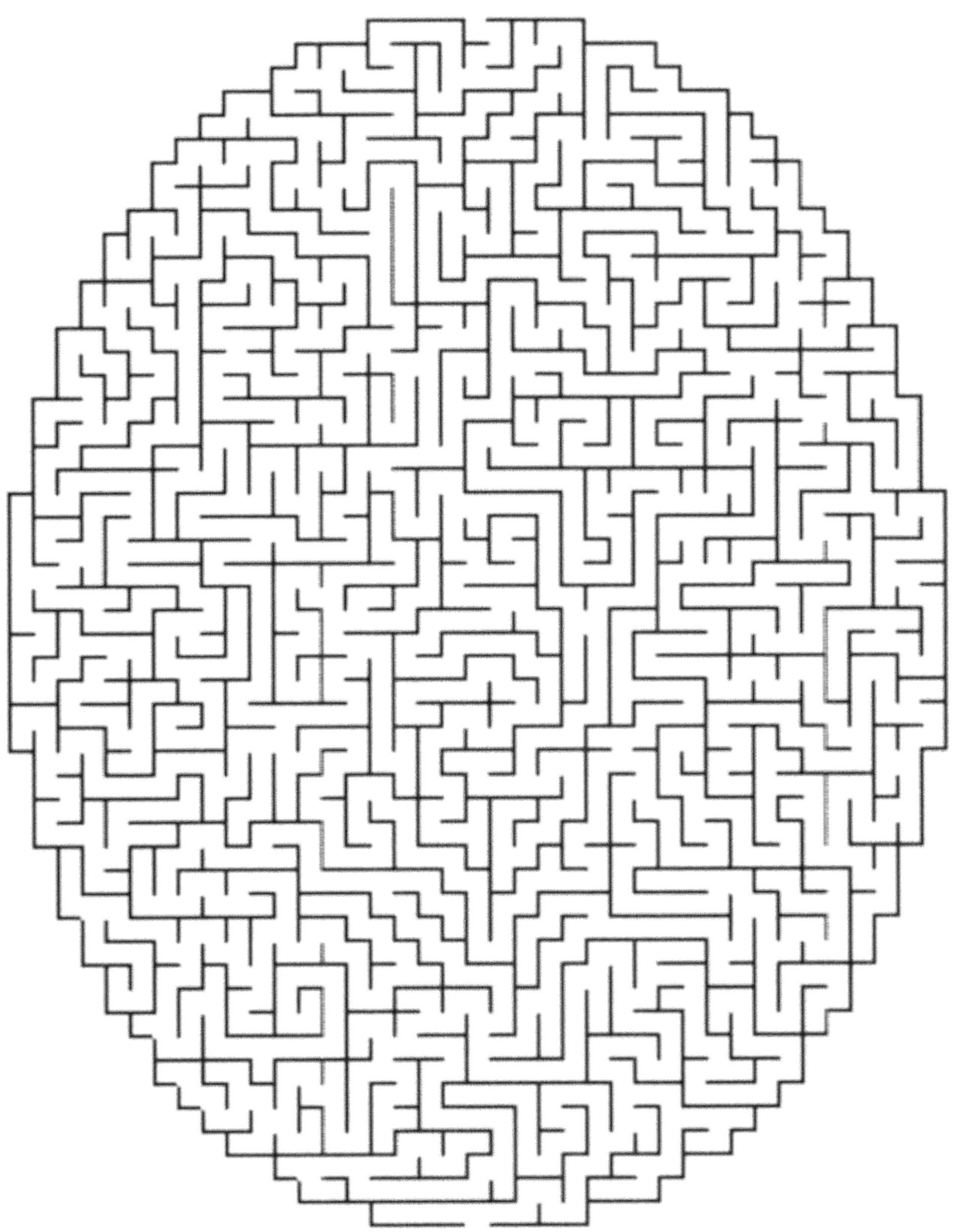

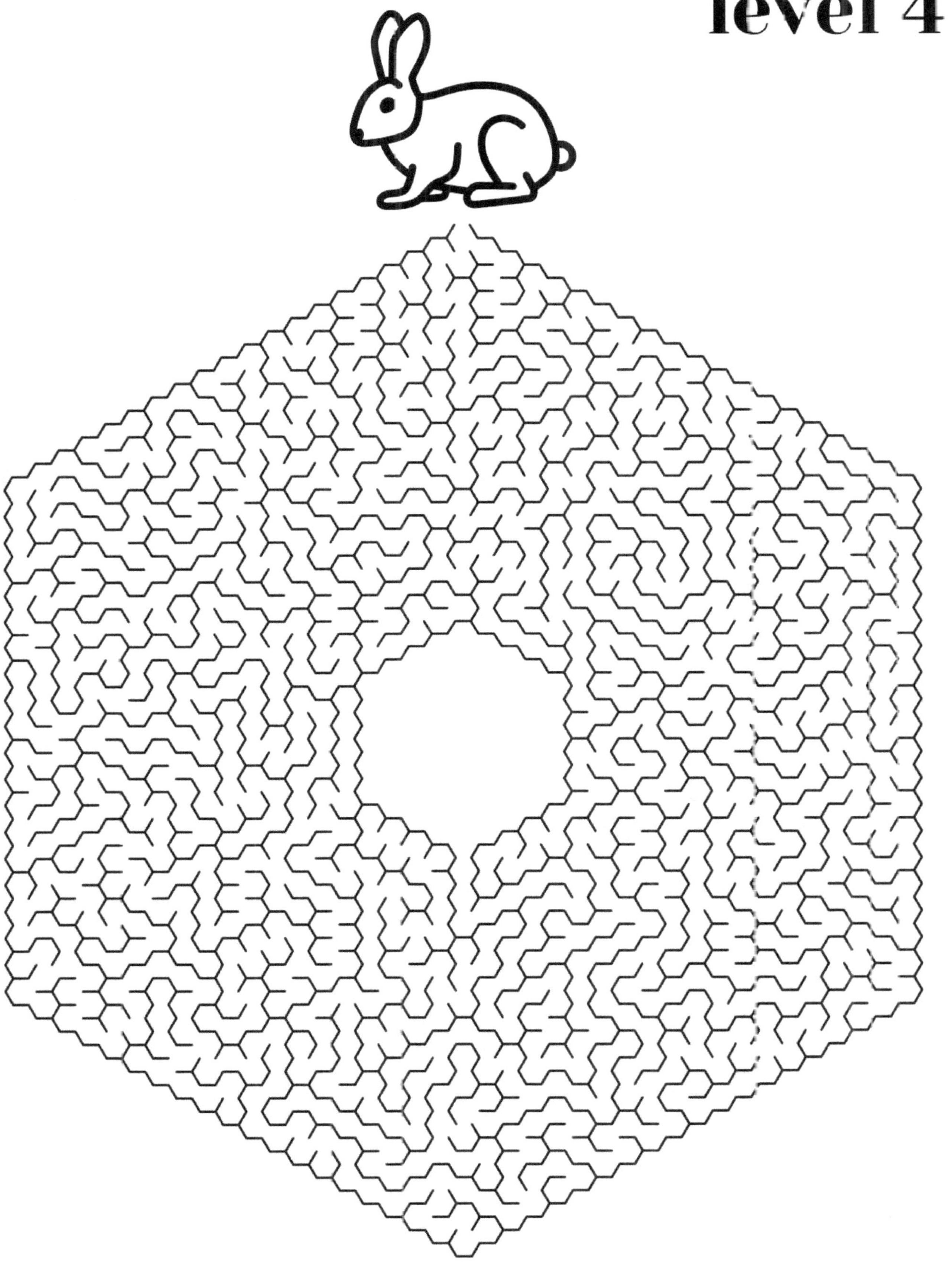

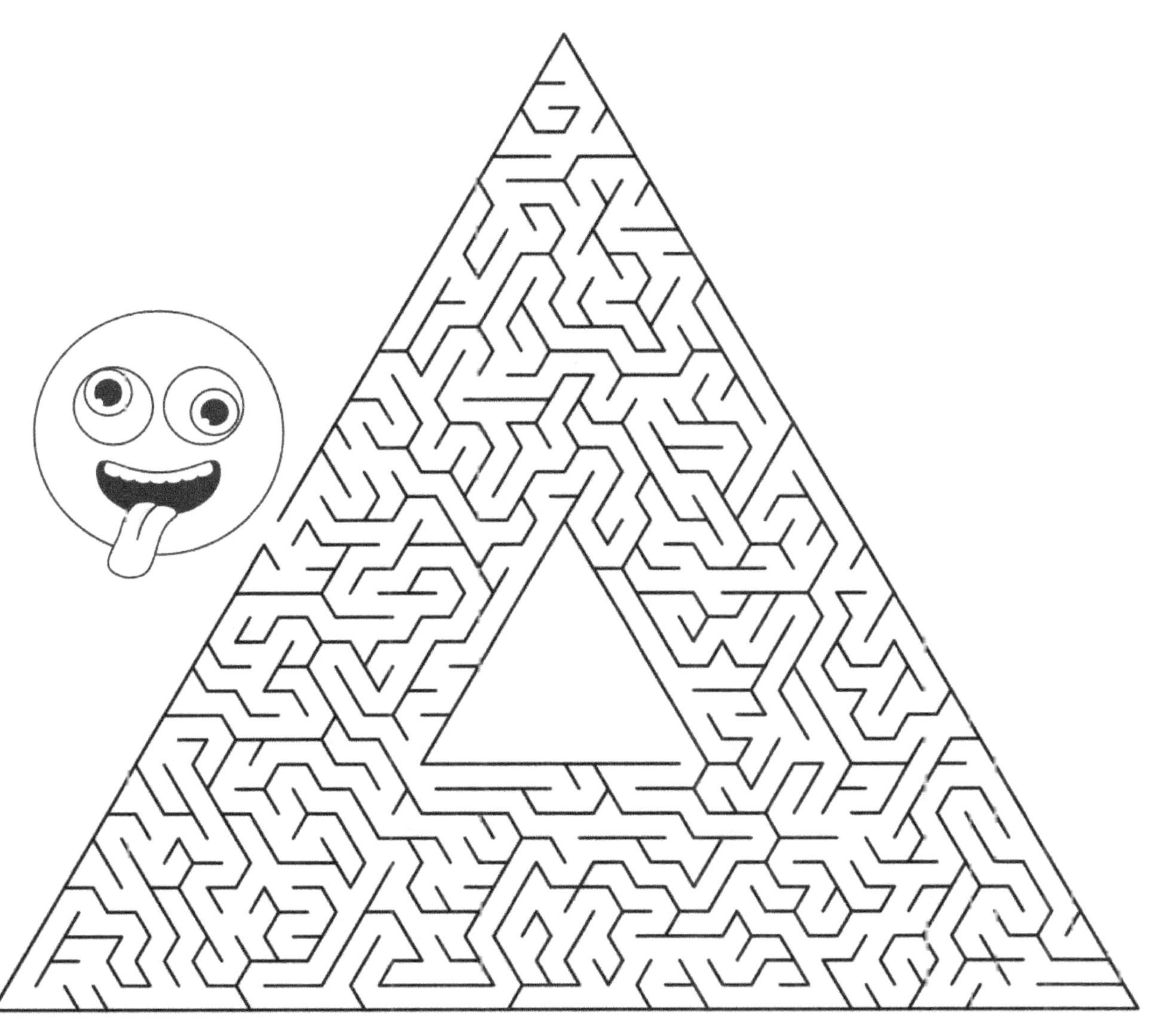

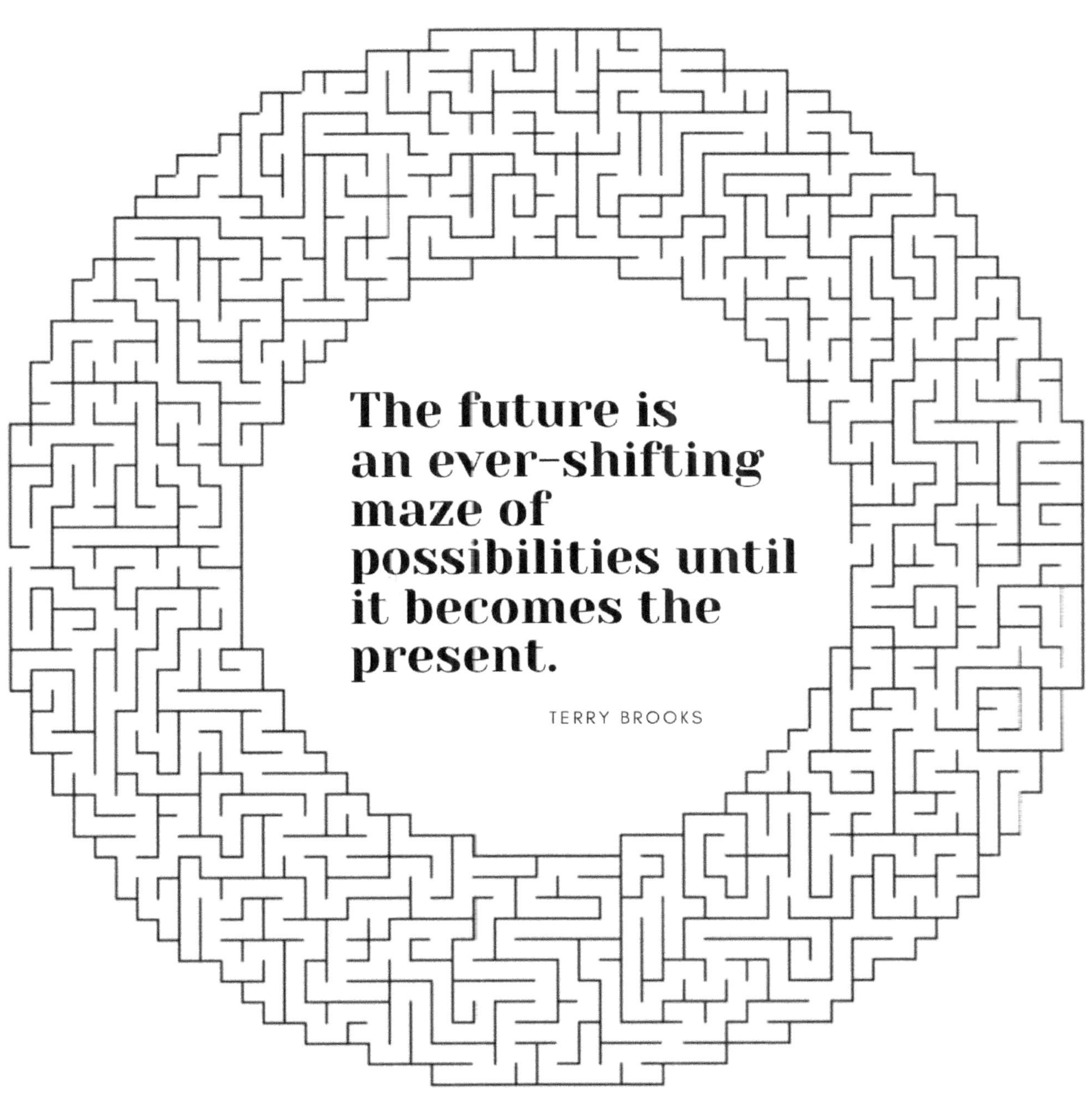
The future is
an ever-shifting
maze of
possibilities until
it becomes the
present.

TERRY BROOKS

level 5

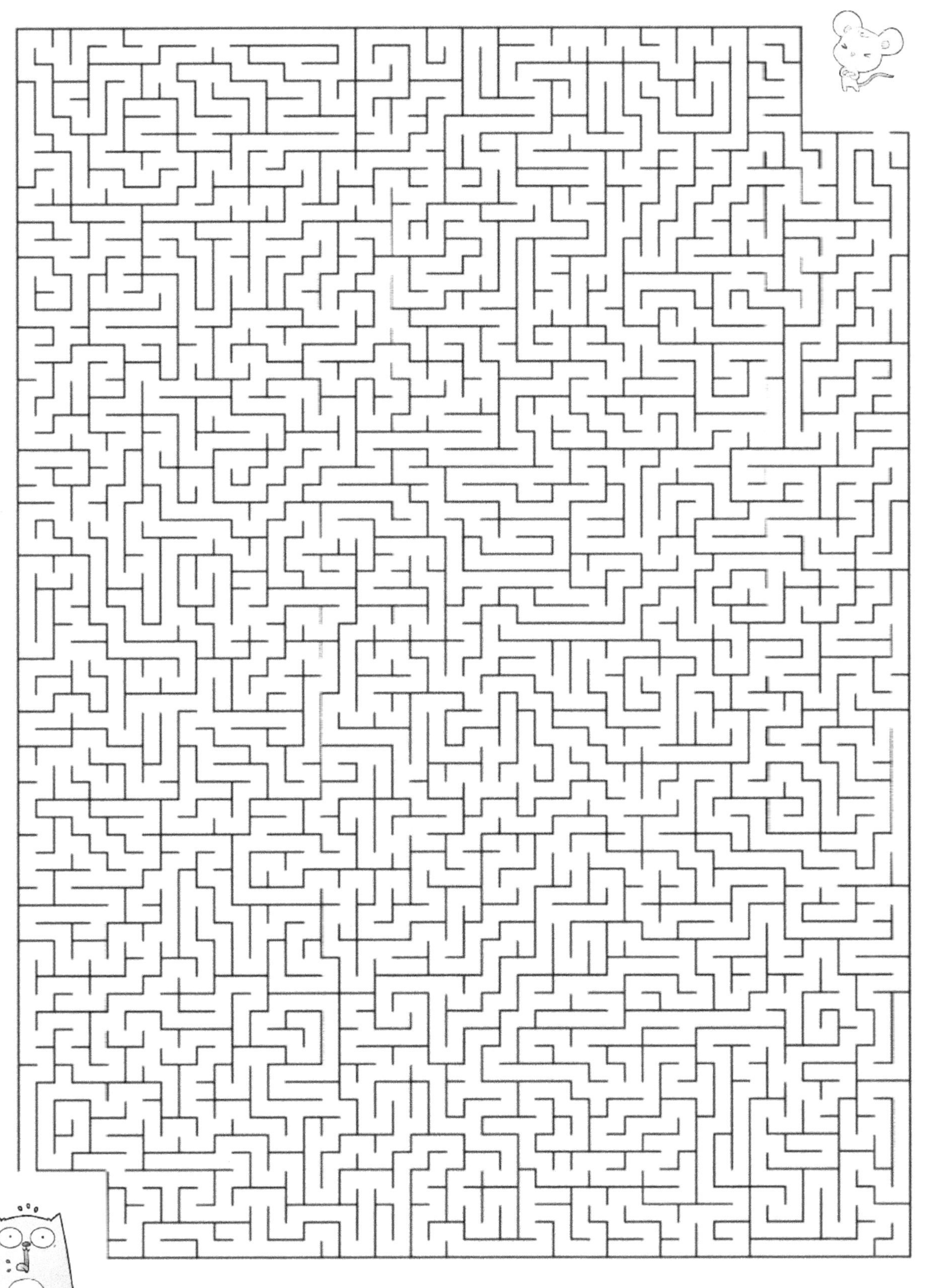

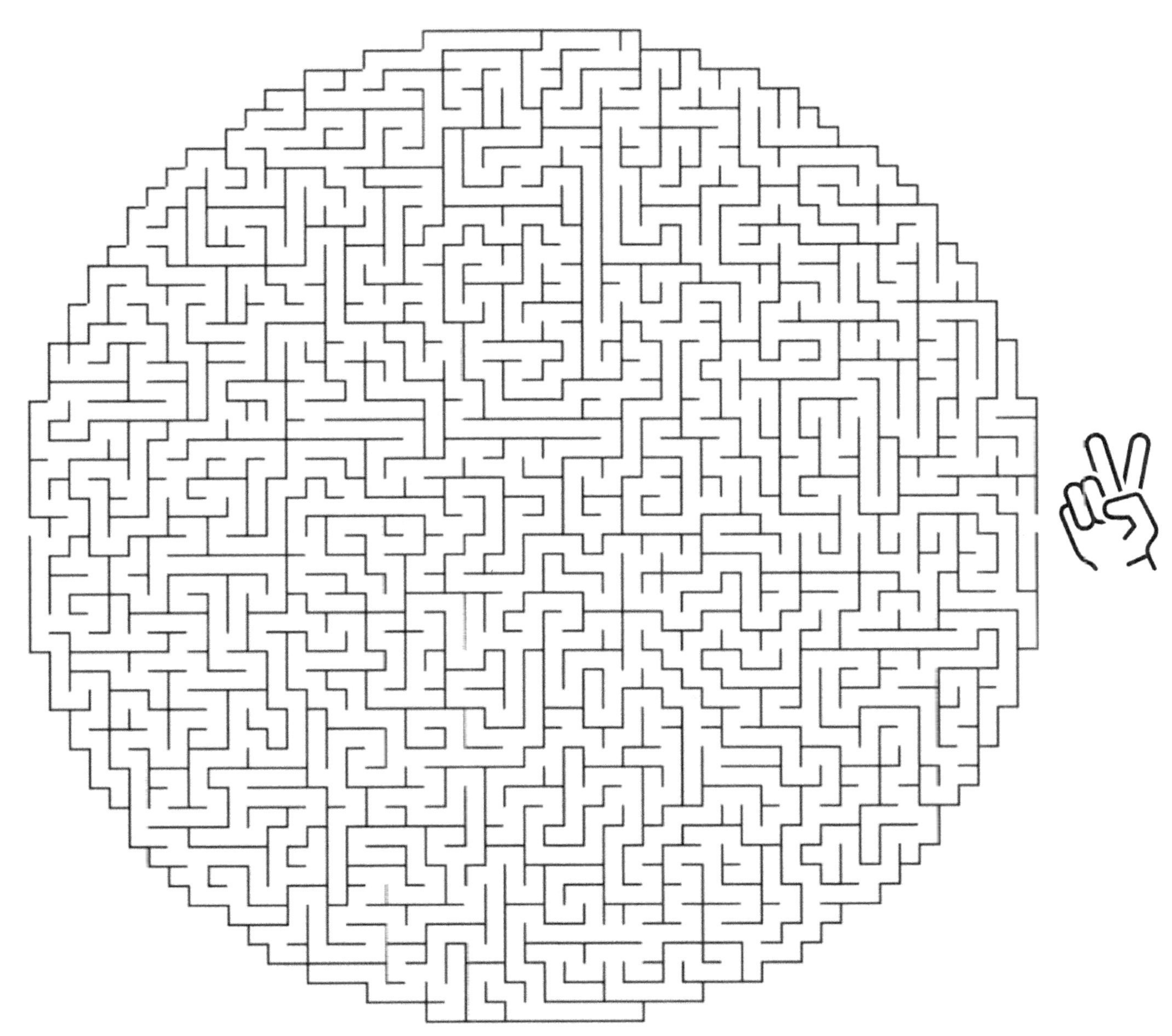

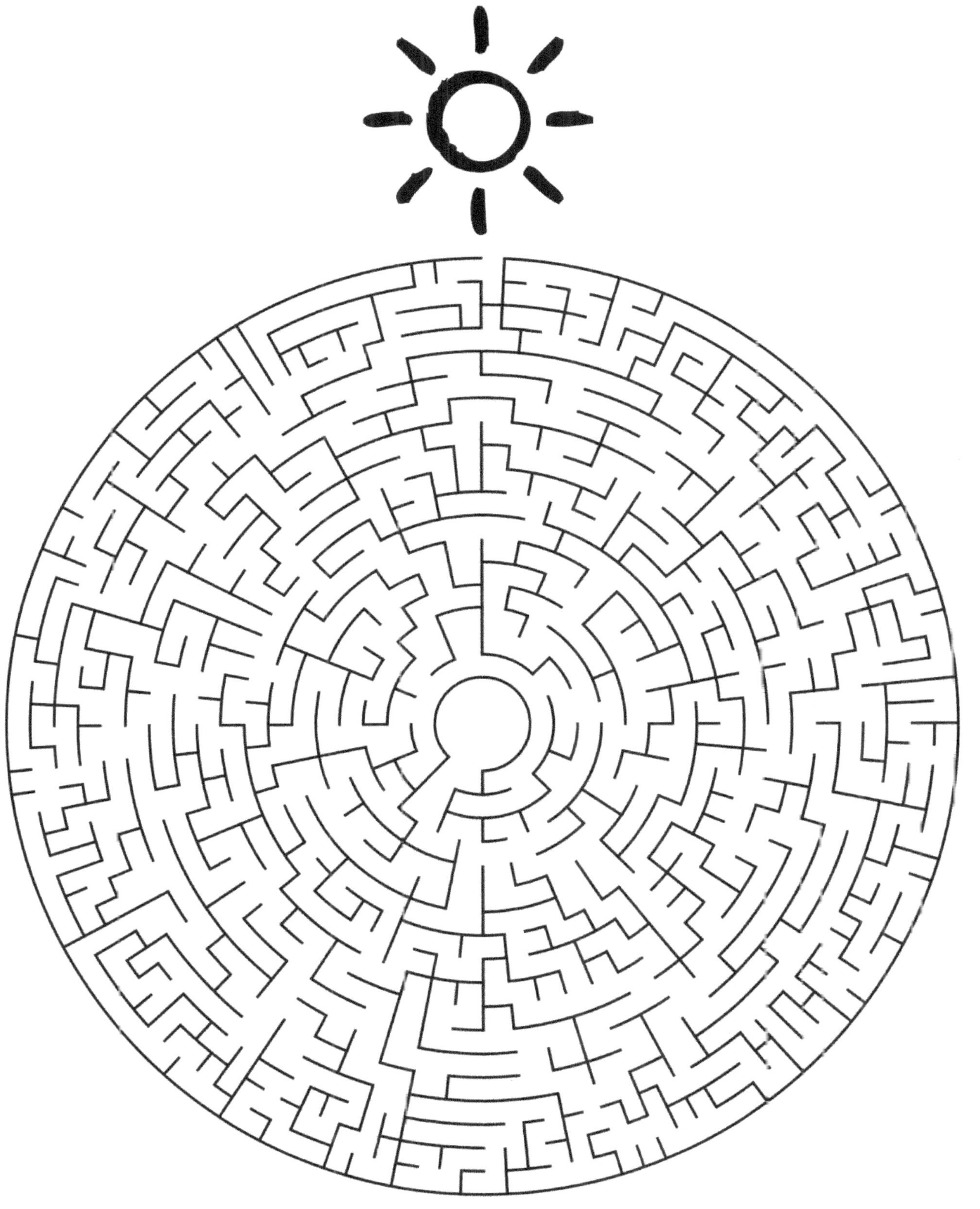

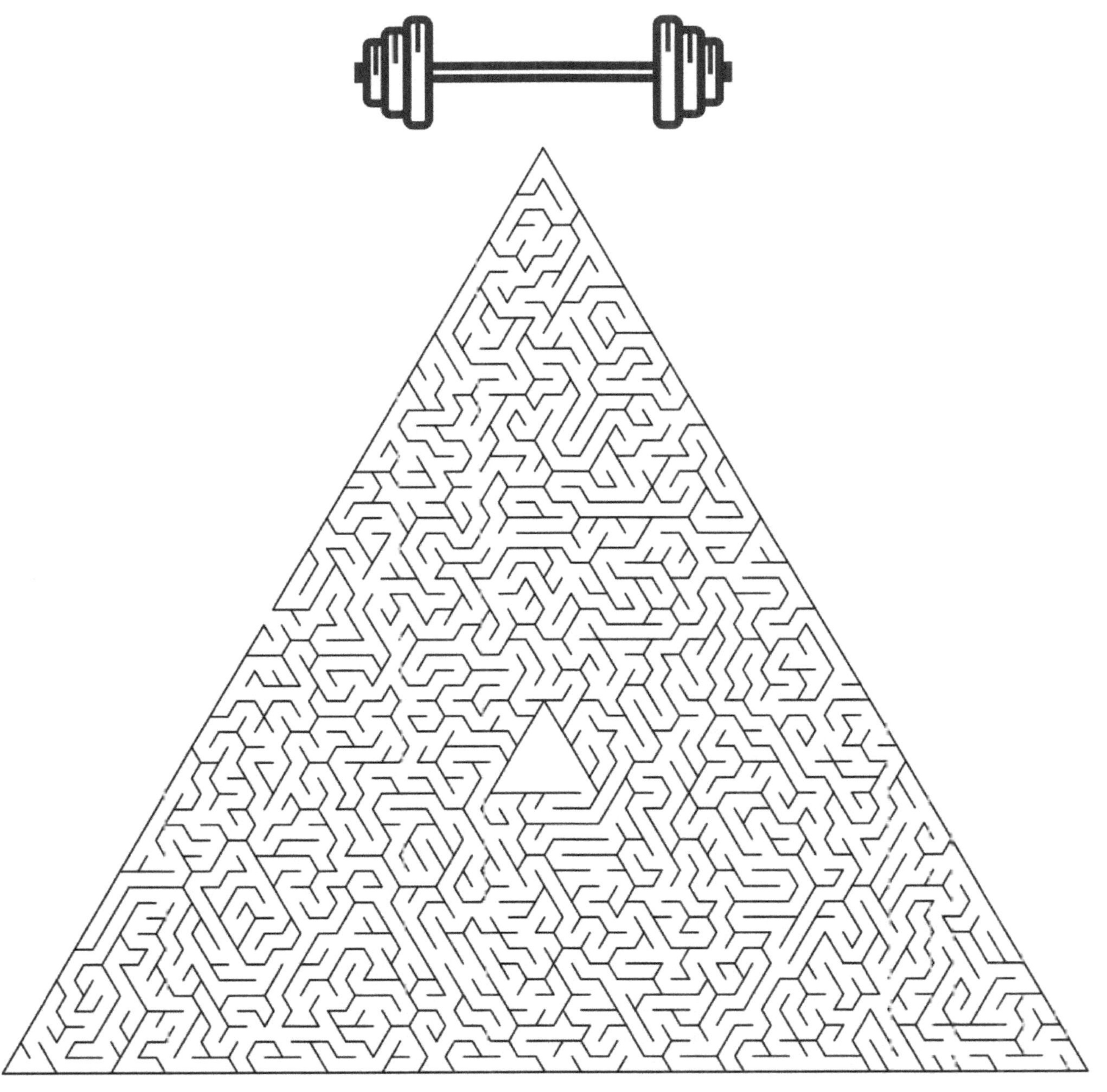

Yes you can! Yes you can!

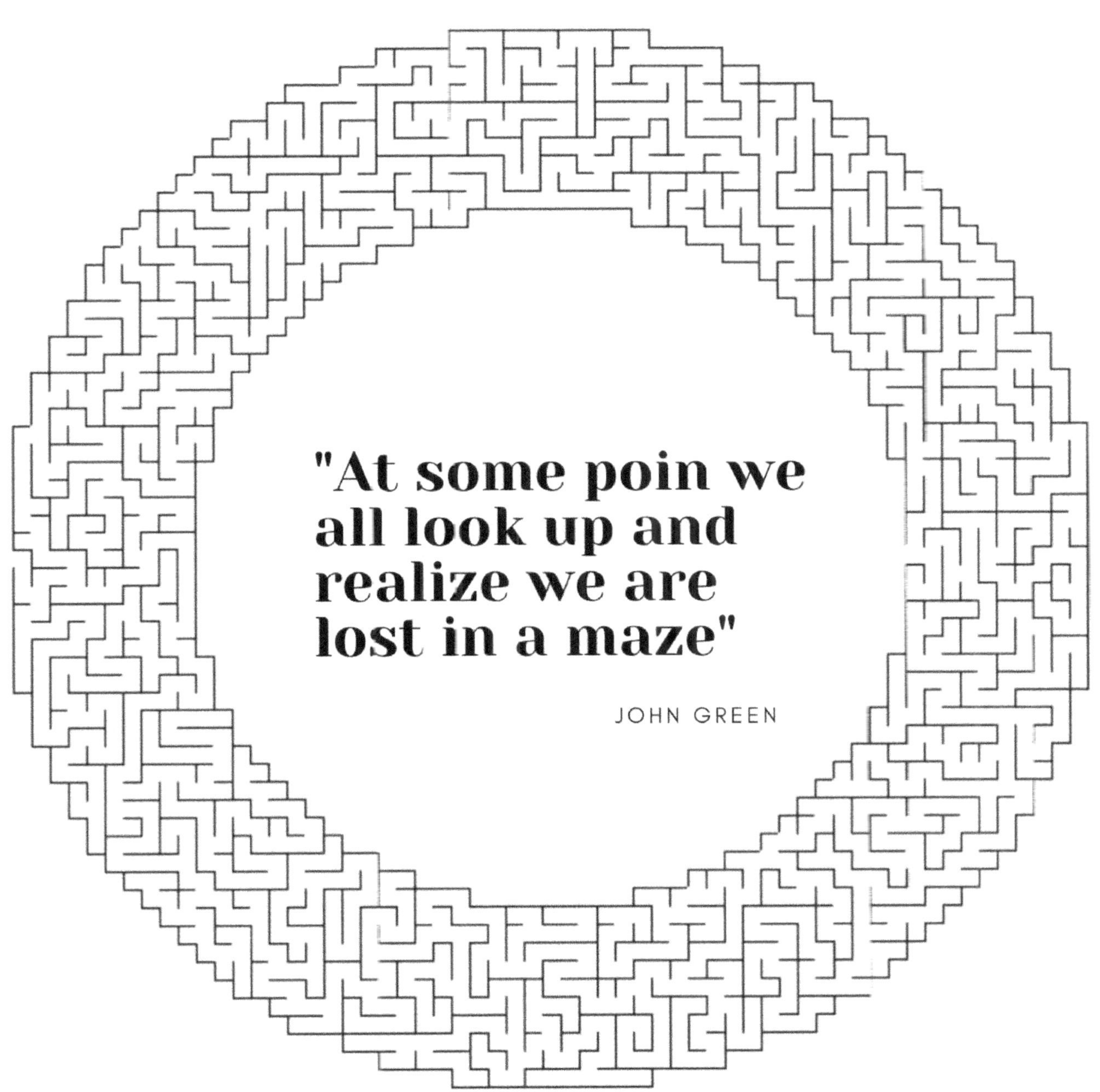
"At some poin we
all look up and
realize we are
lost in a maze"

JOHN GREEN

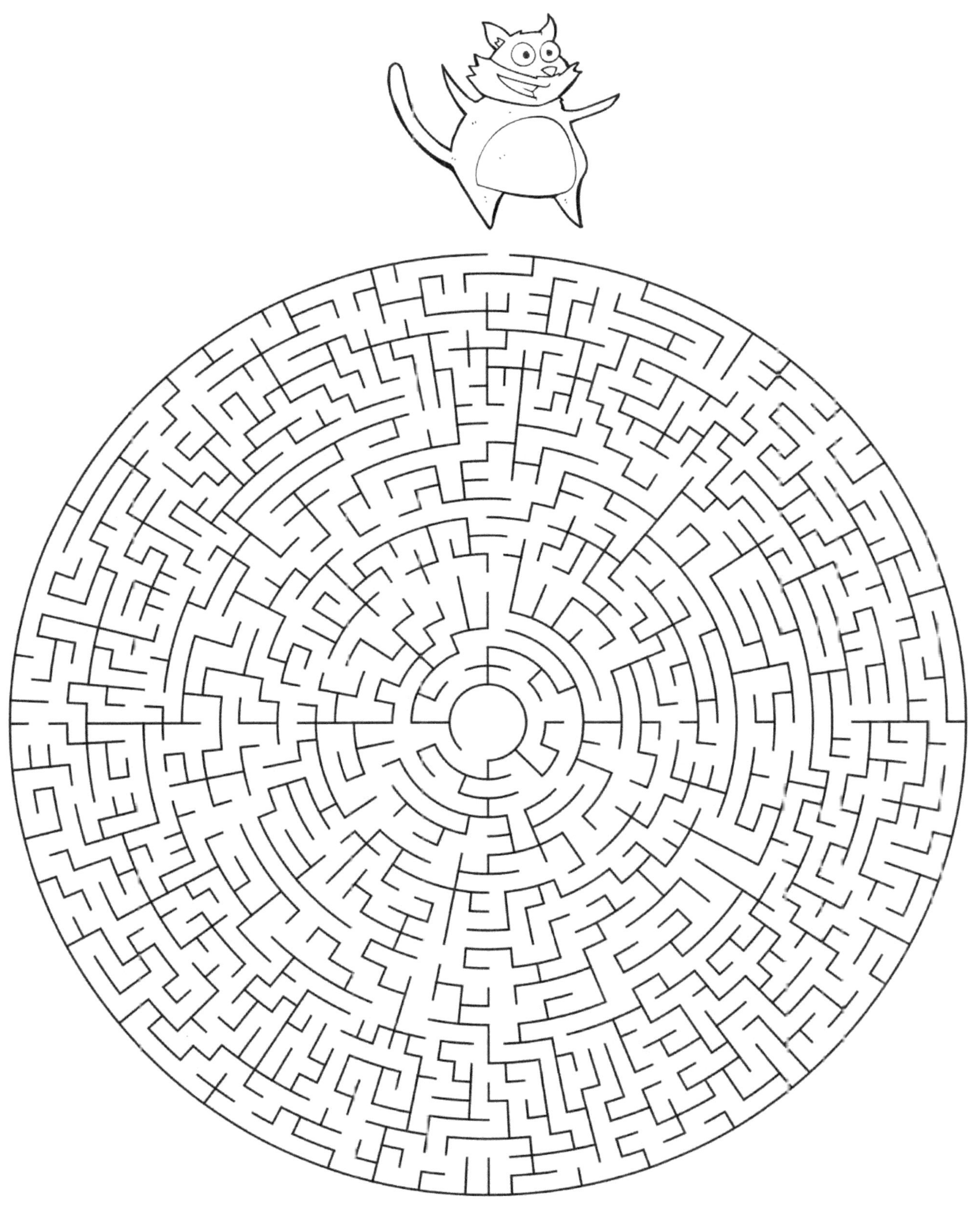

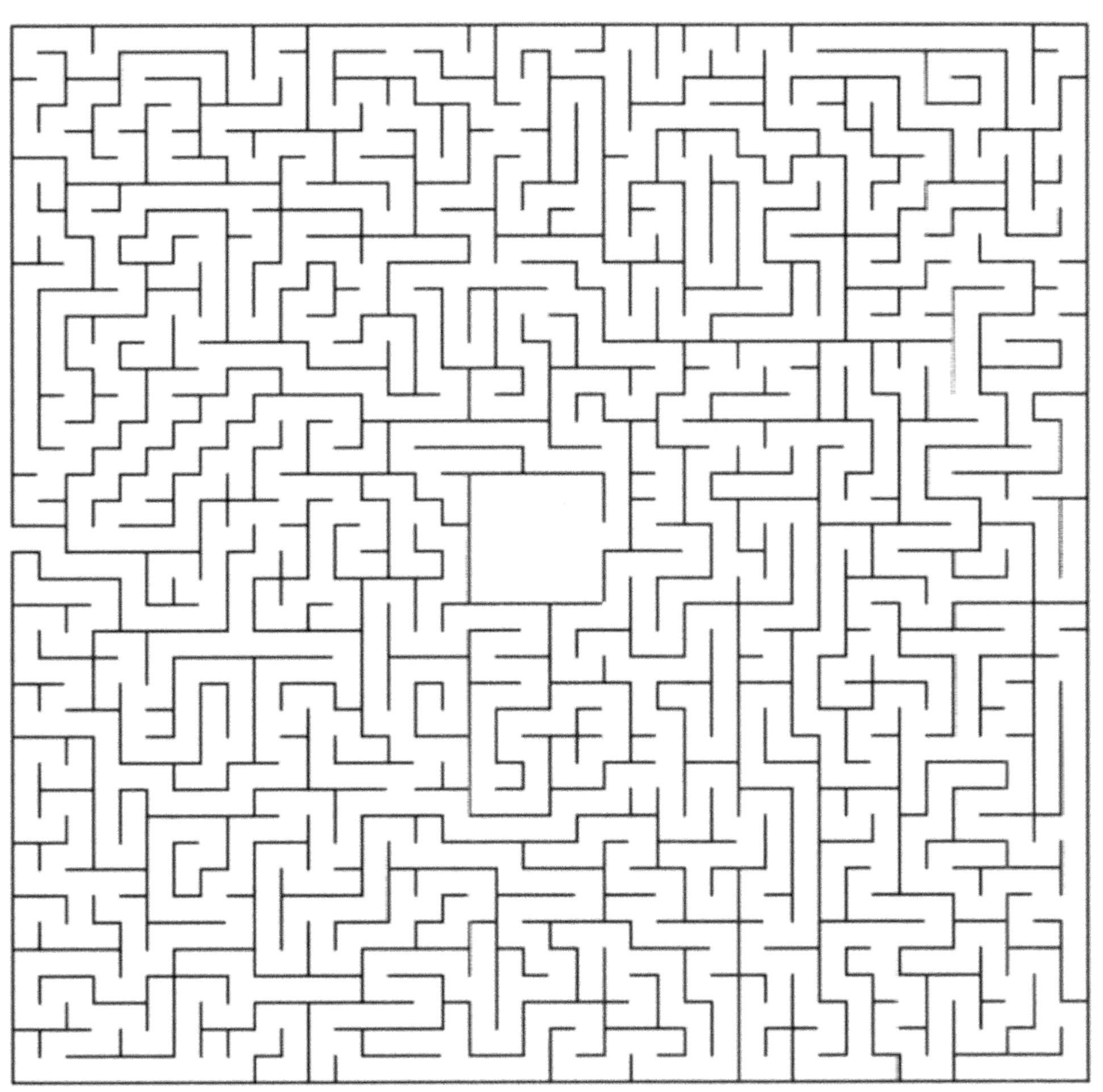

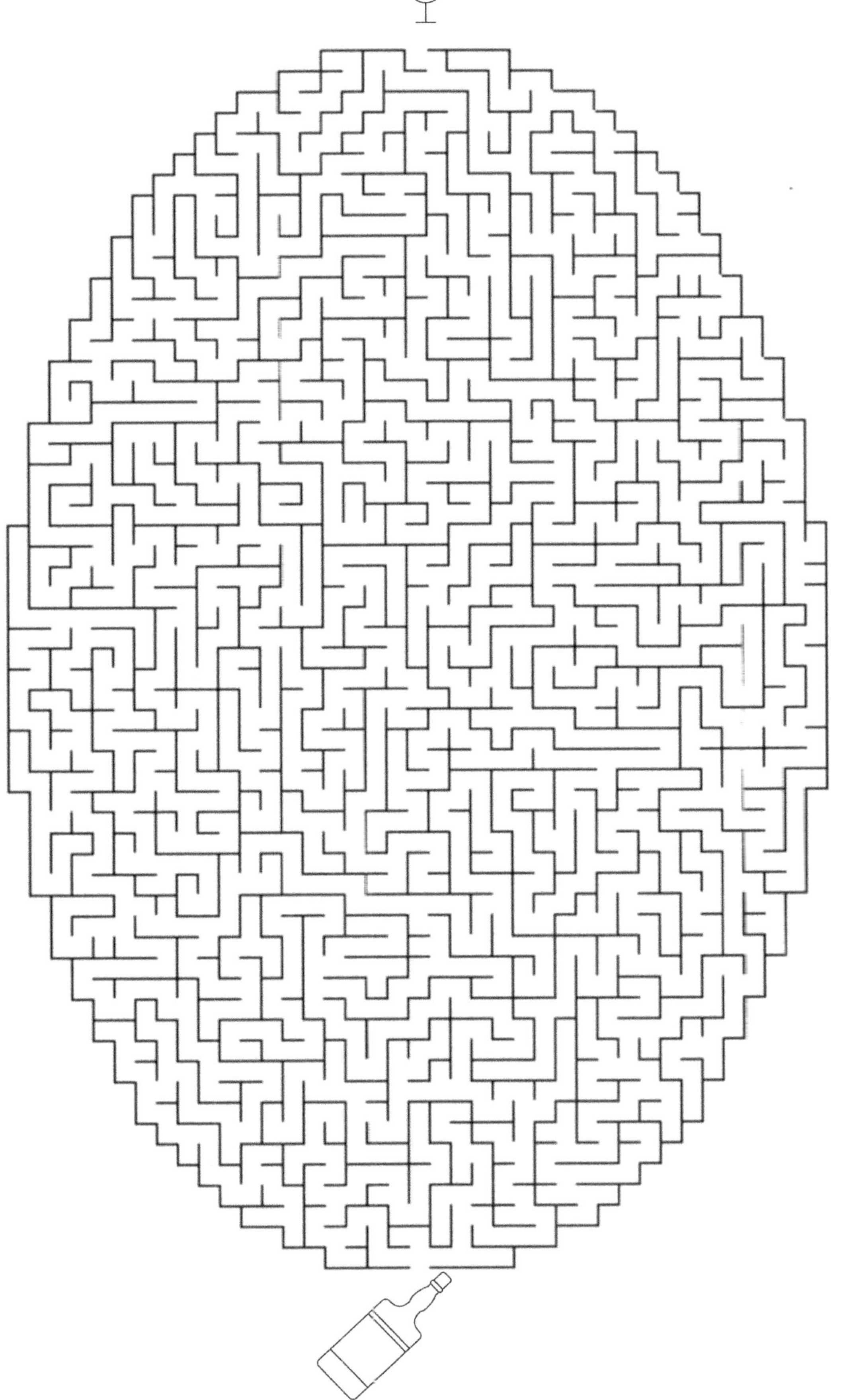

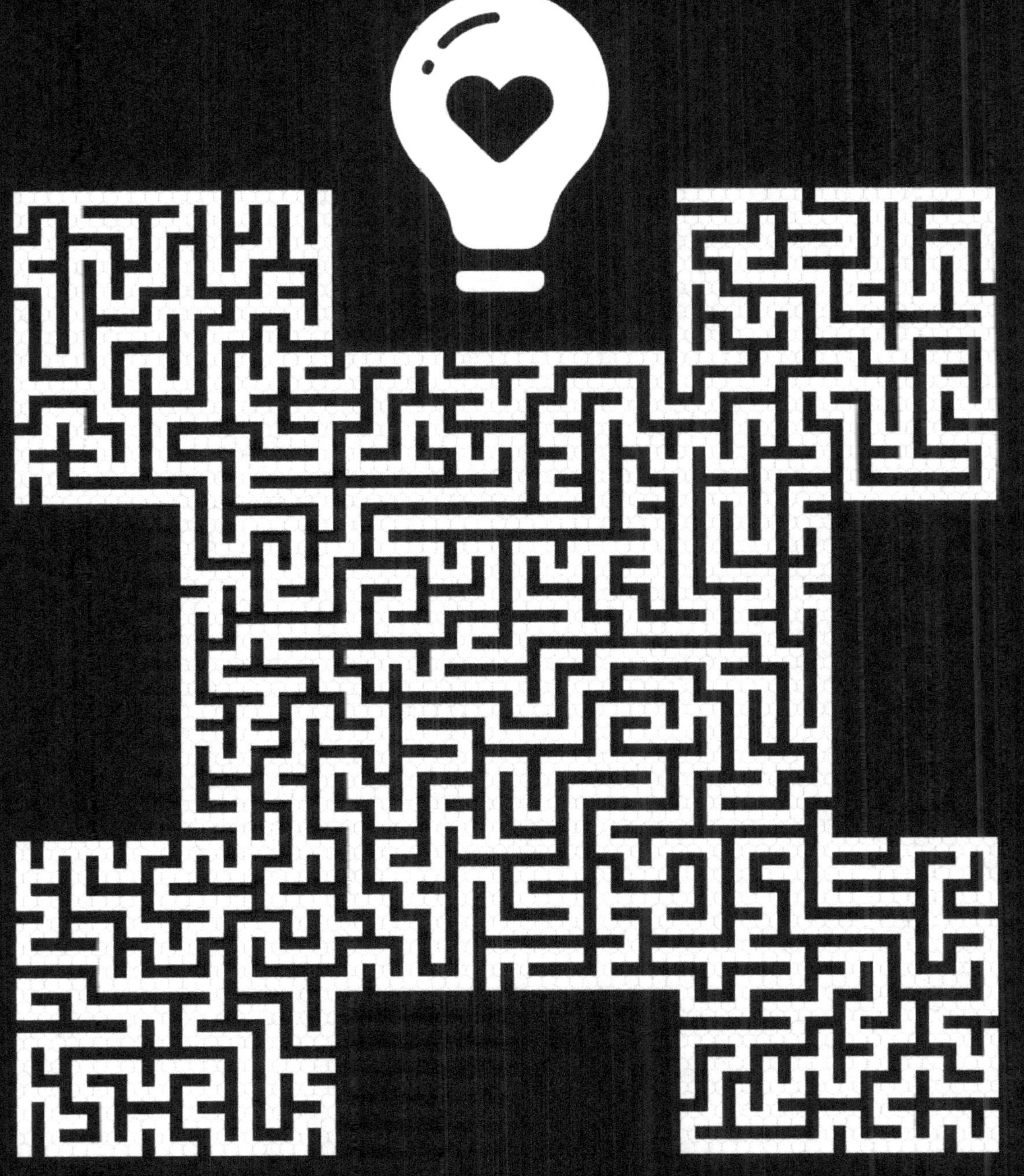

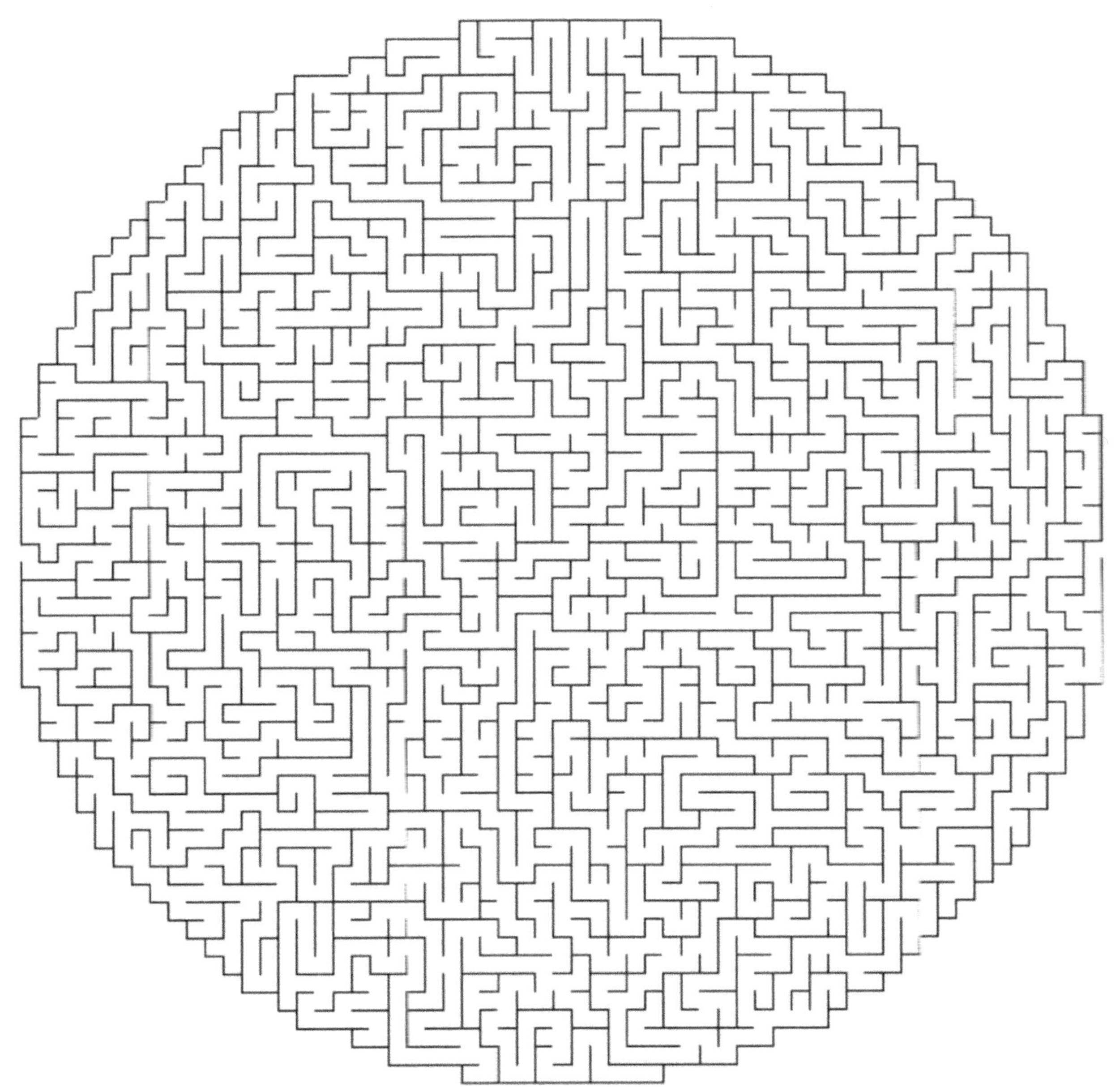

It seems like you don't have better things to do in your life. Good luck!

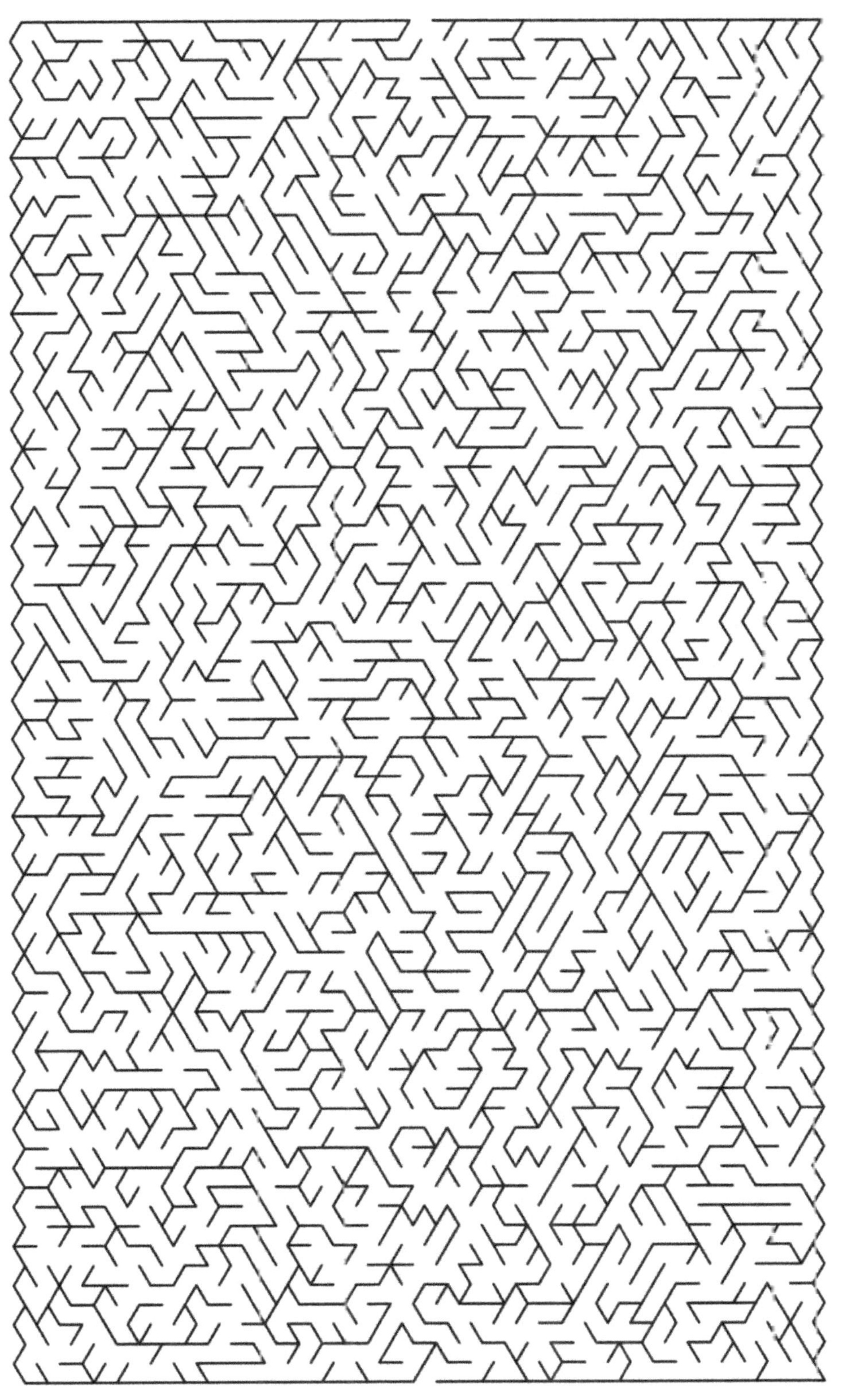

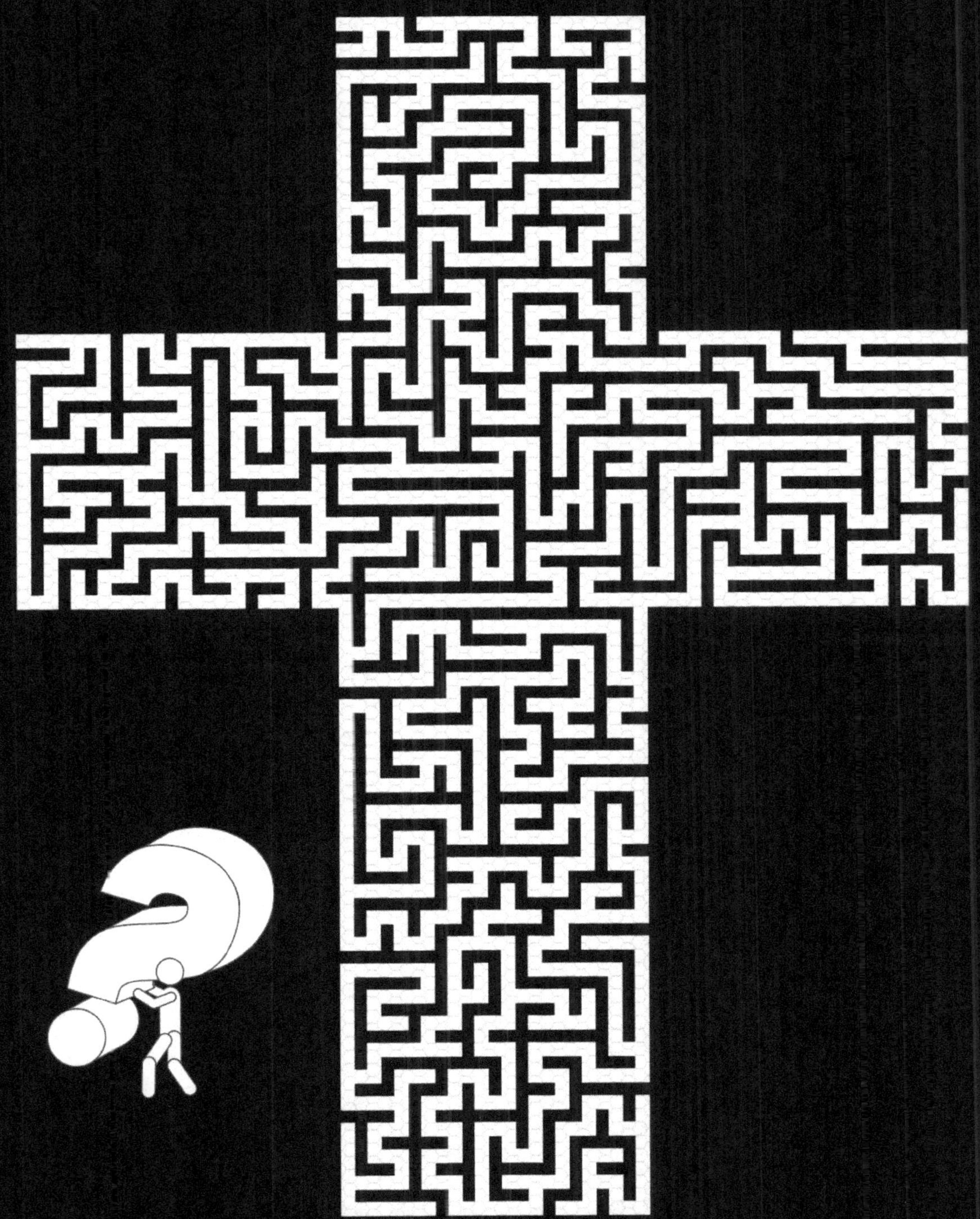

level 5

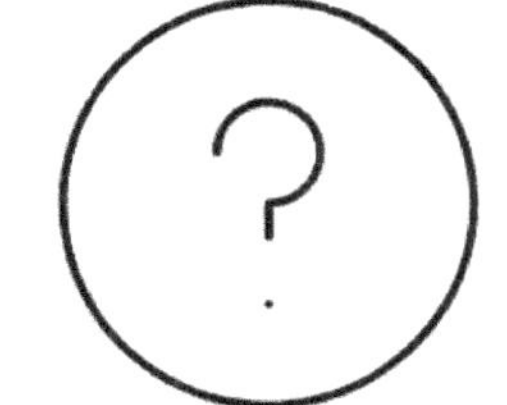

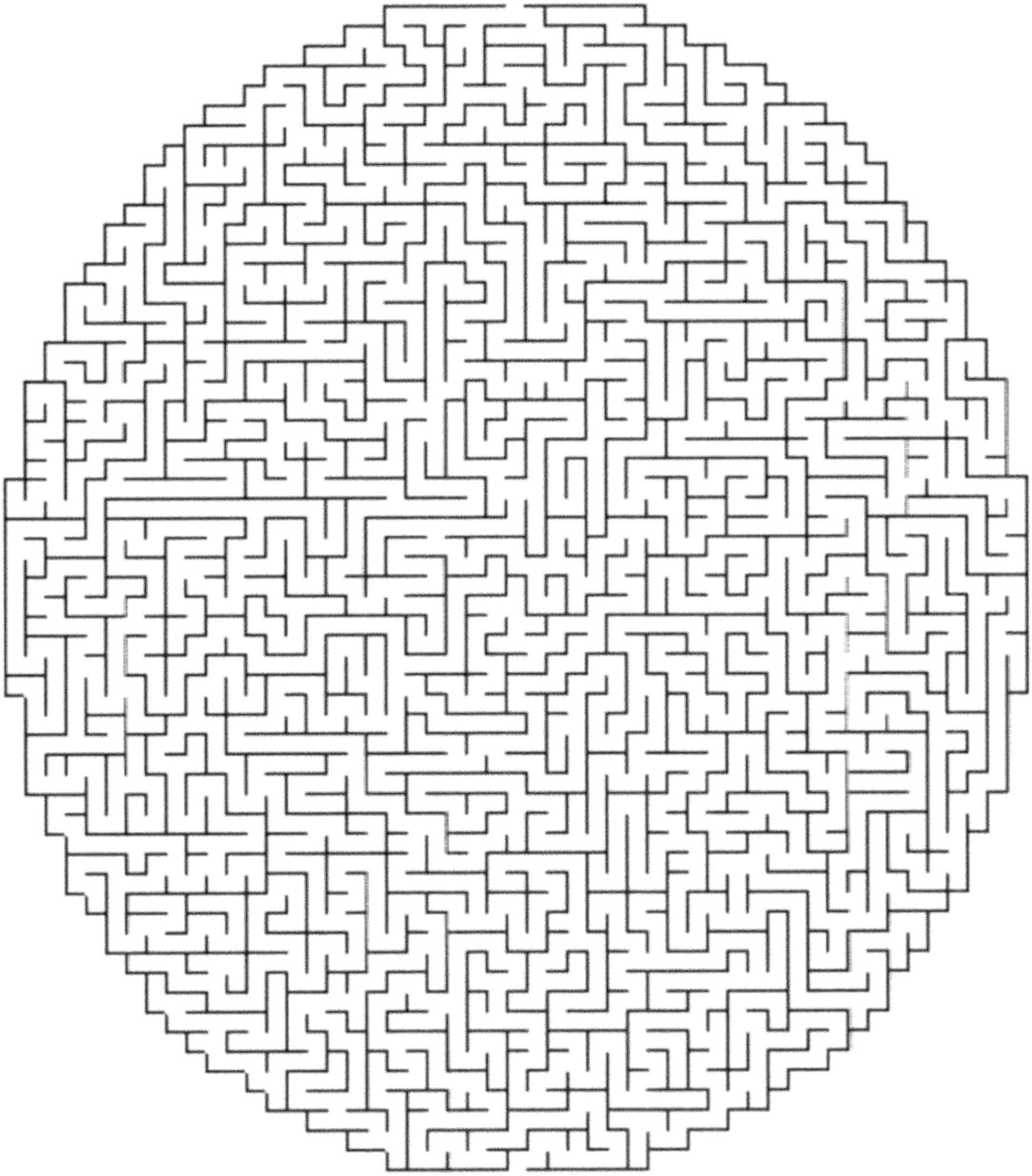

level 5

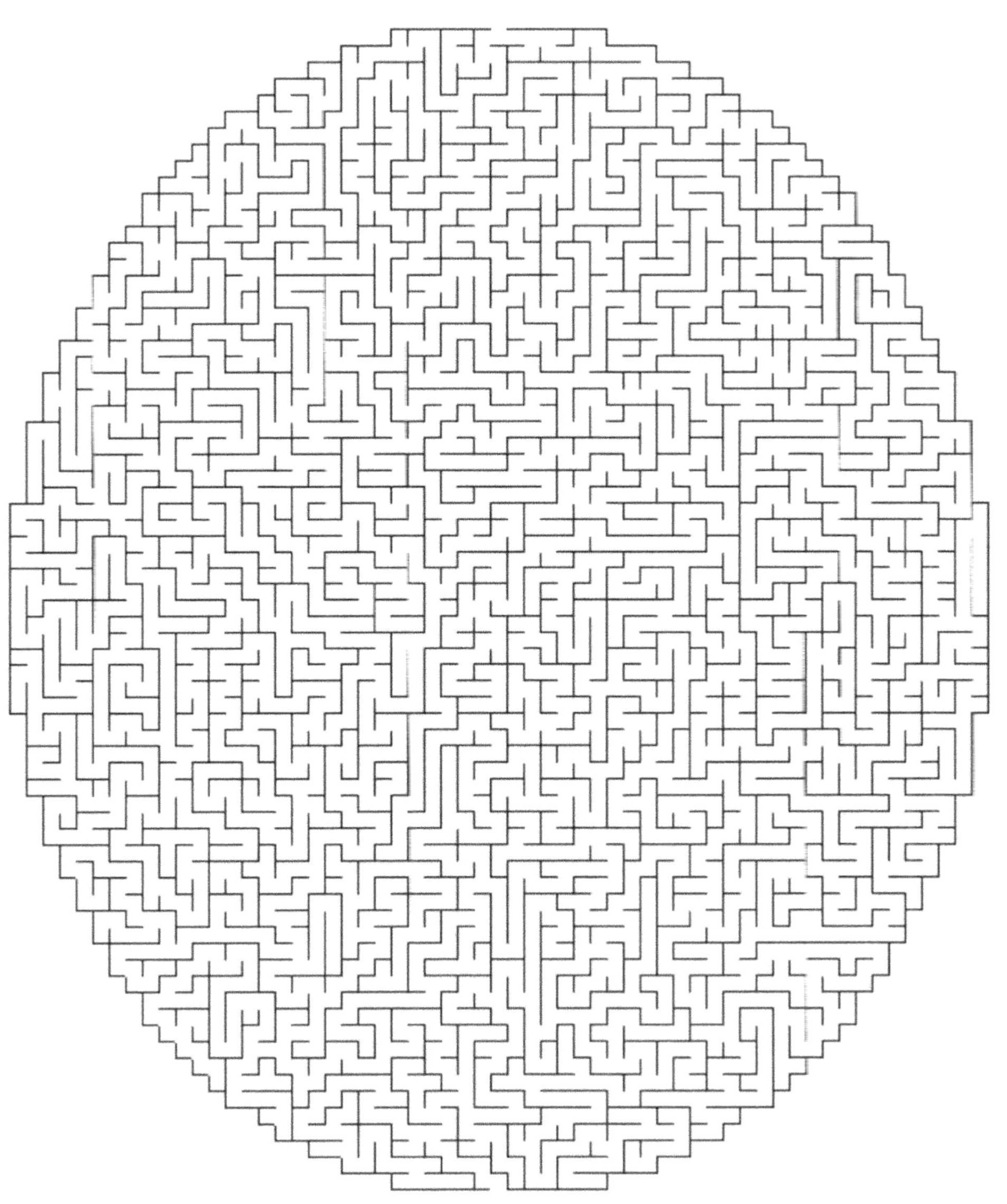

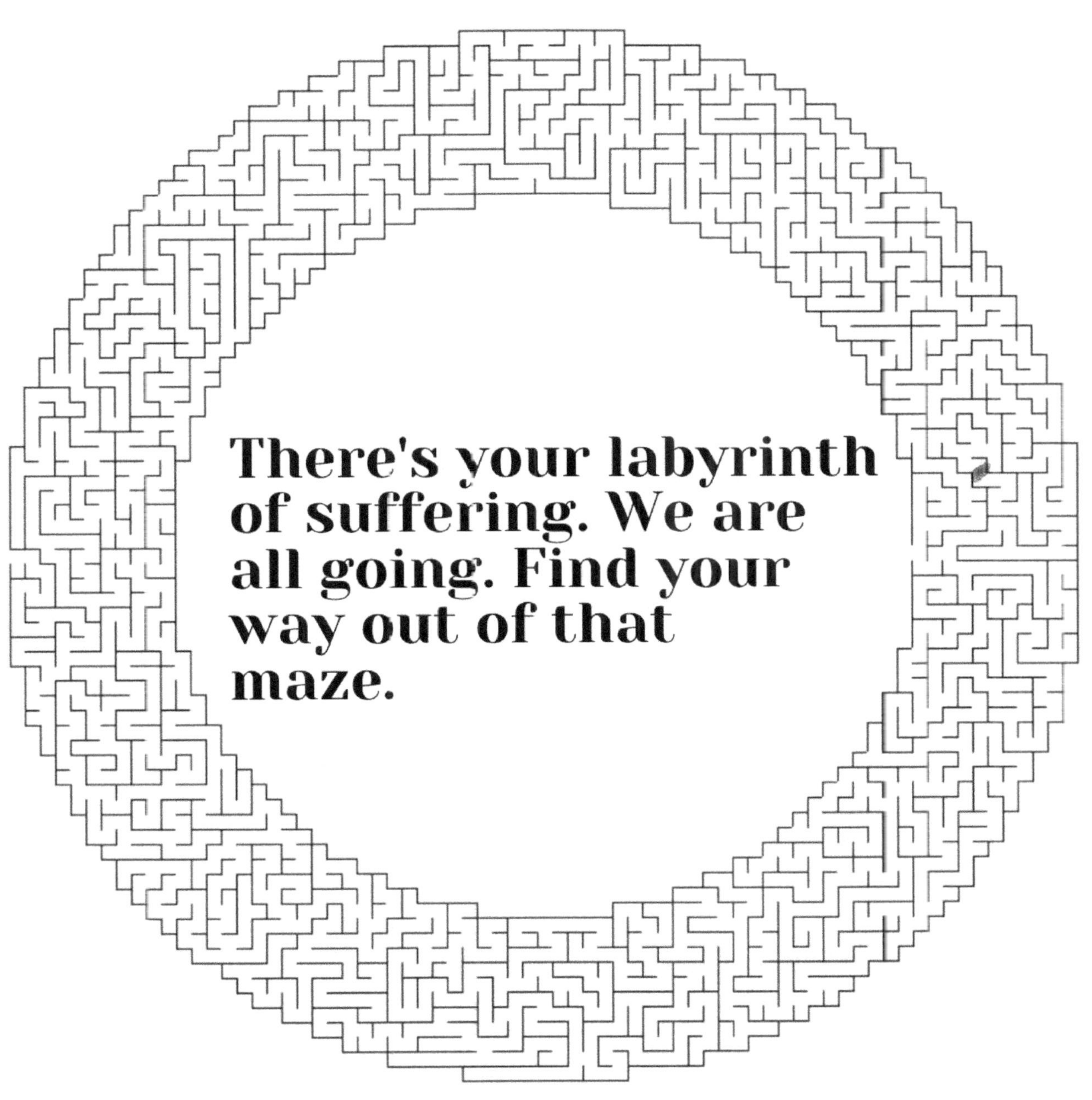

There's your labyrinth
of suffering. We are
all going. Find your
way out of that
maze.

level 6

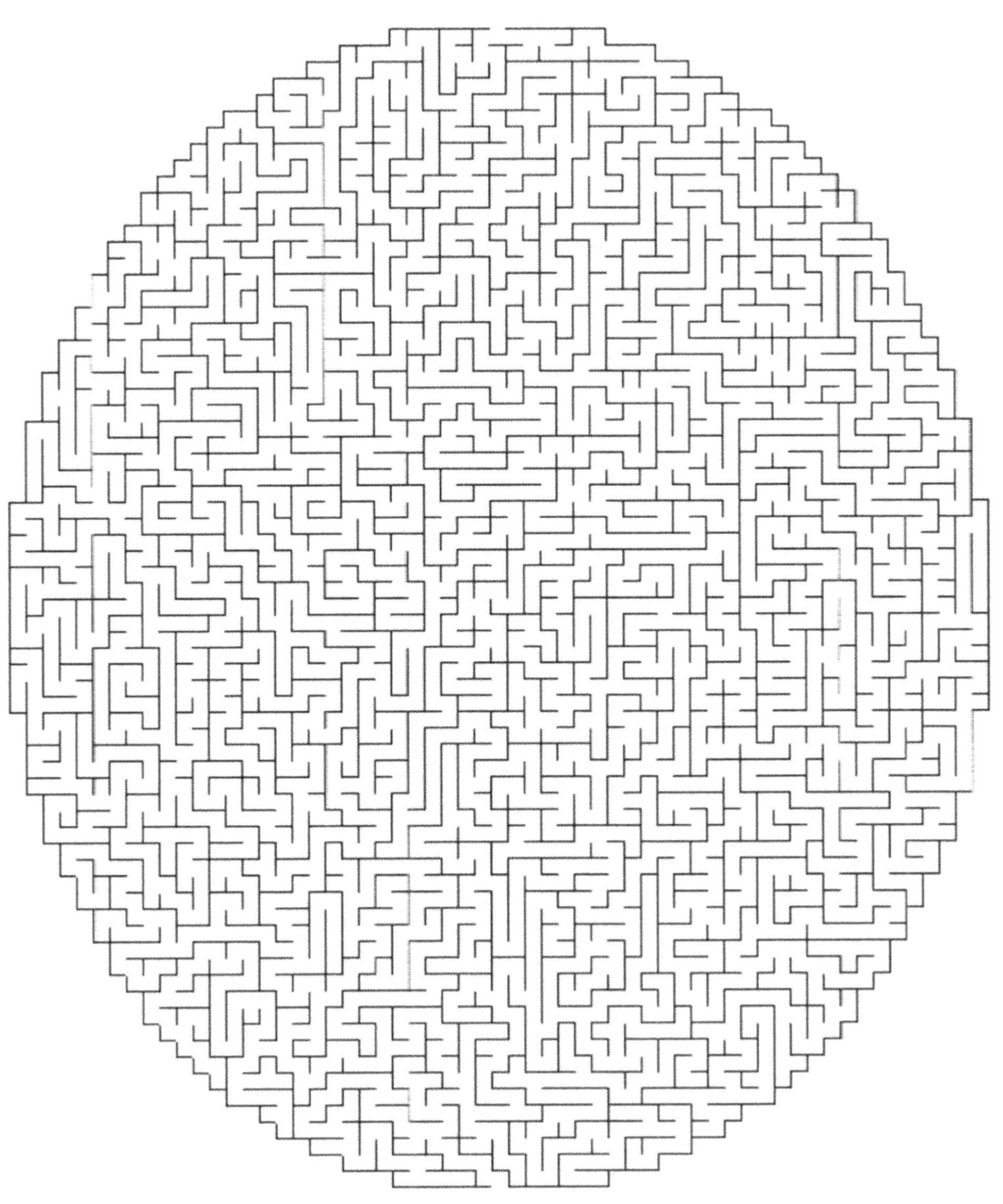

level 6

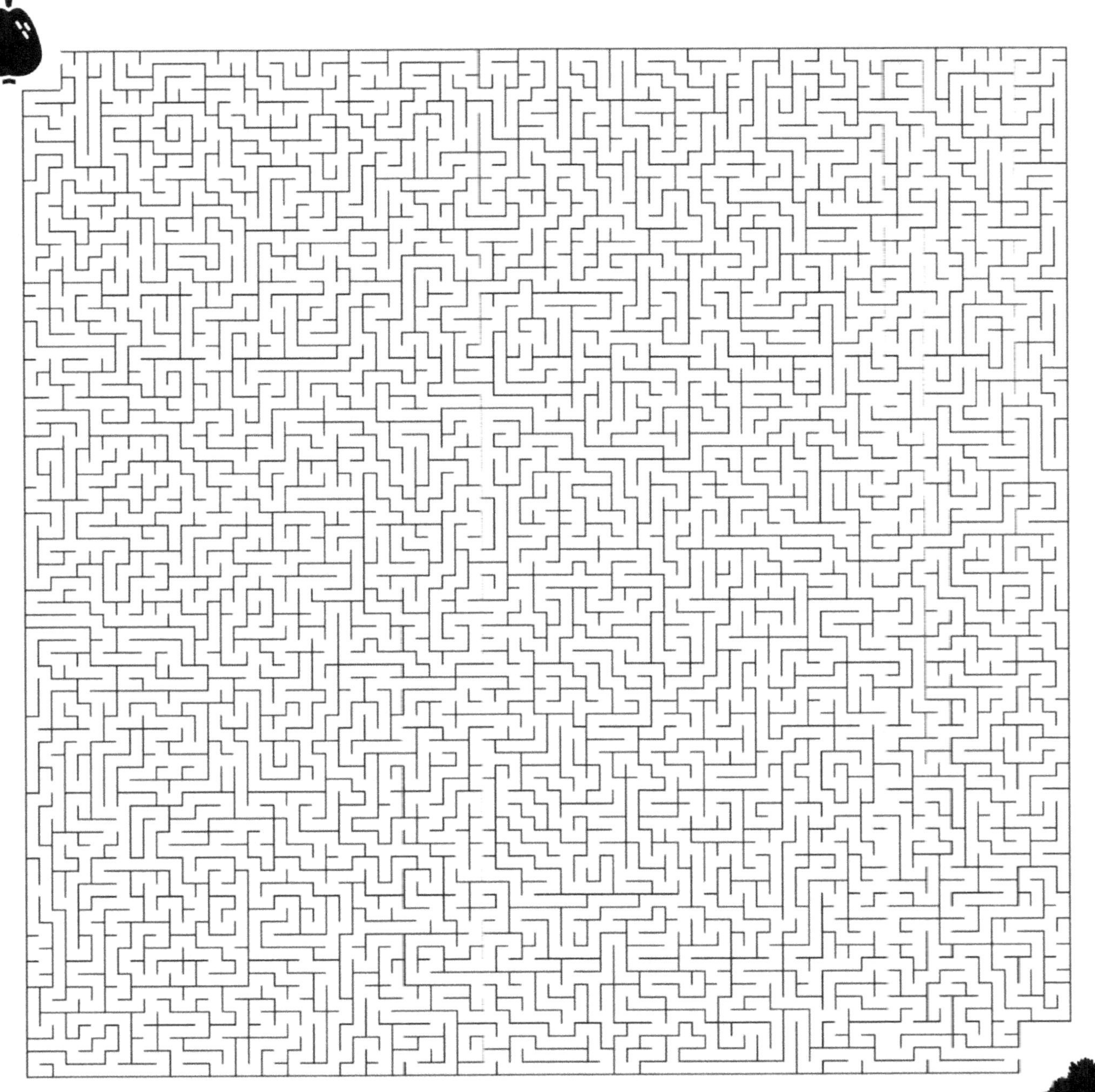

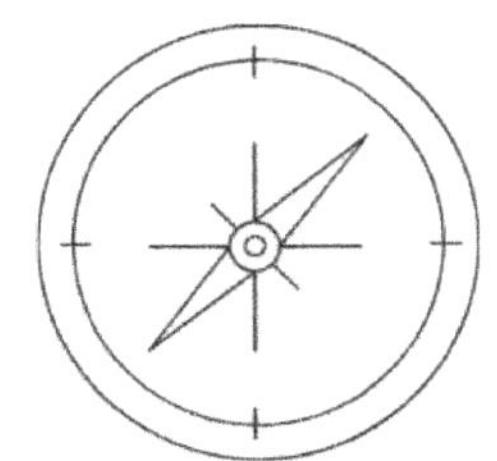

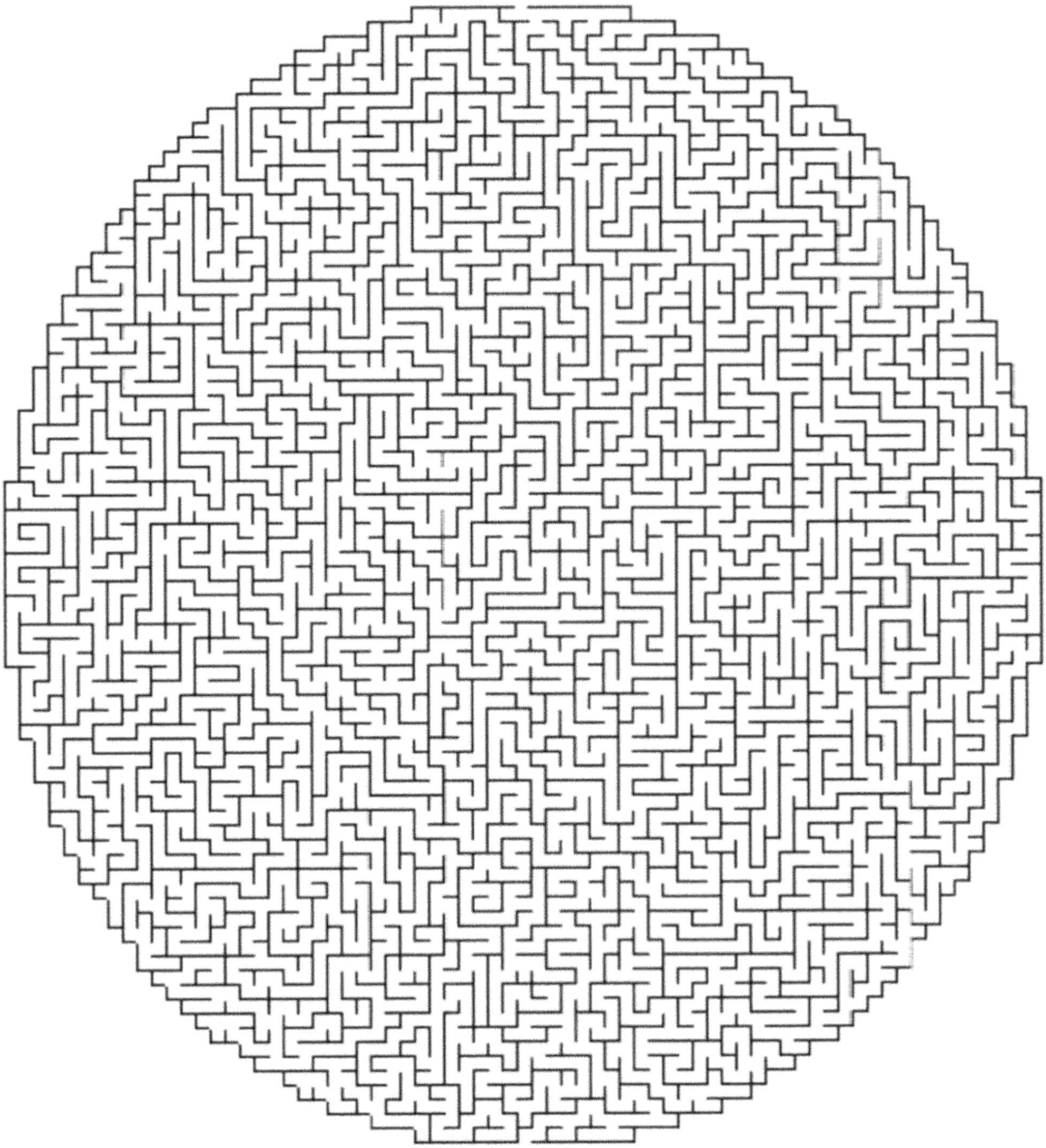

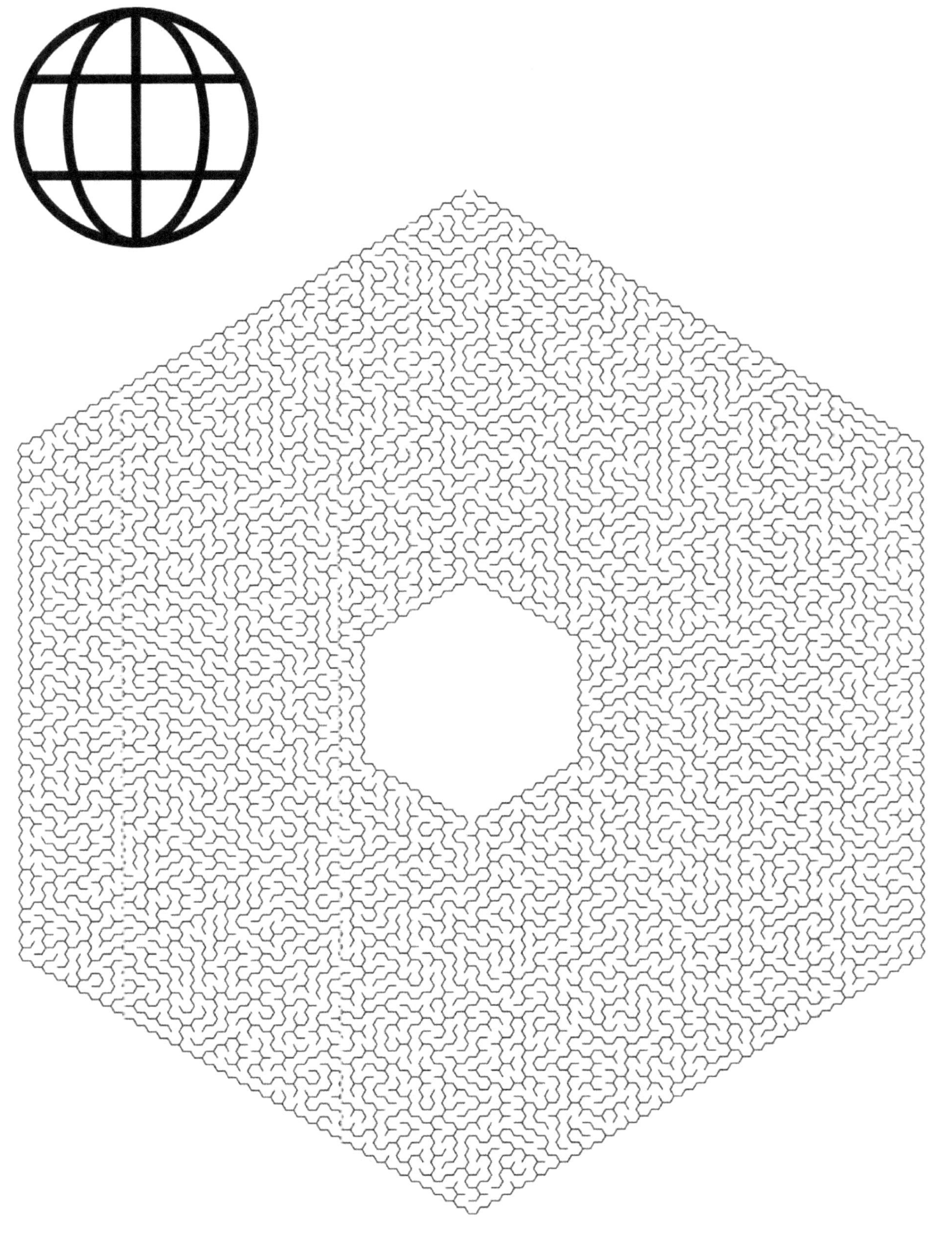

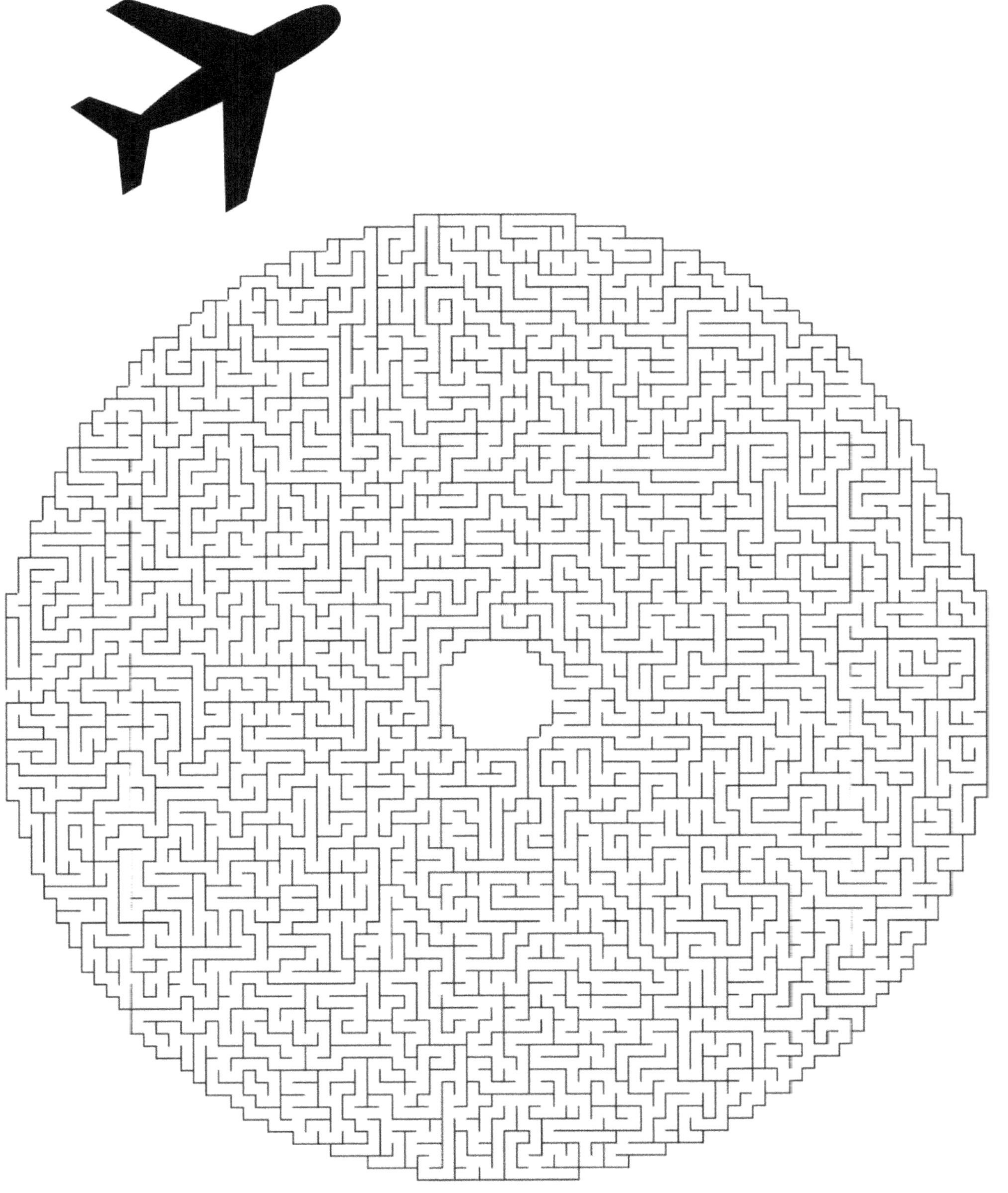

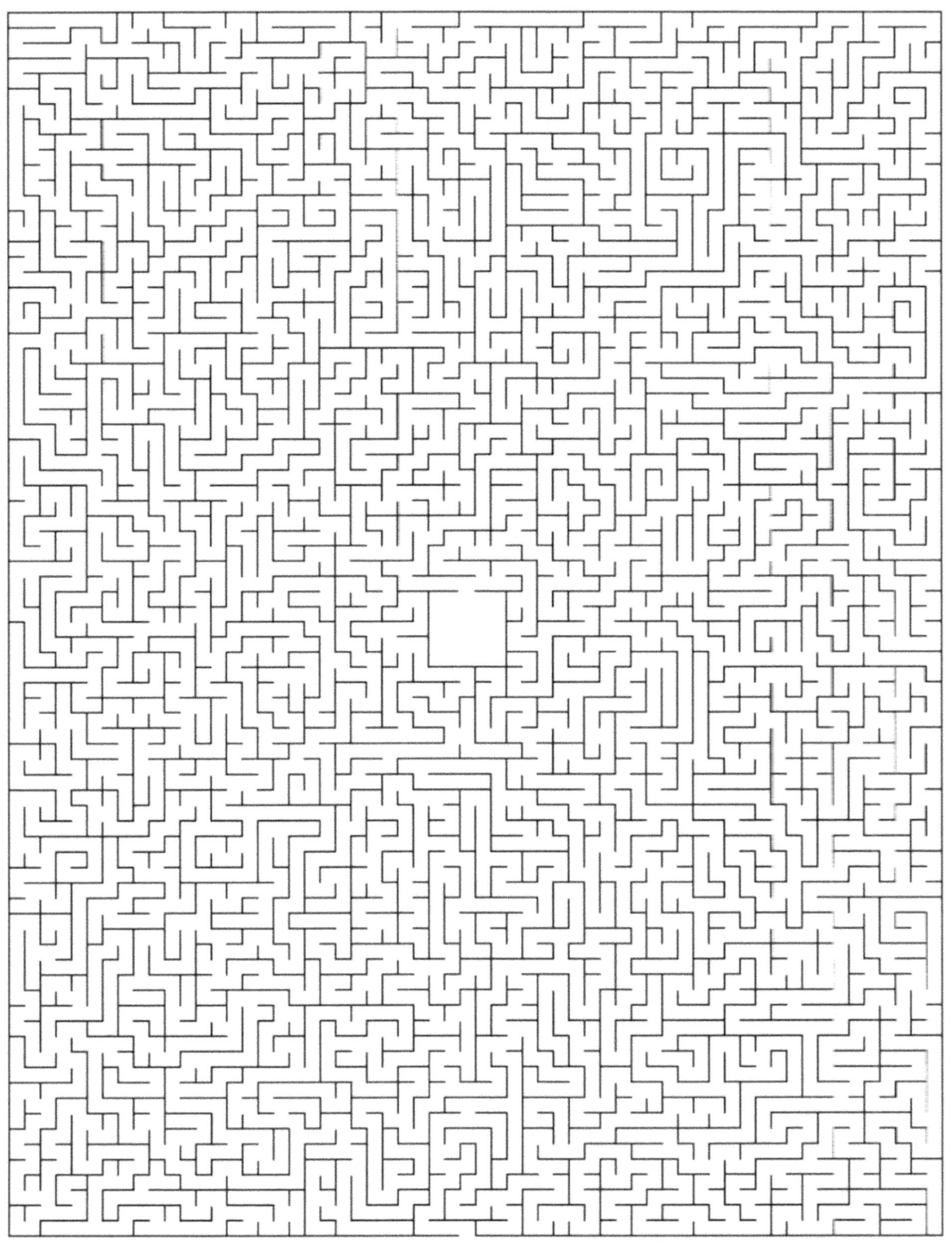

level 6

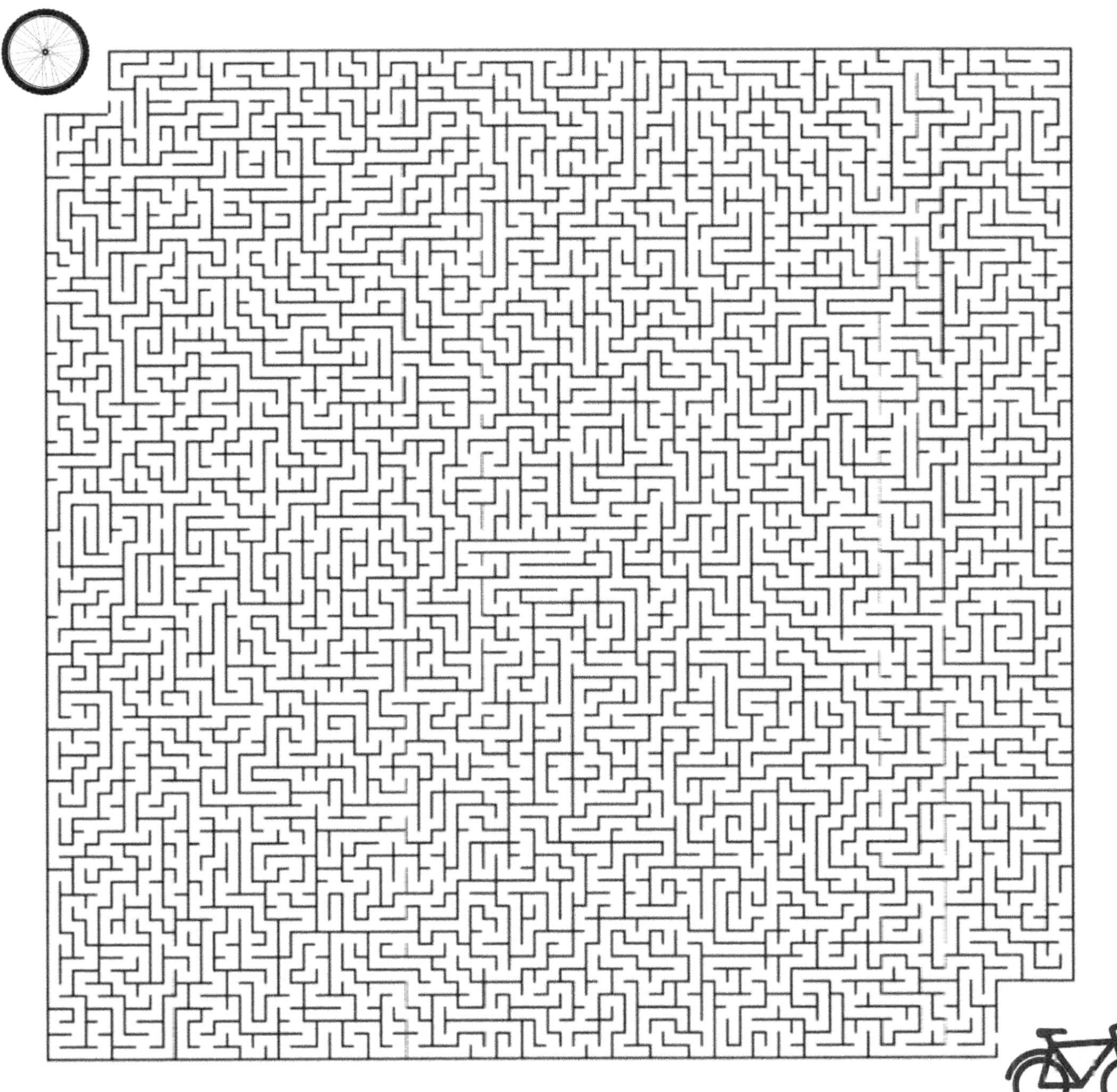

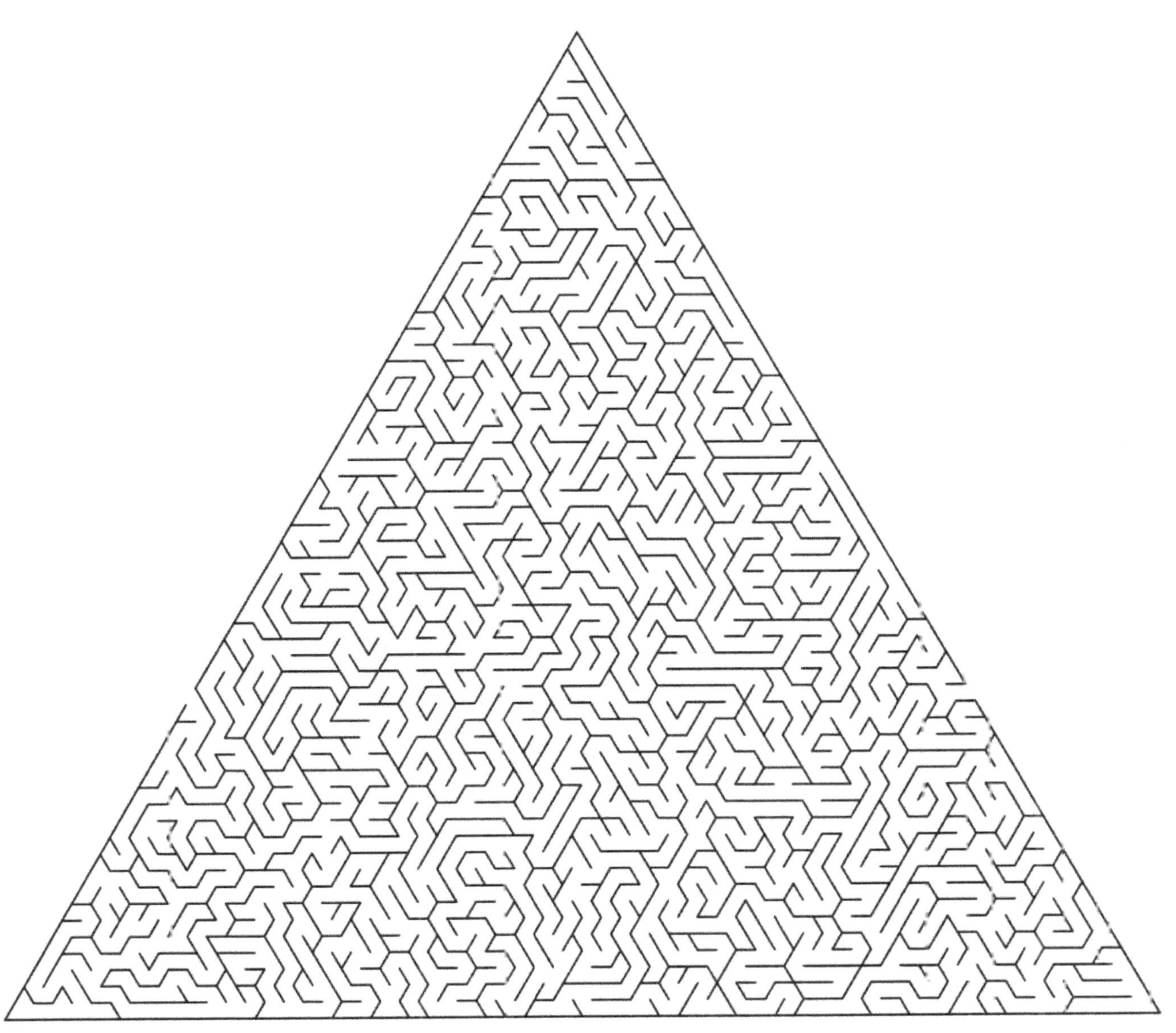

How the fuck to do it?!

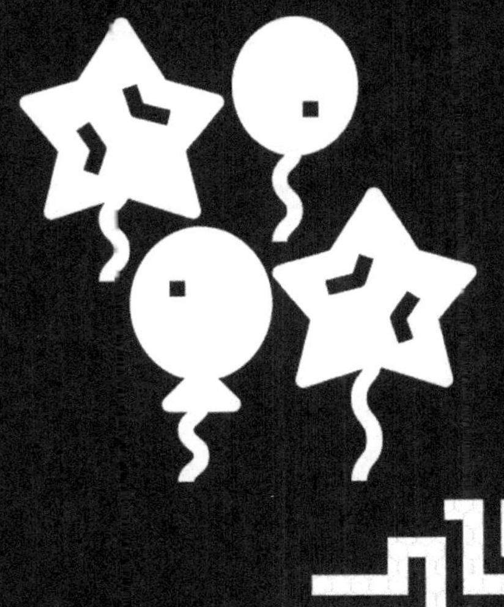

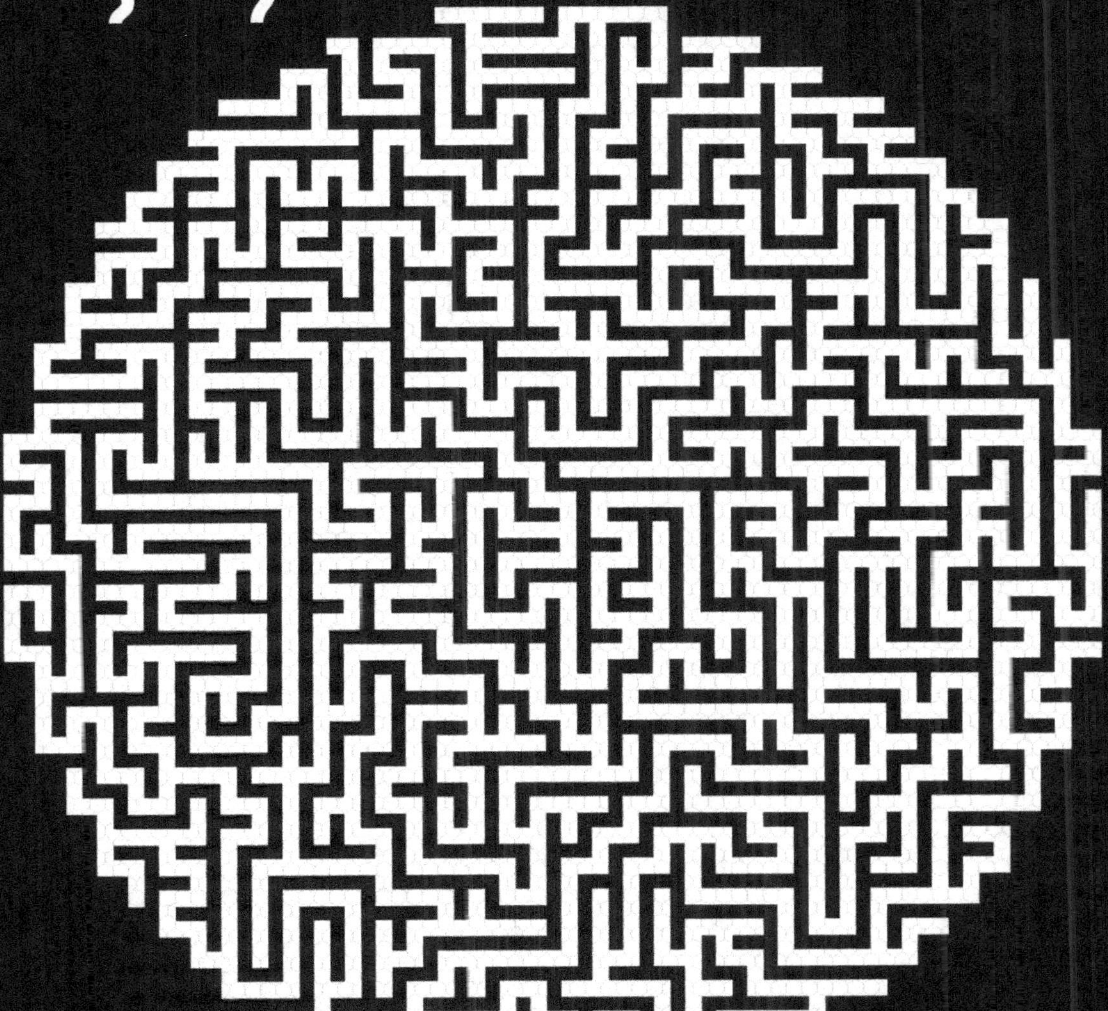

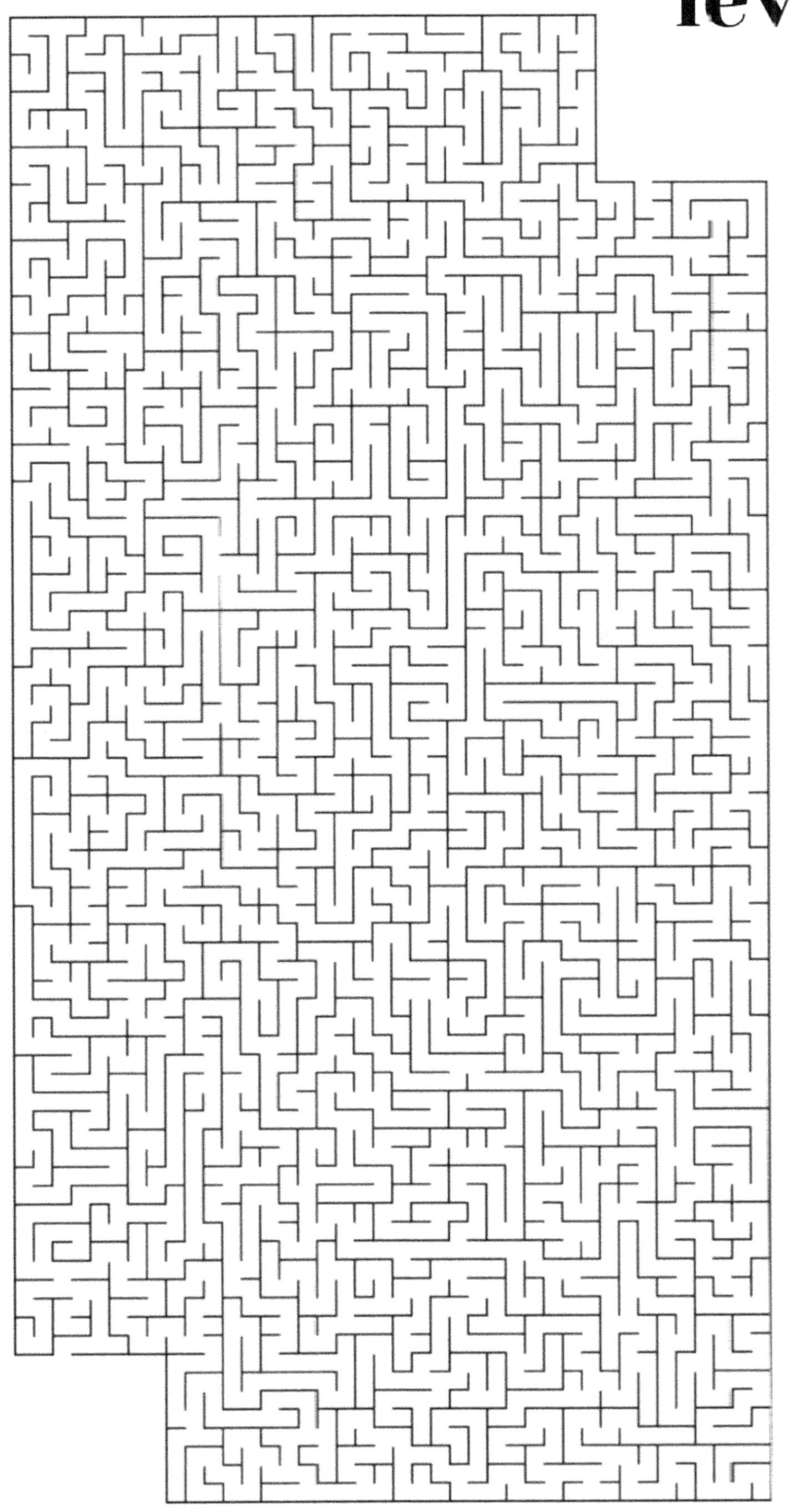

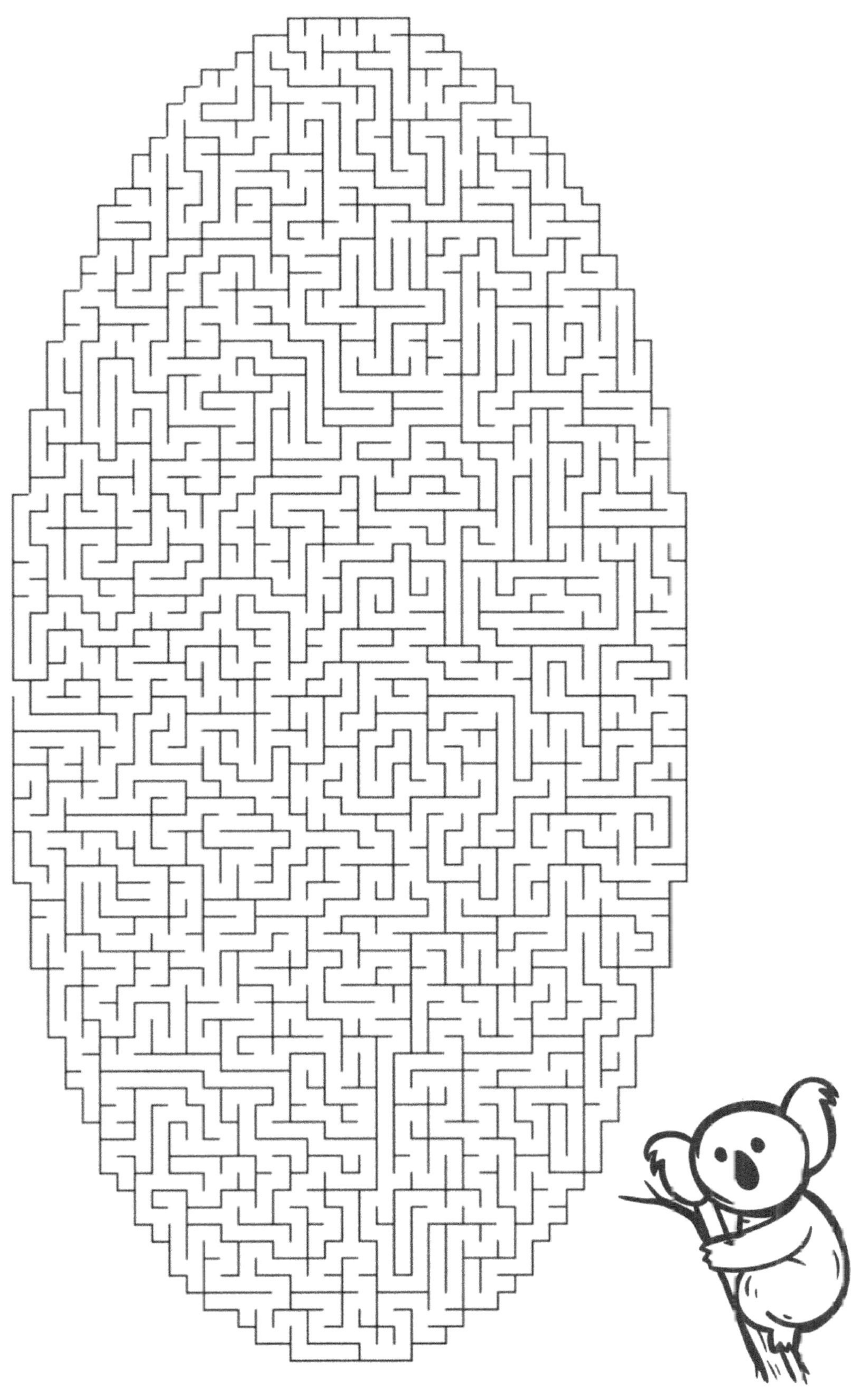

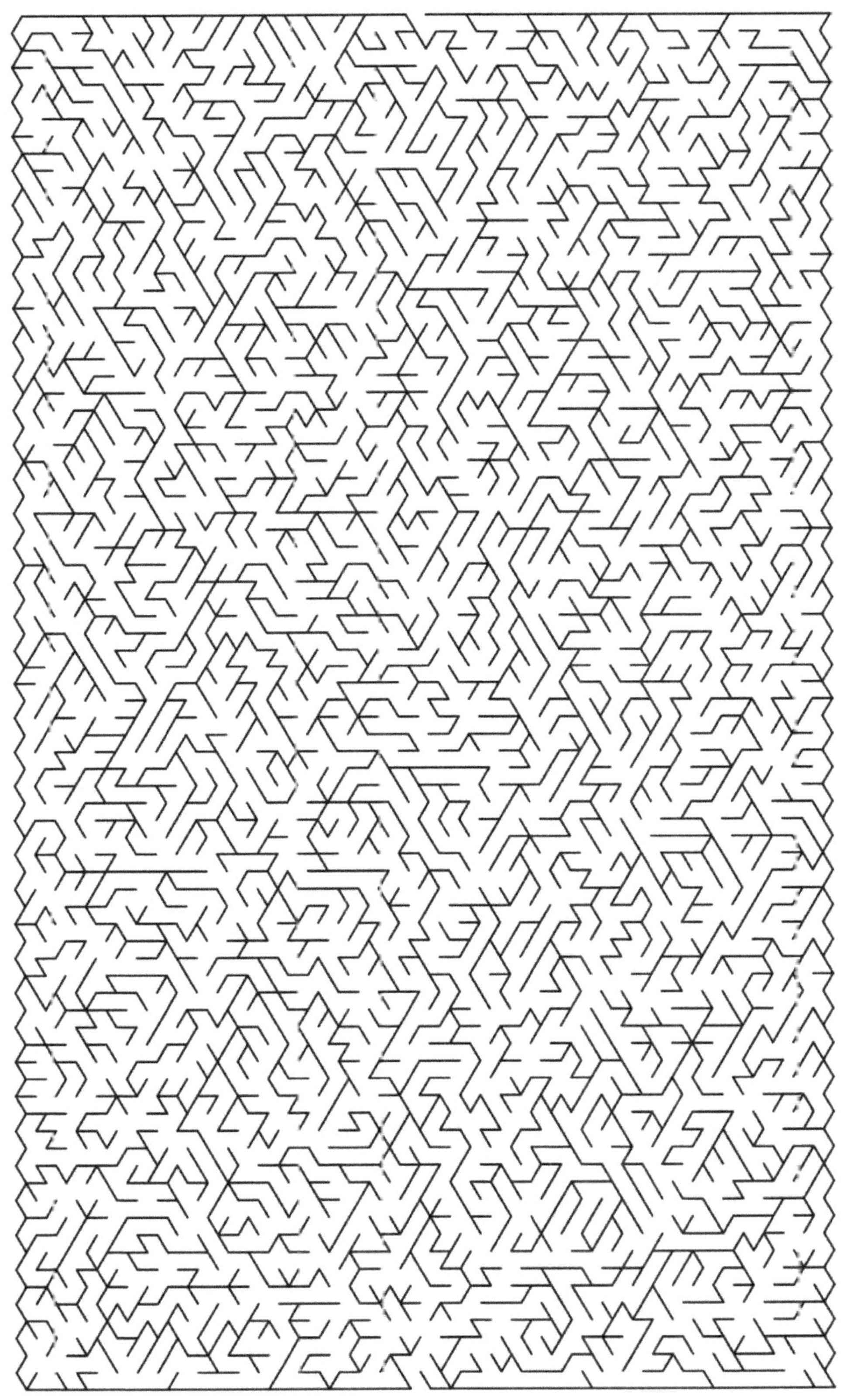

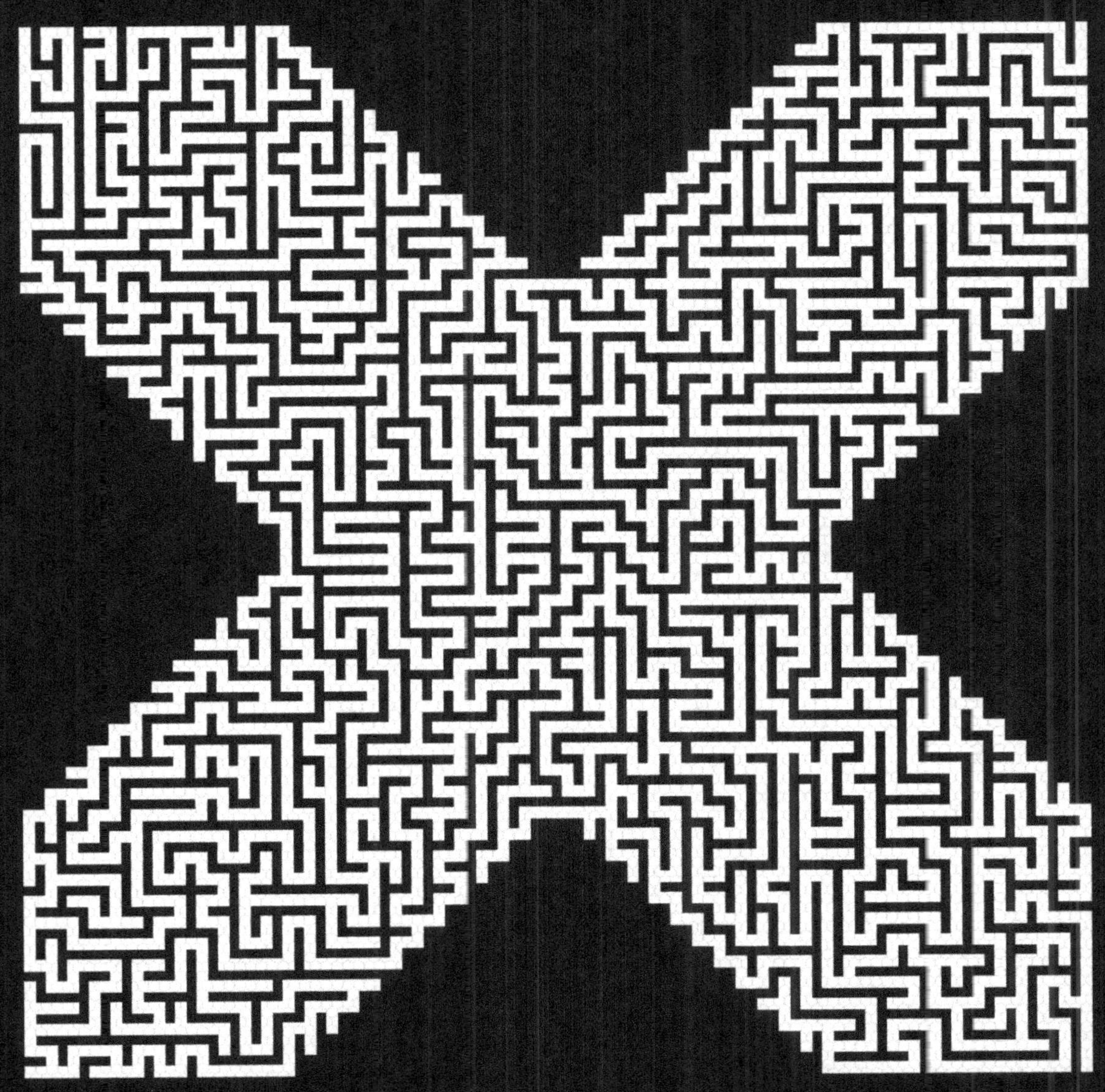

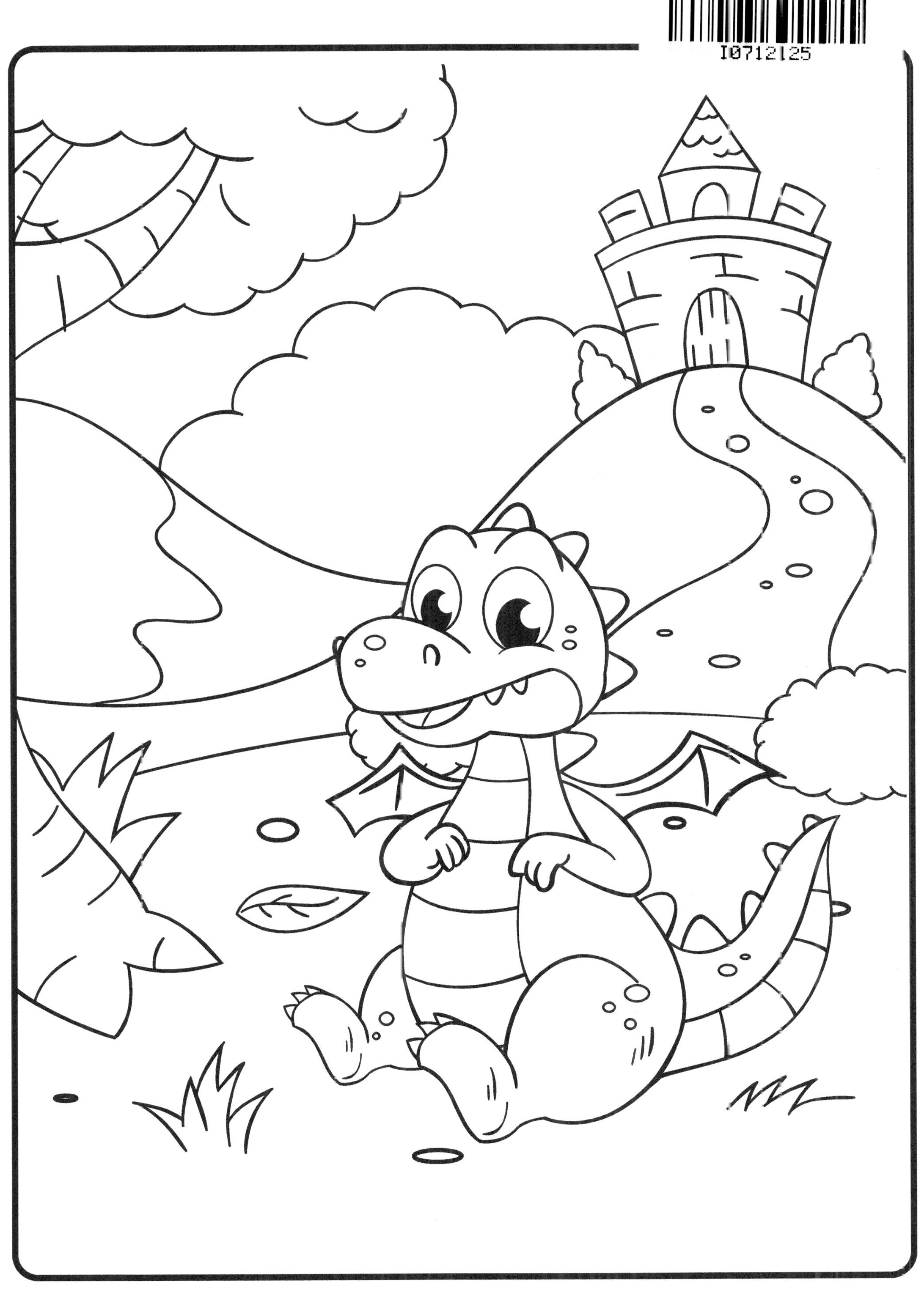
I0712125

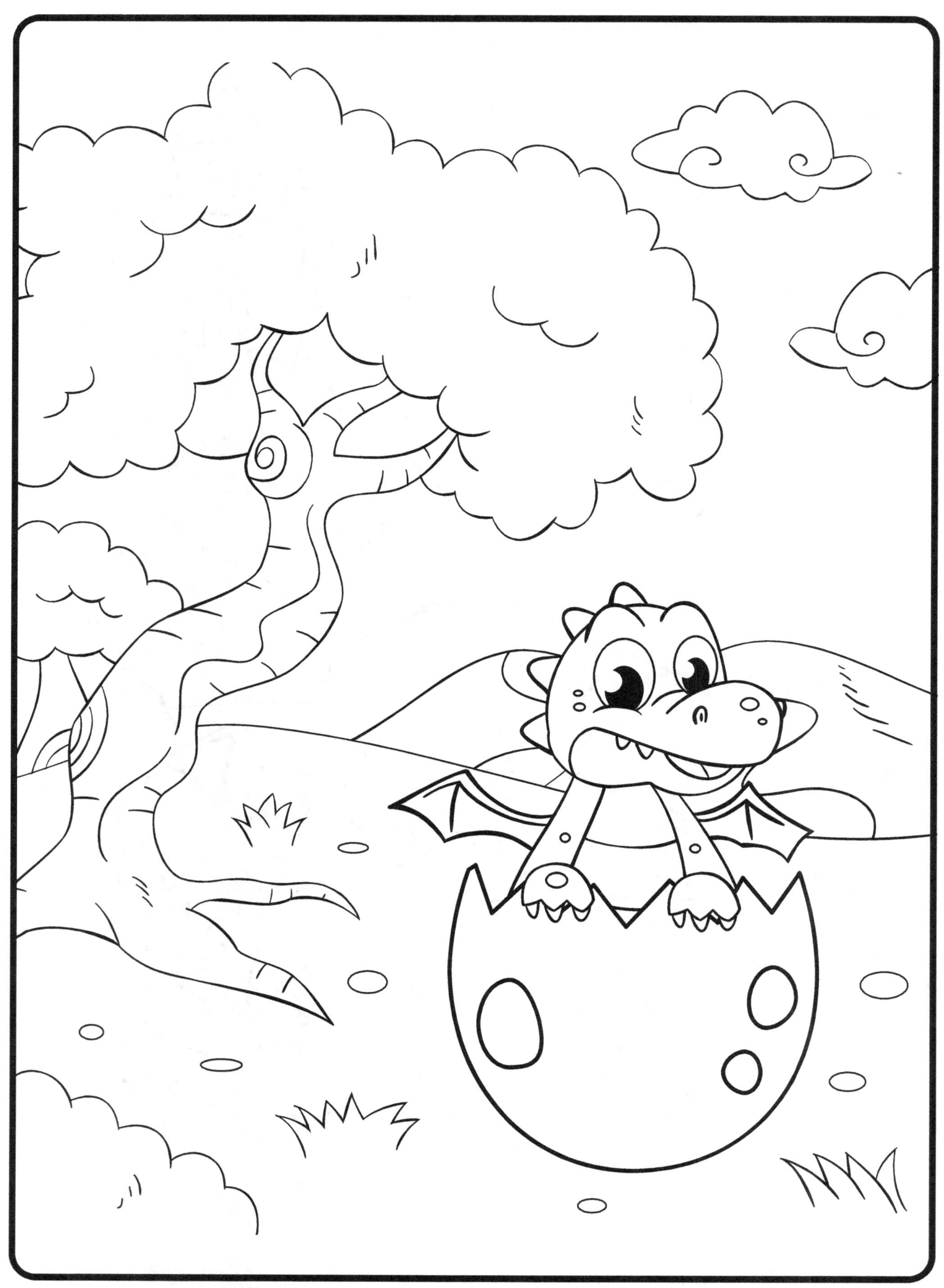

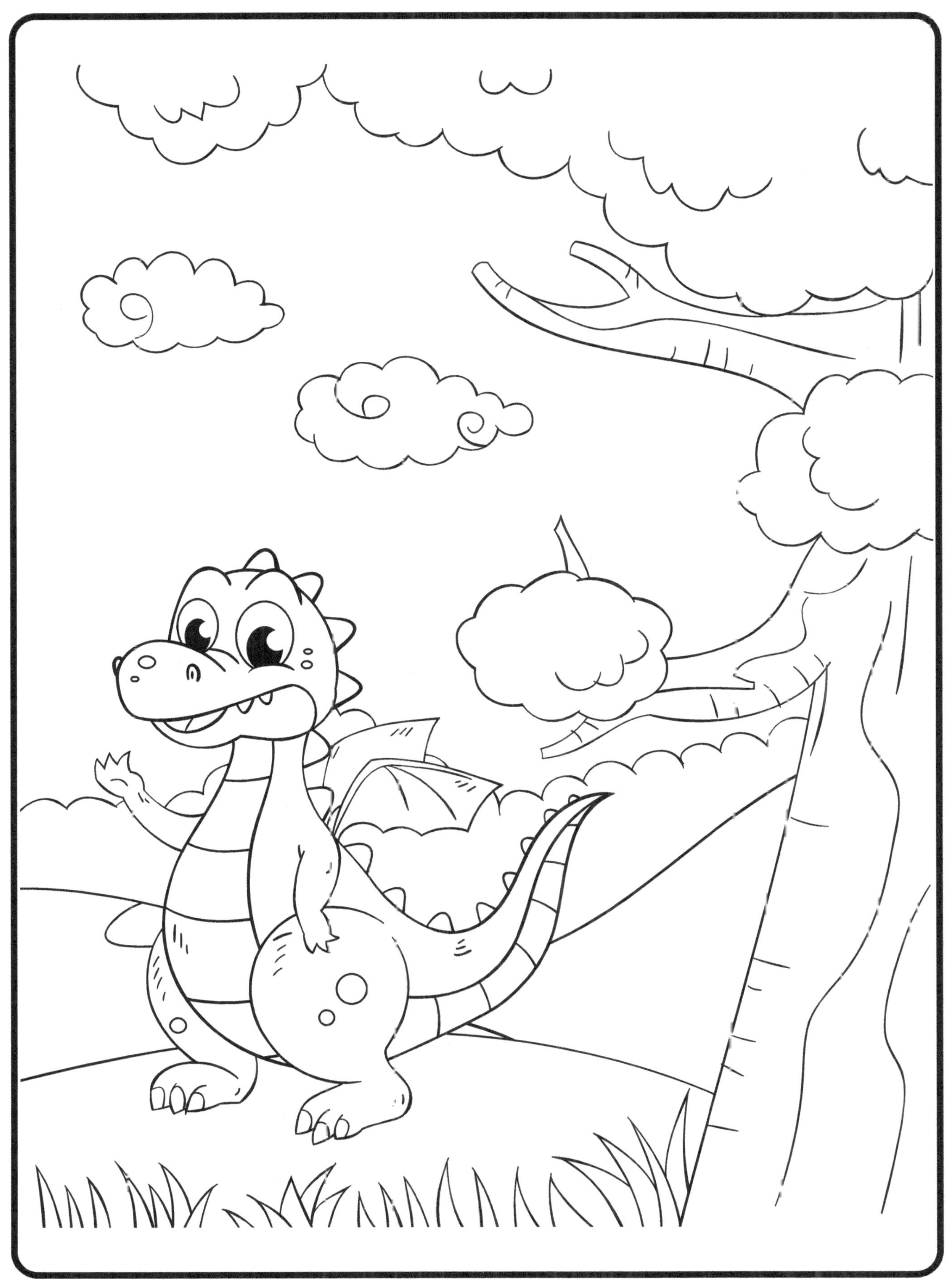

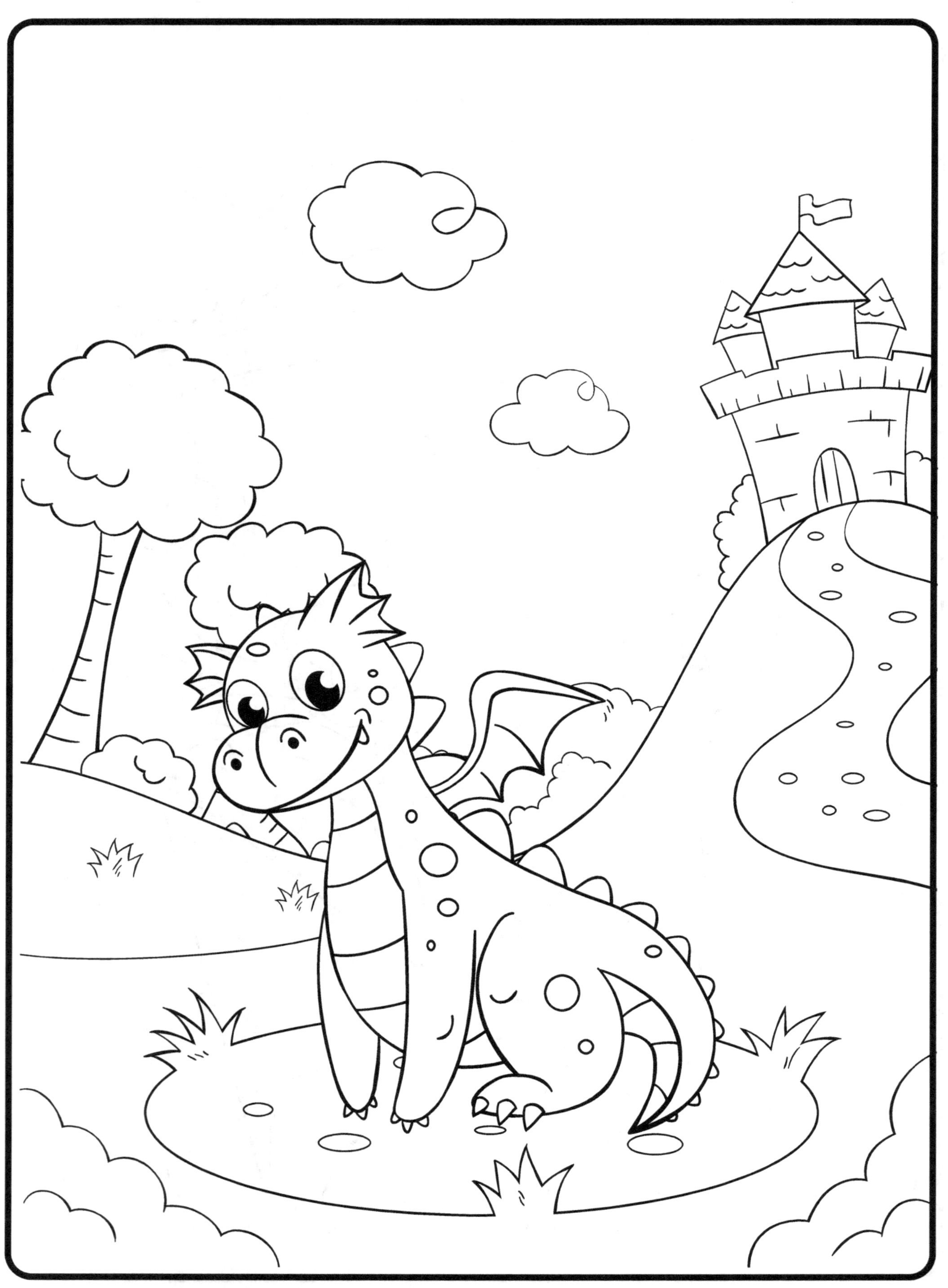

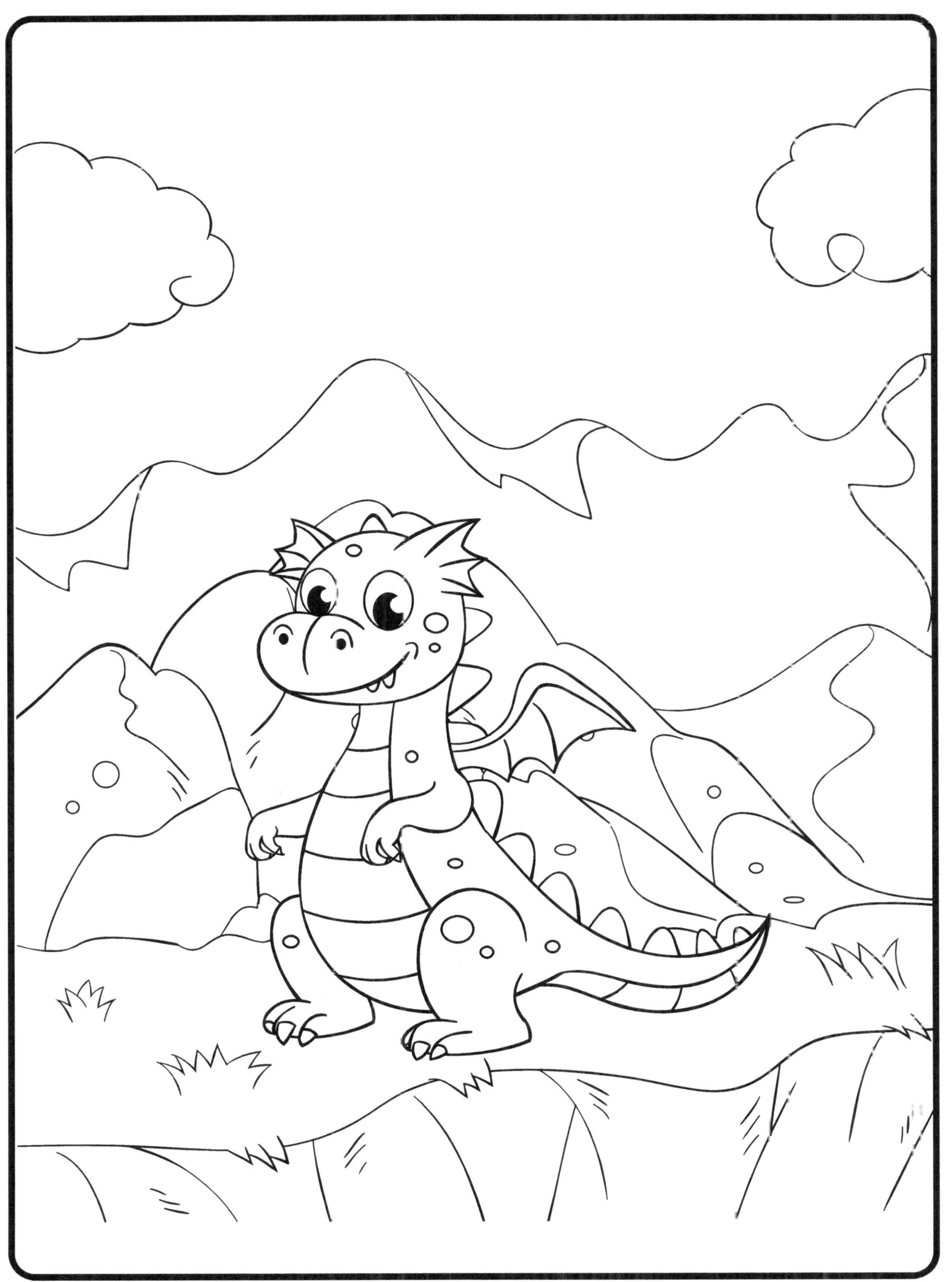

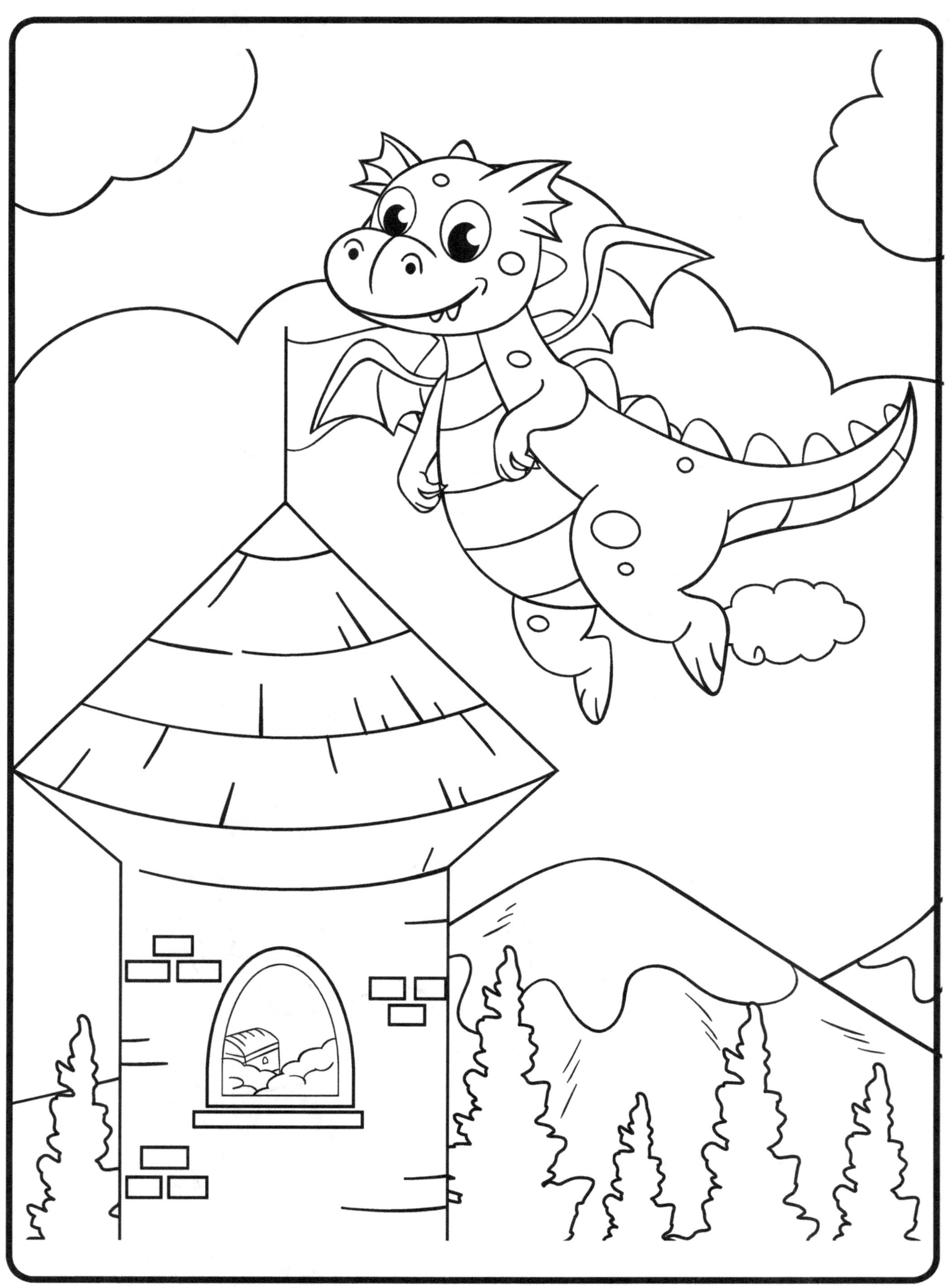

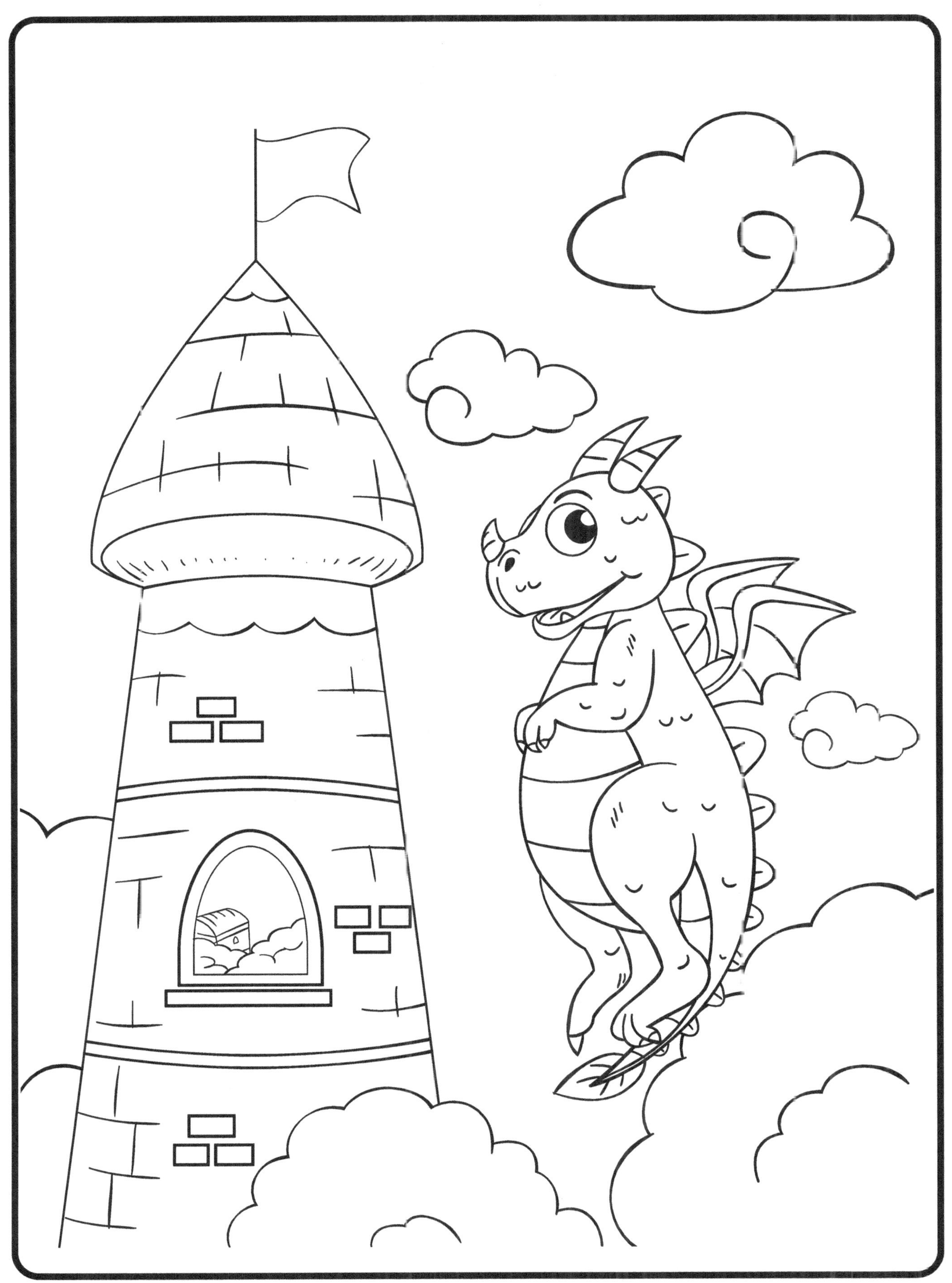

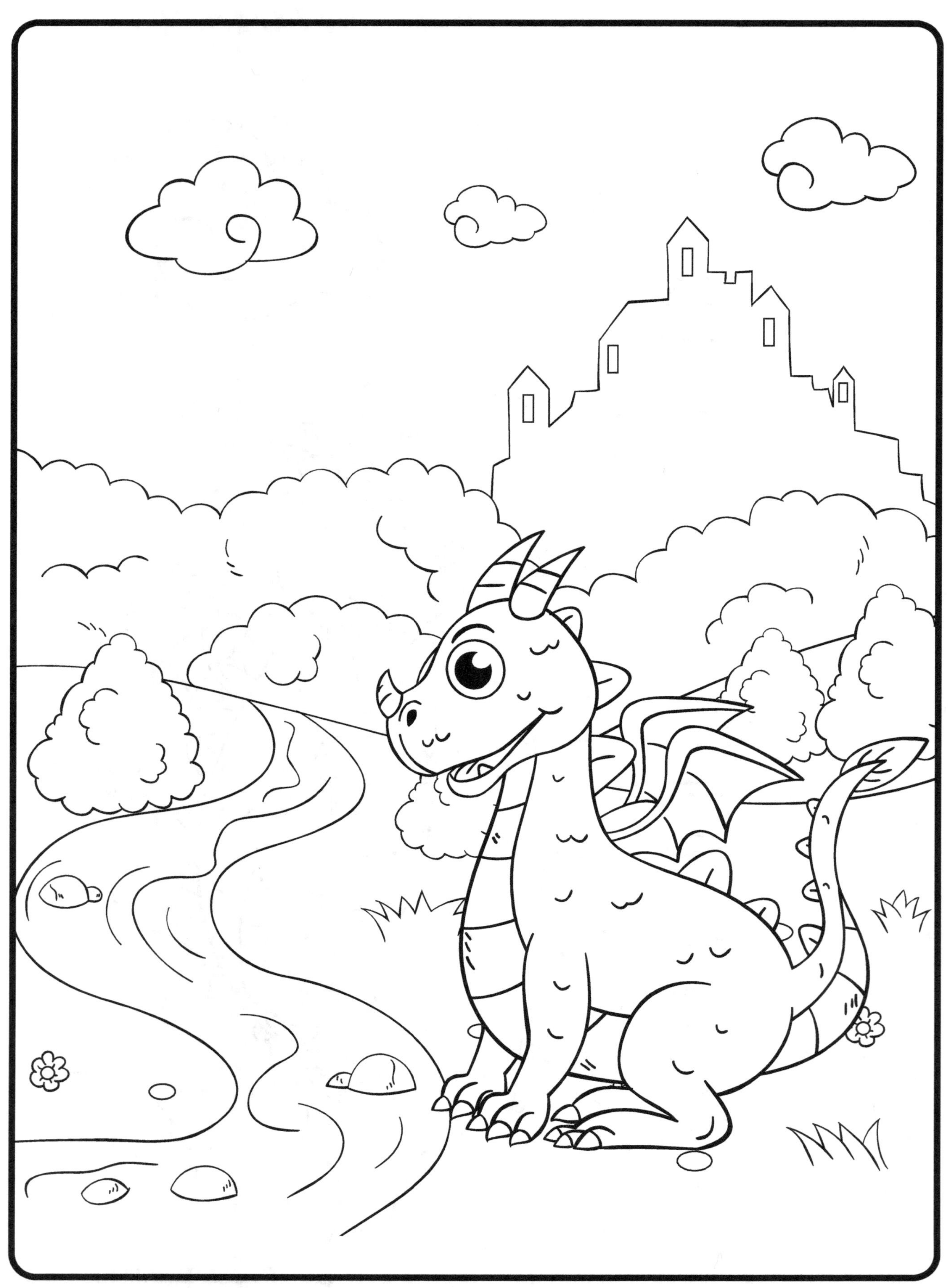

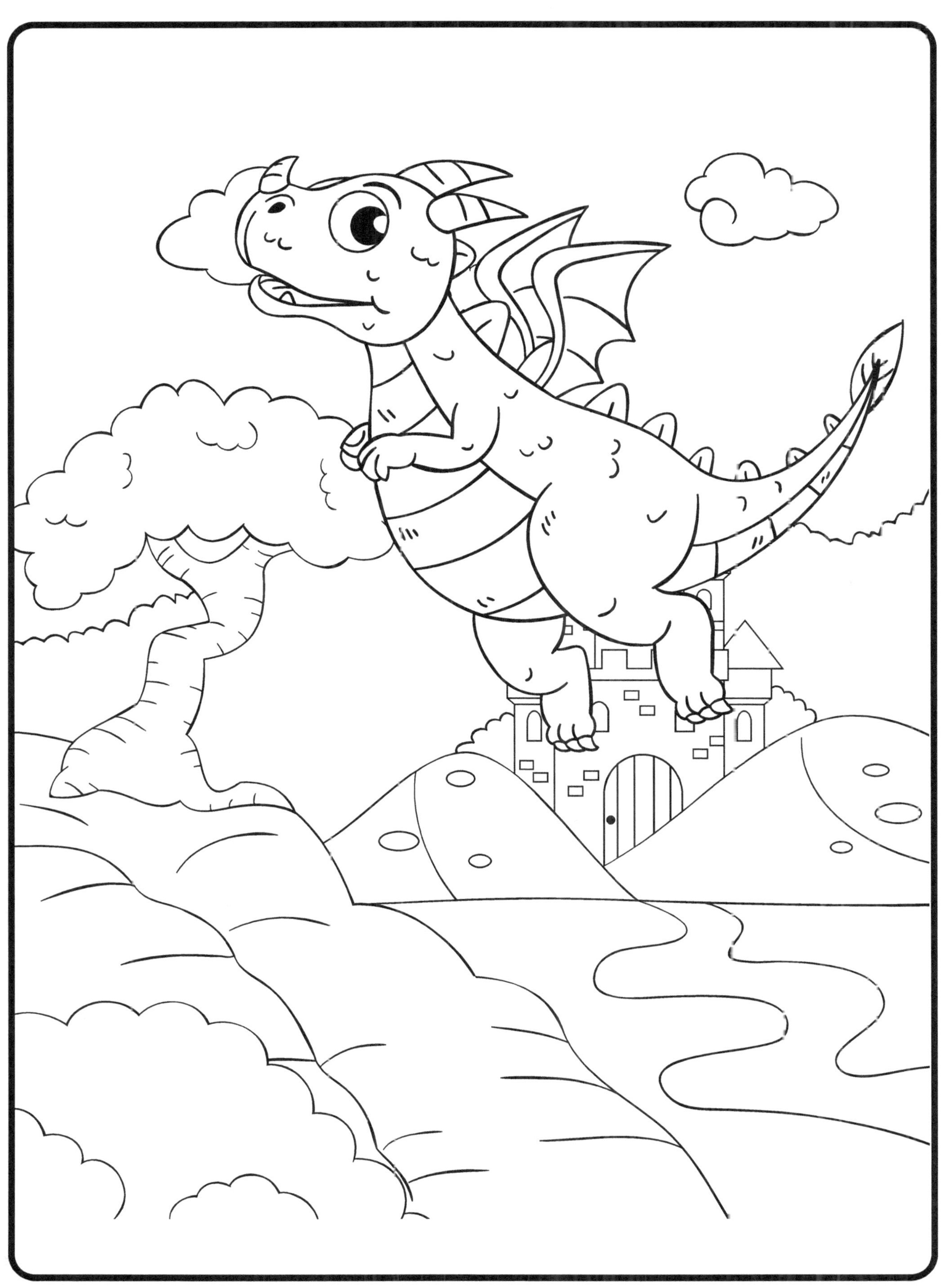

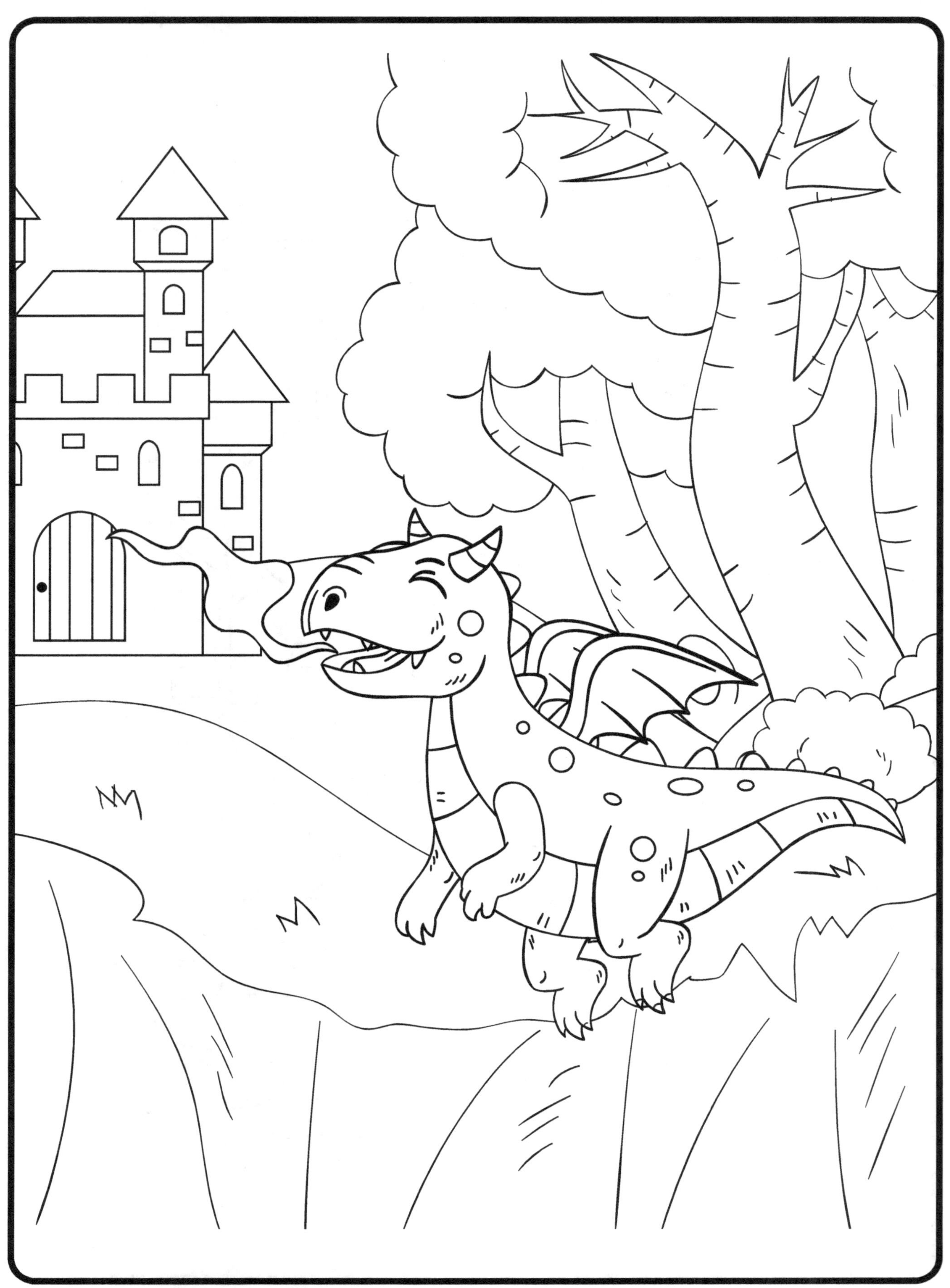

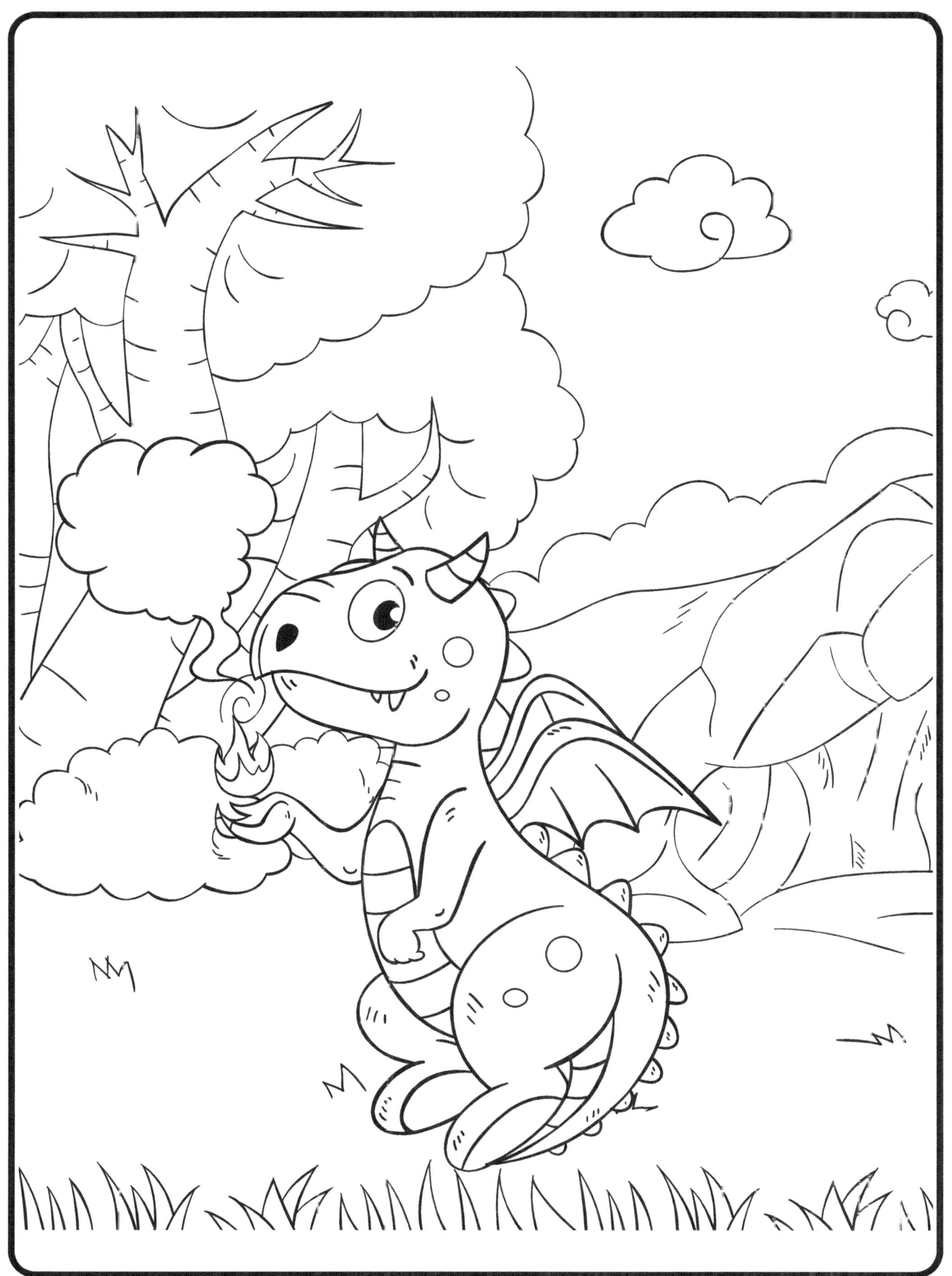

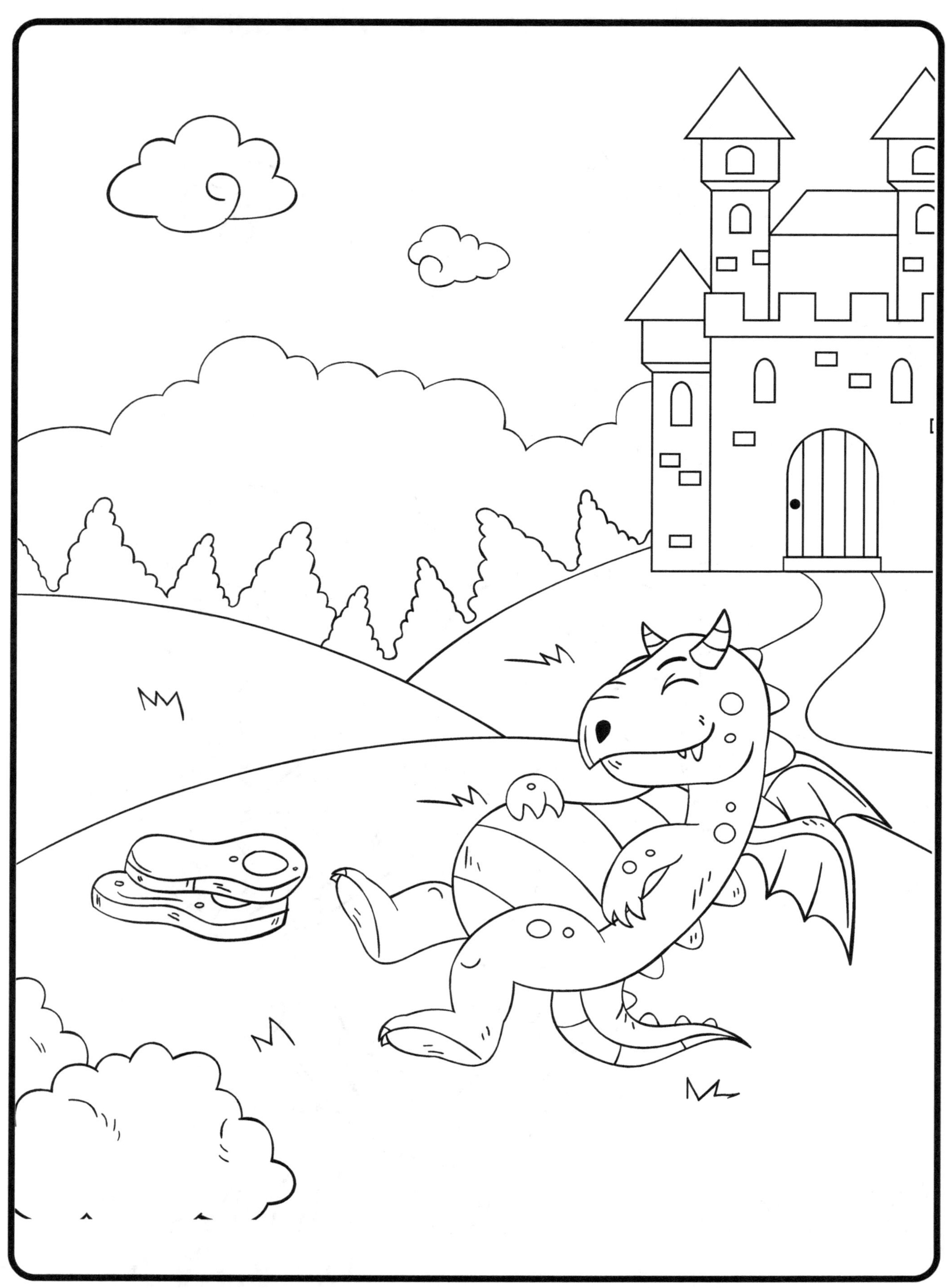

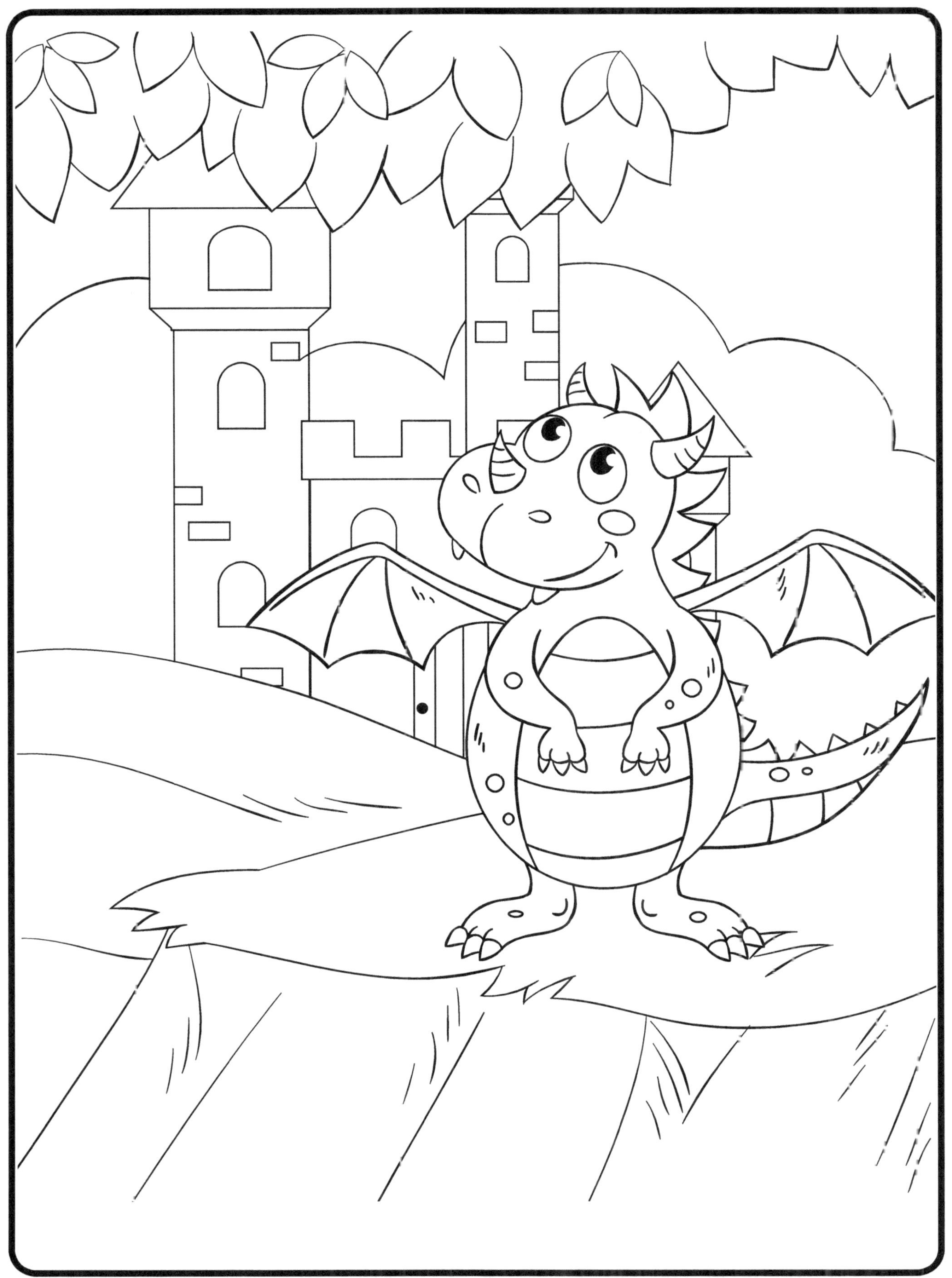

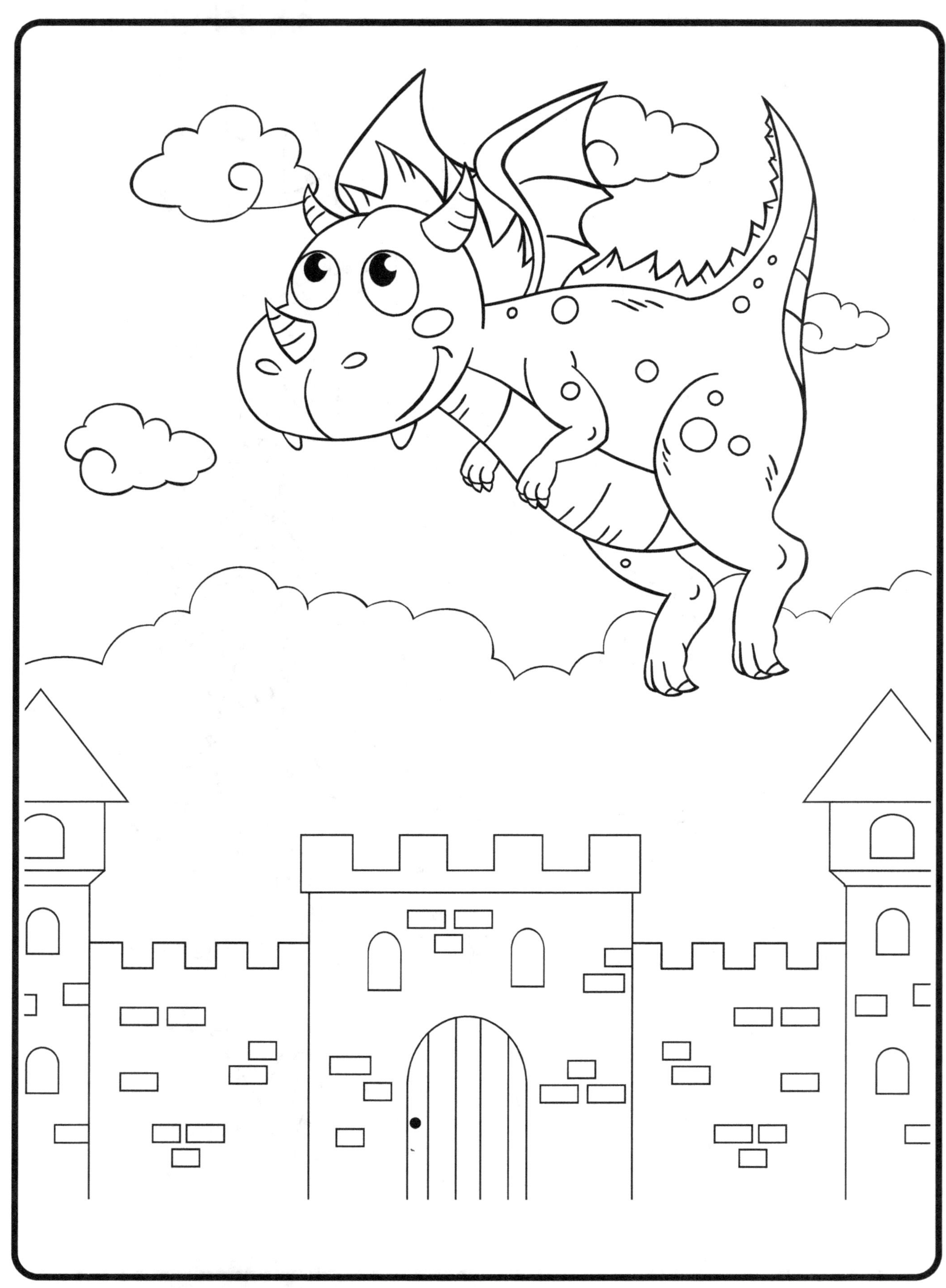

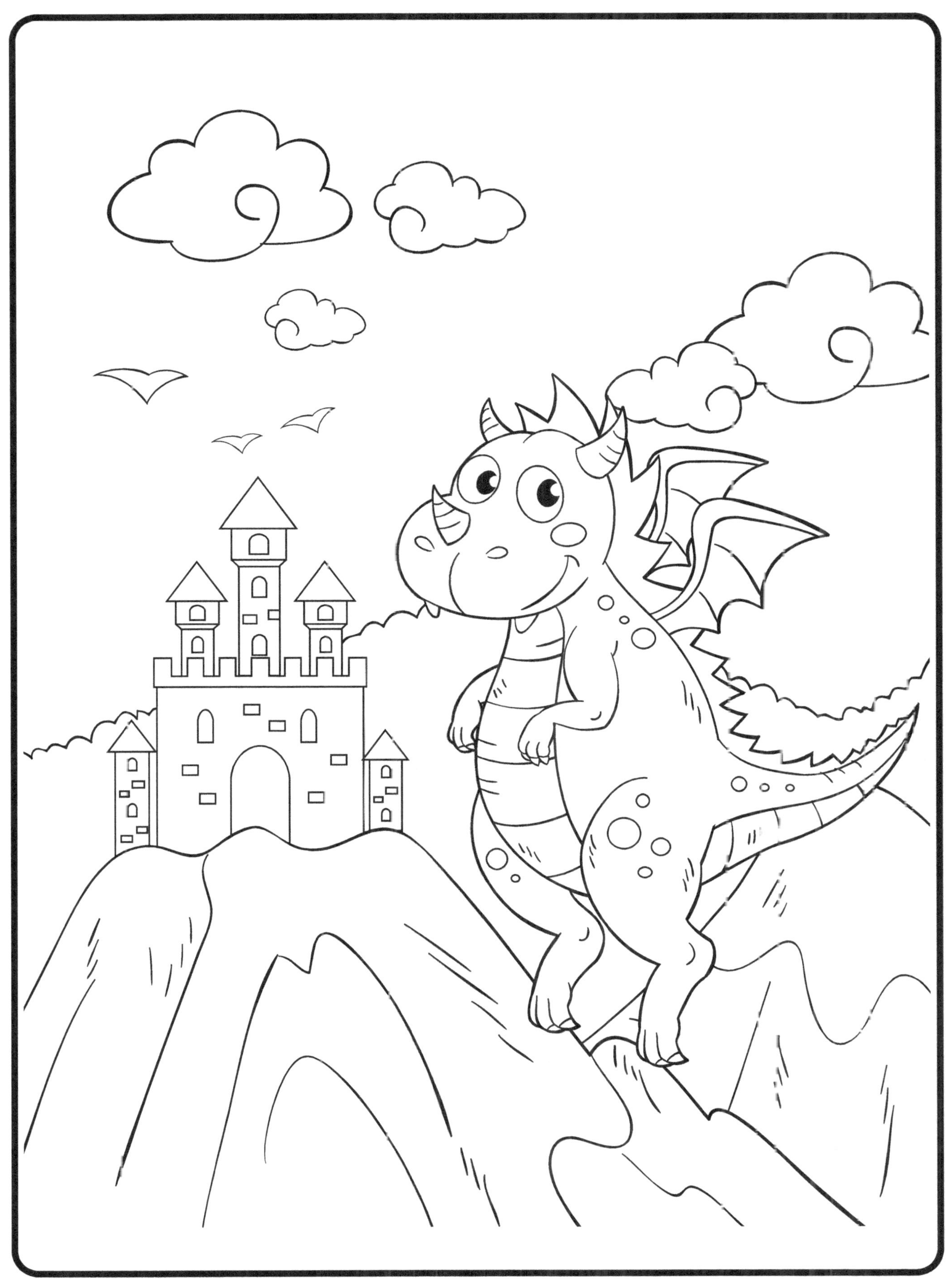

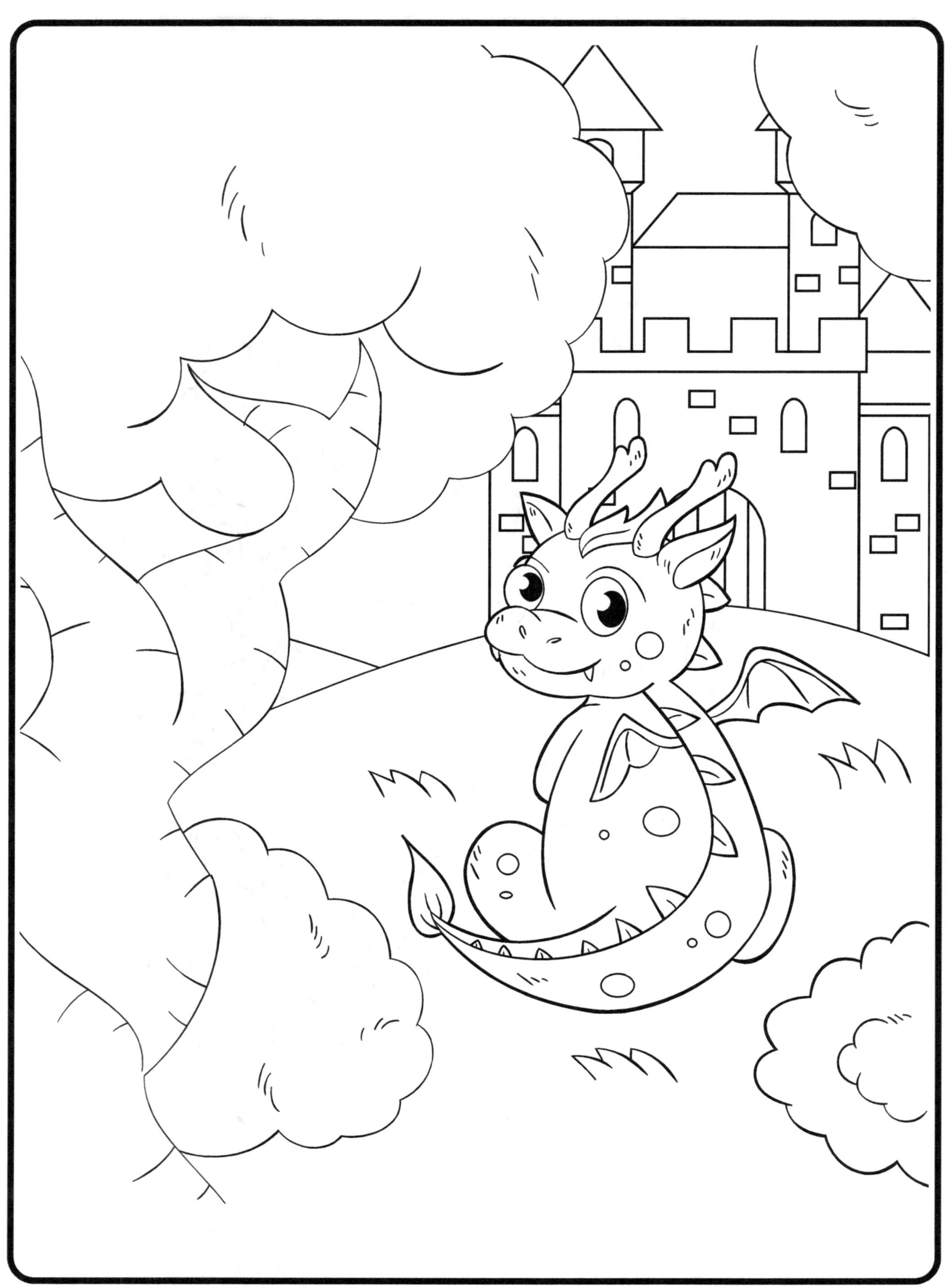

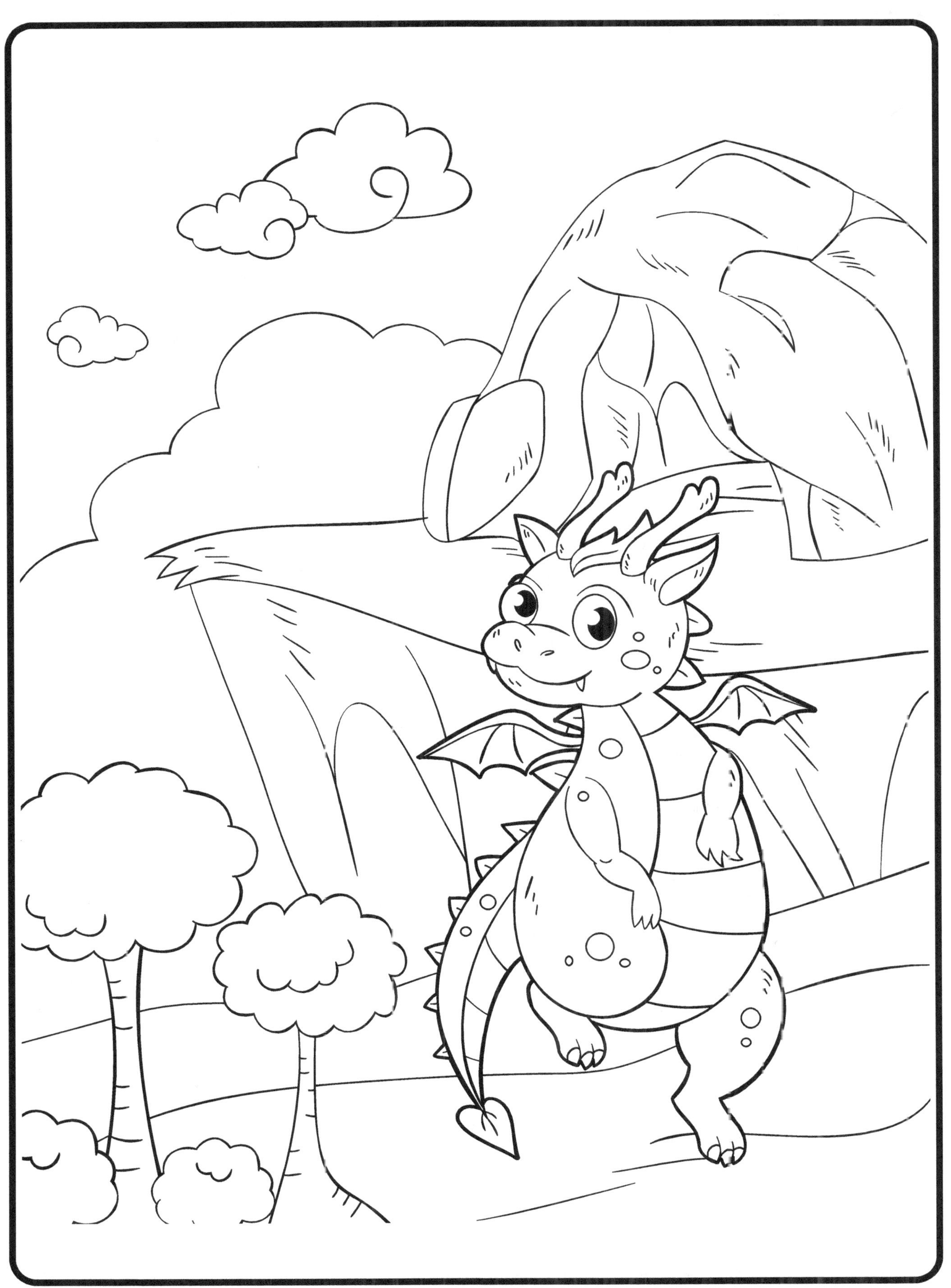

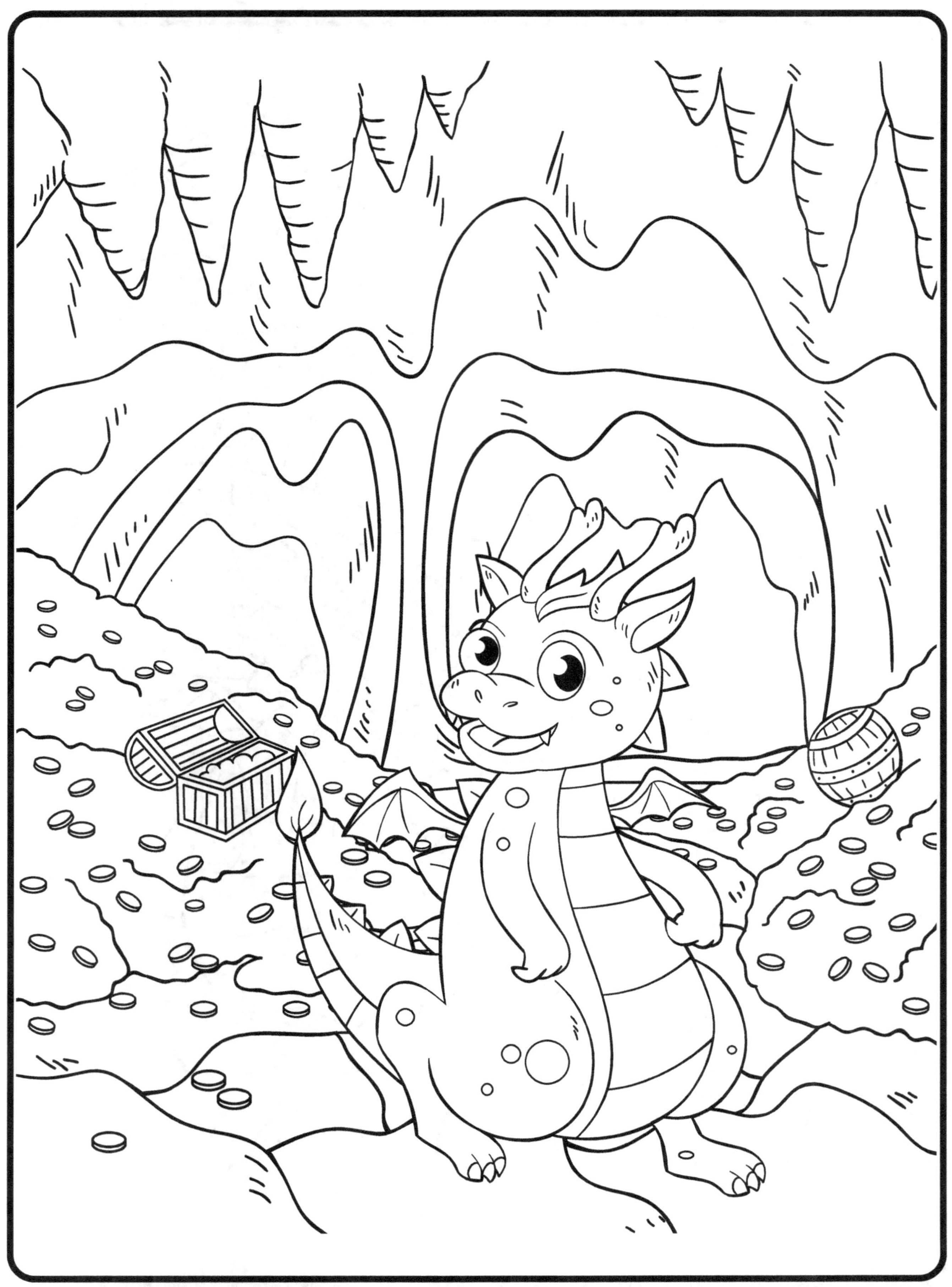

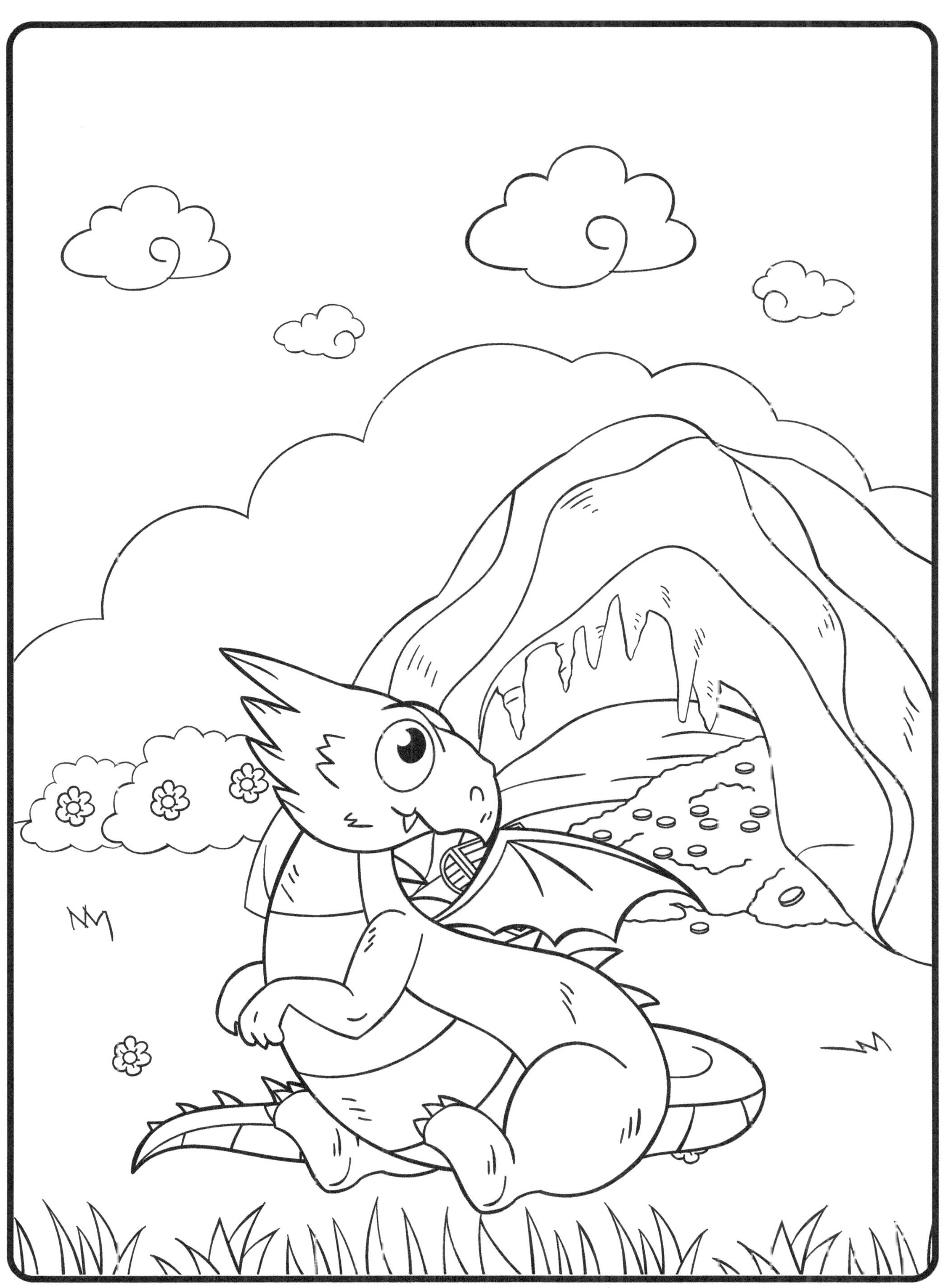

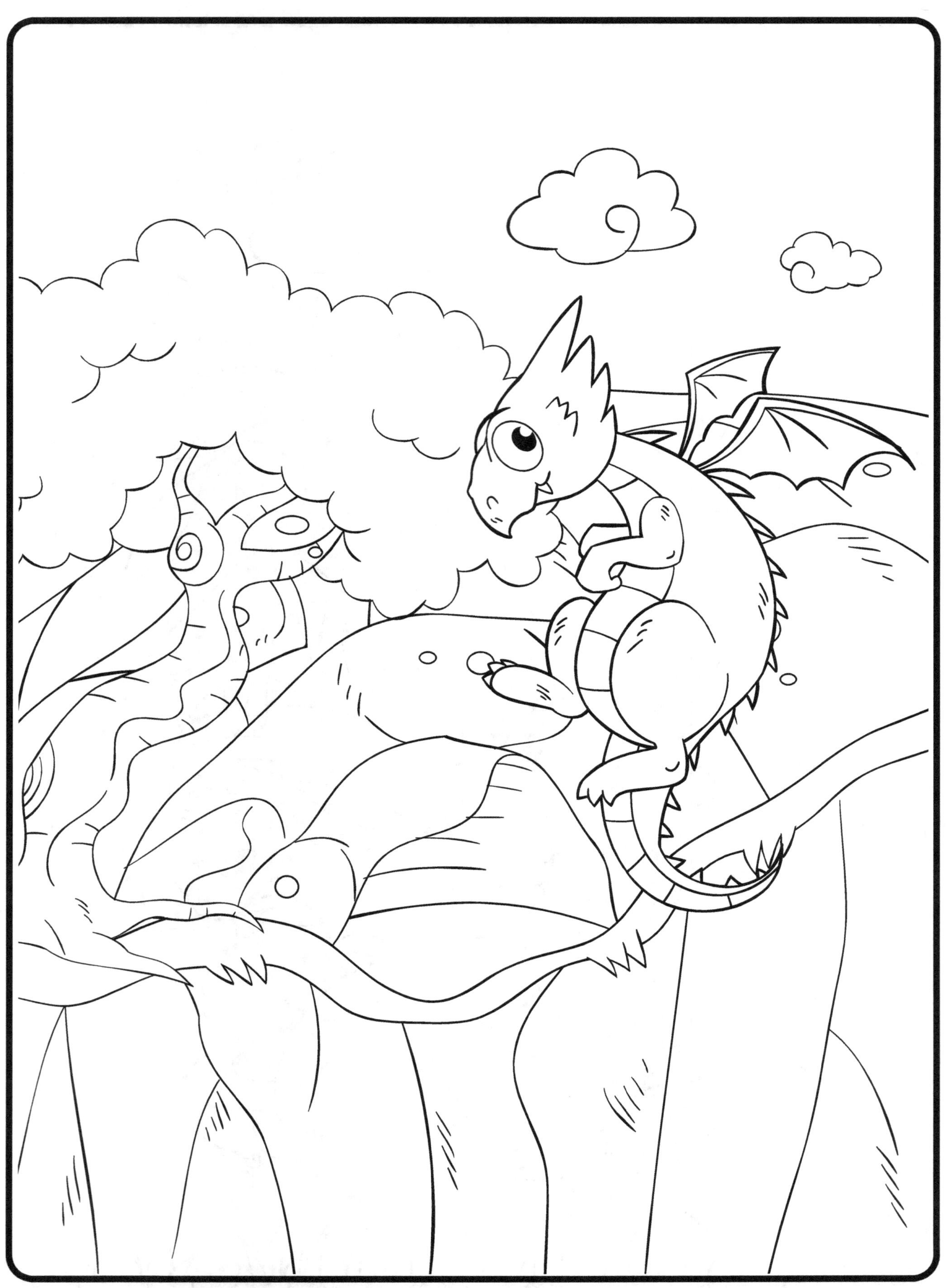

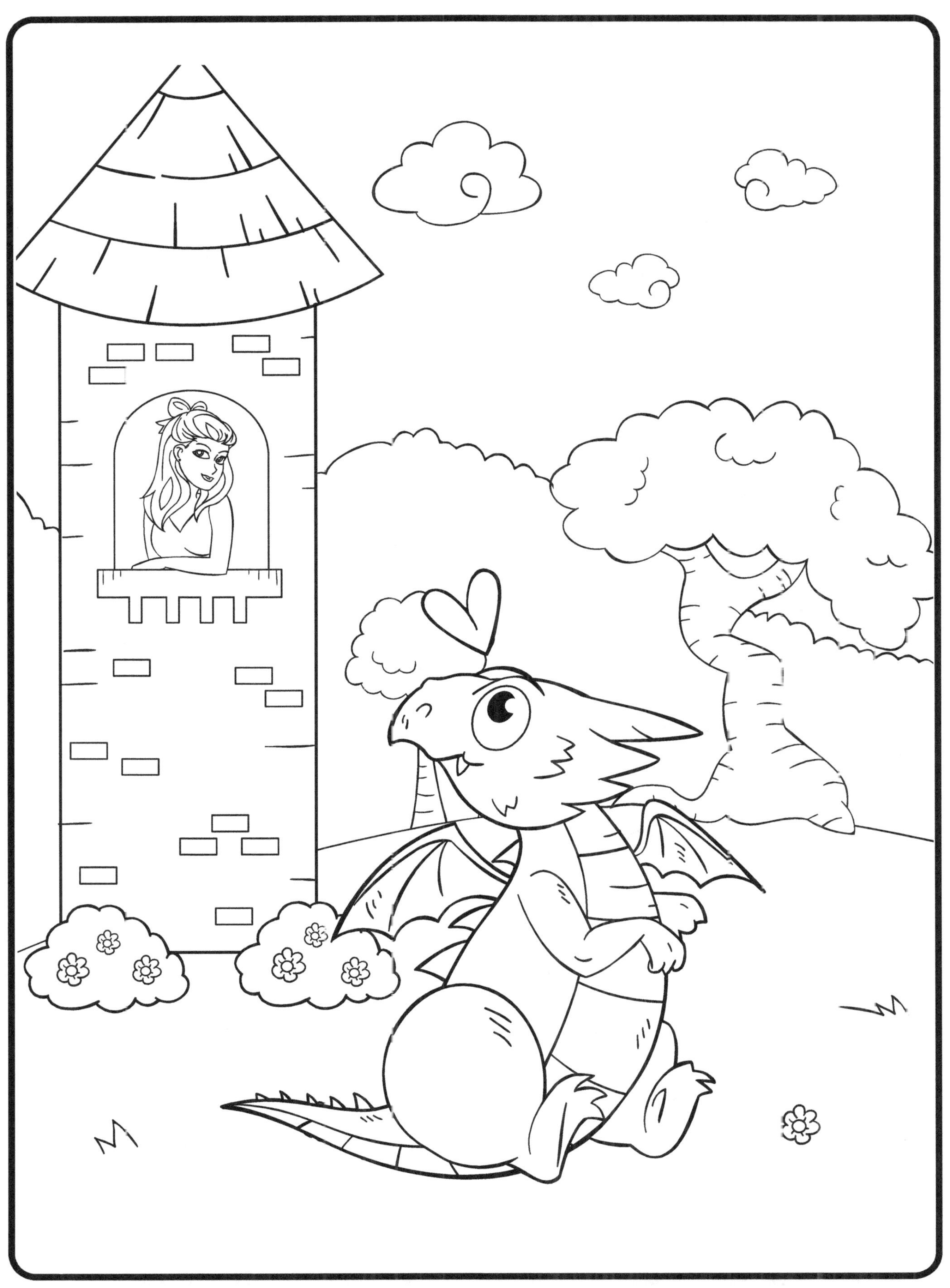

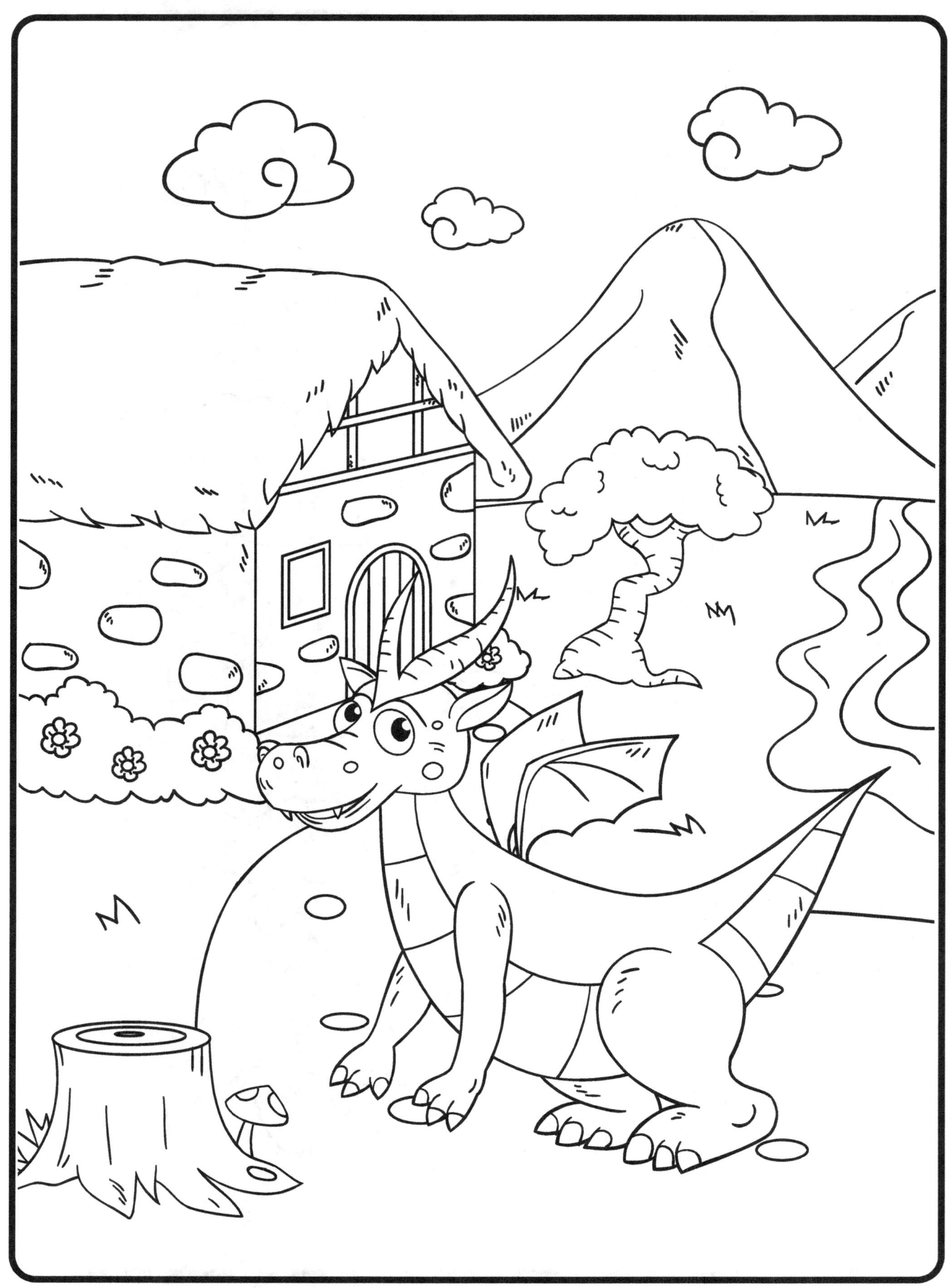

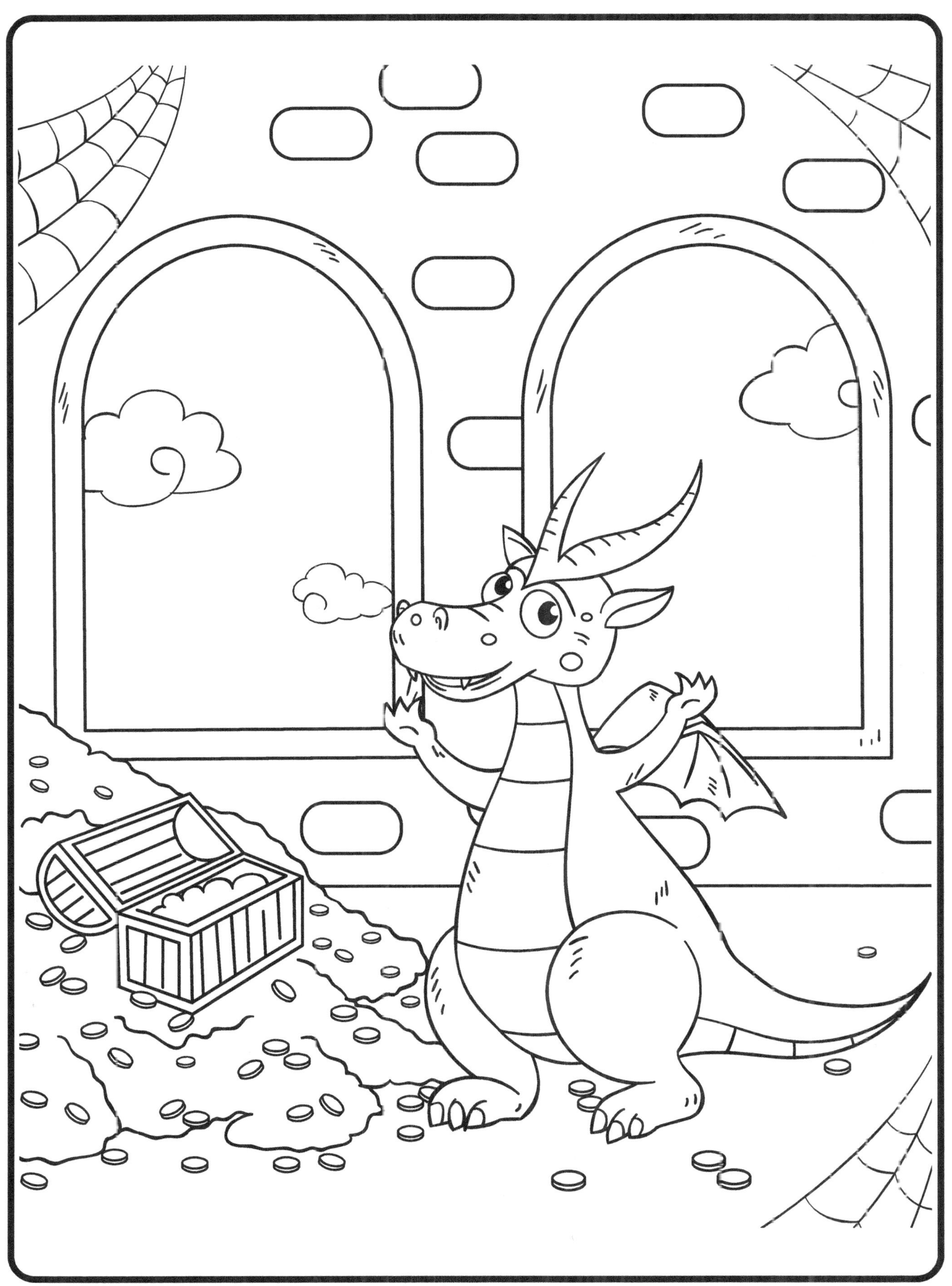

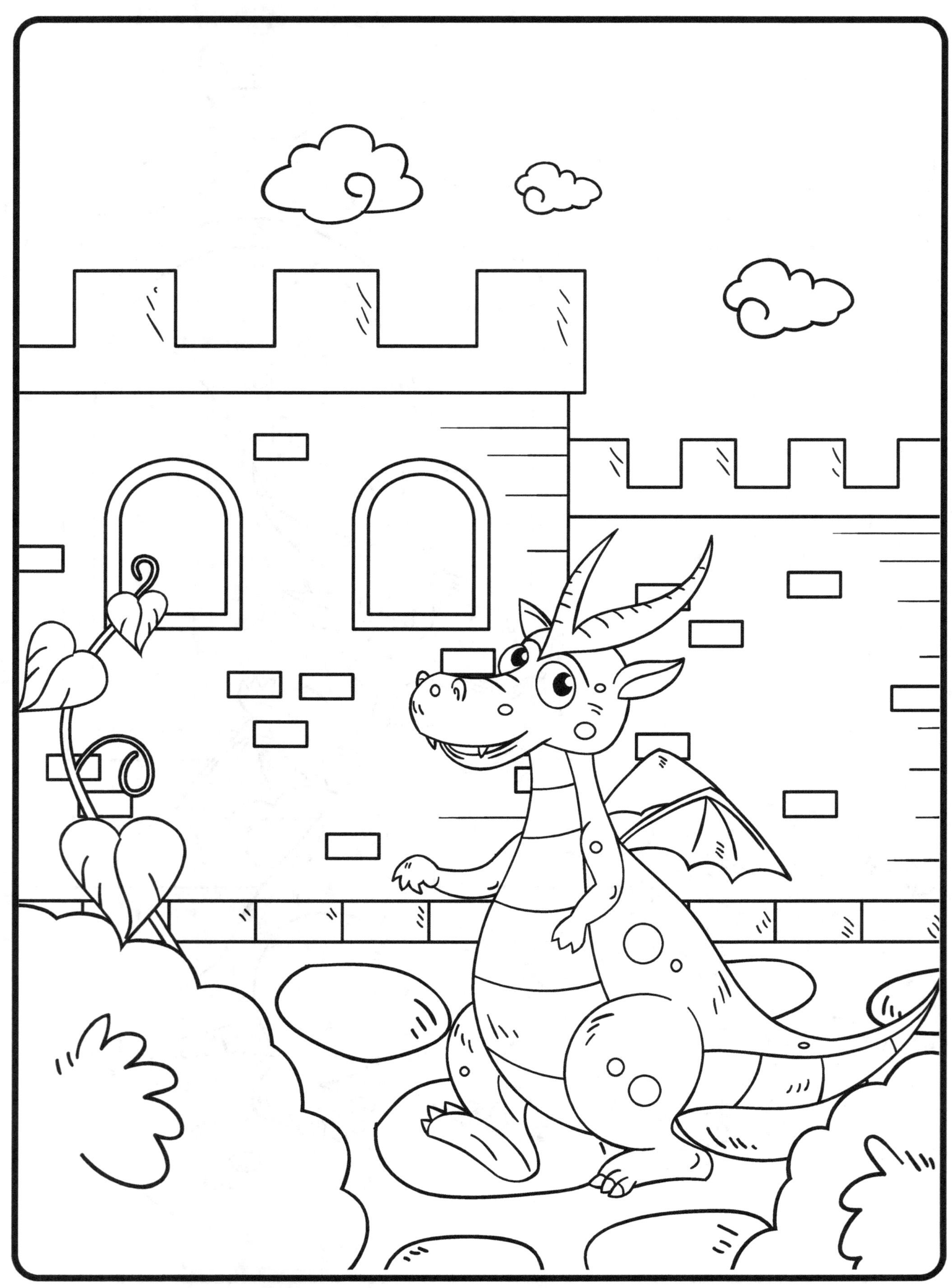

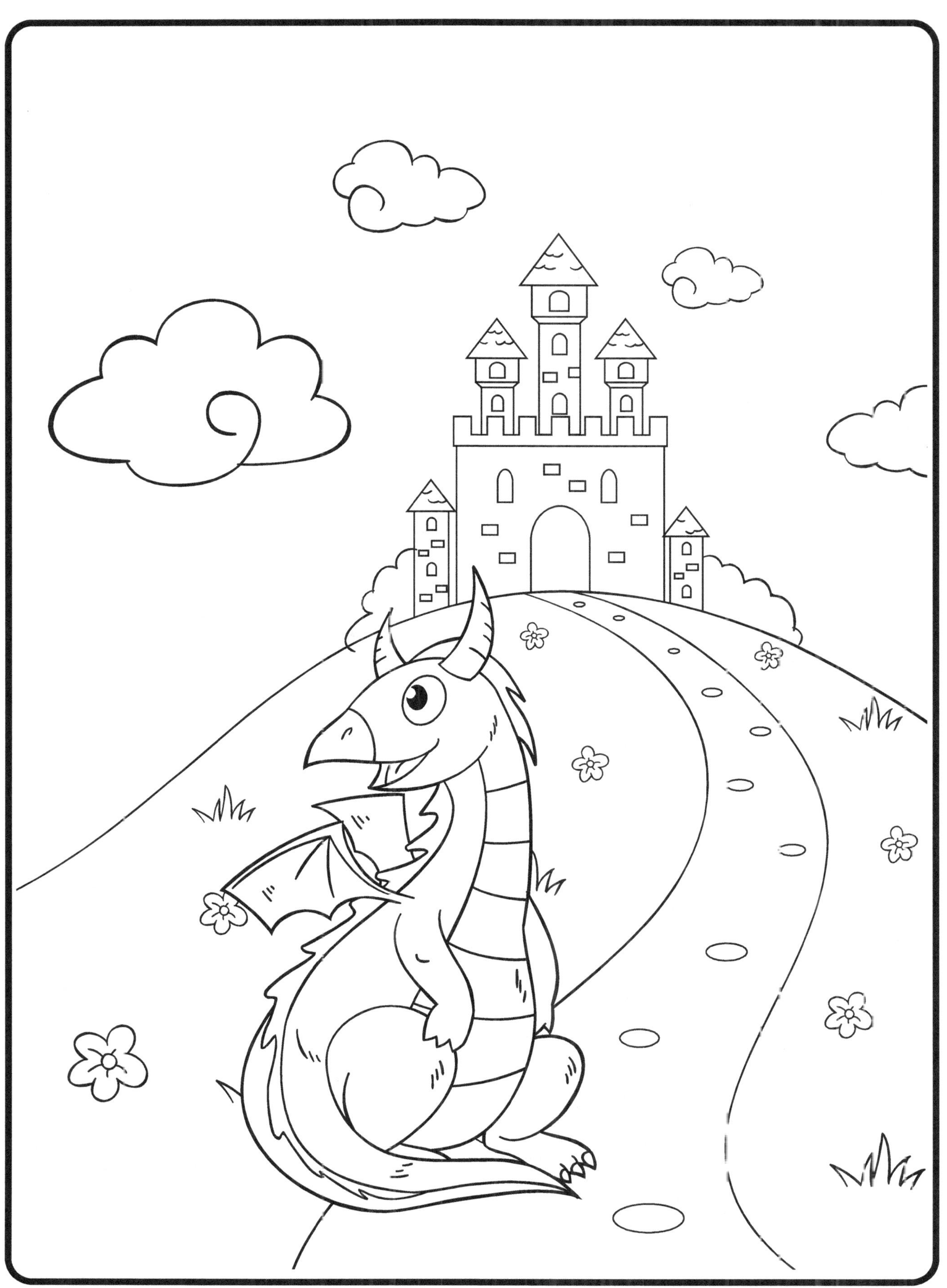

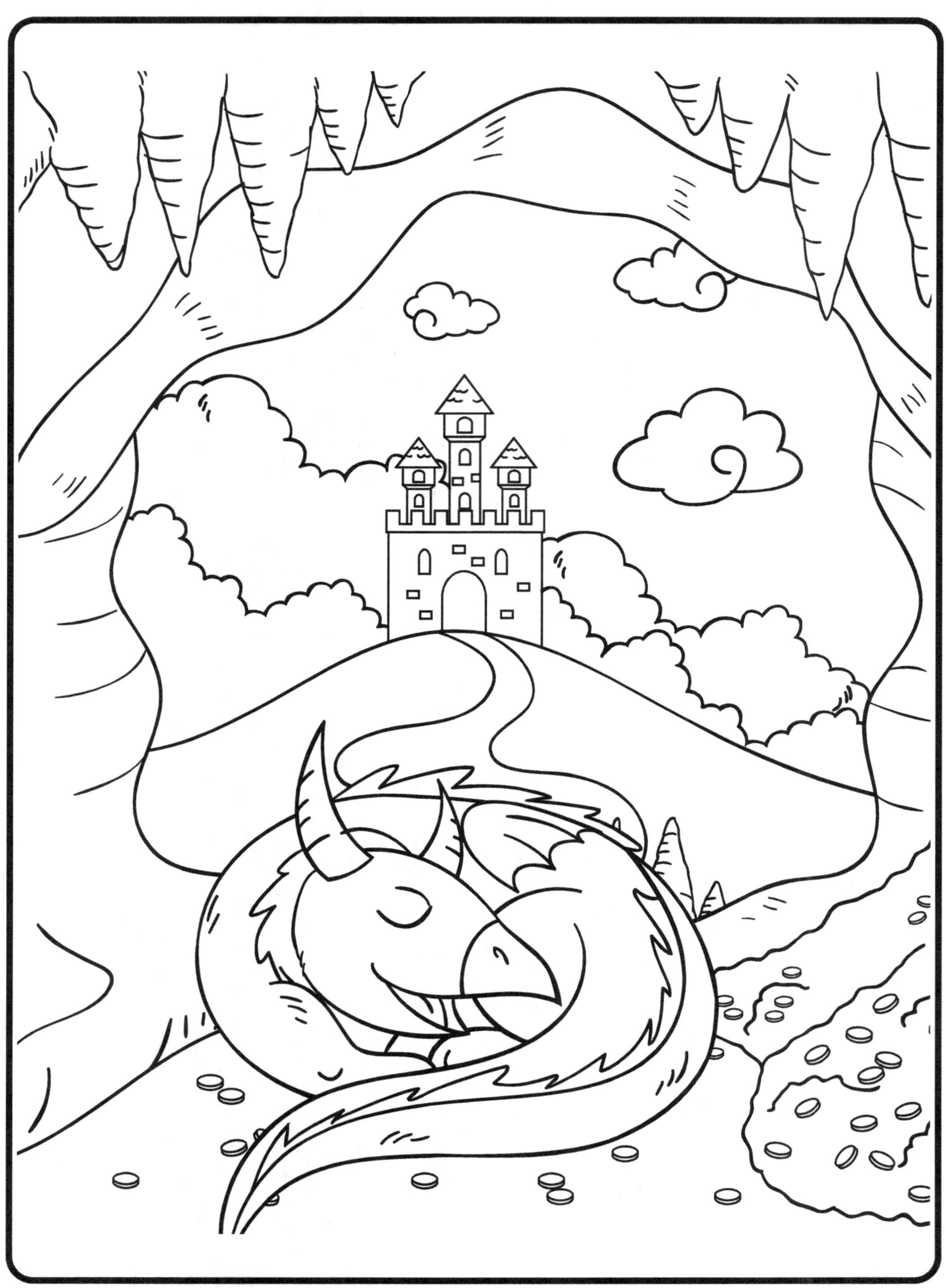

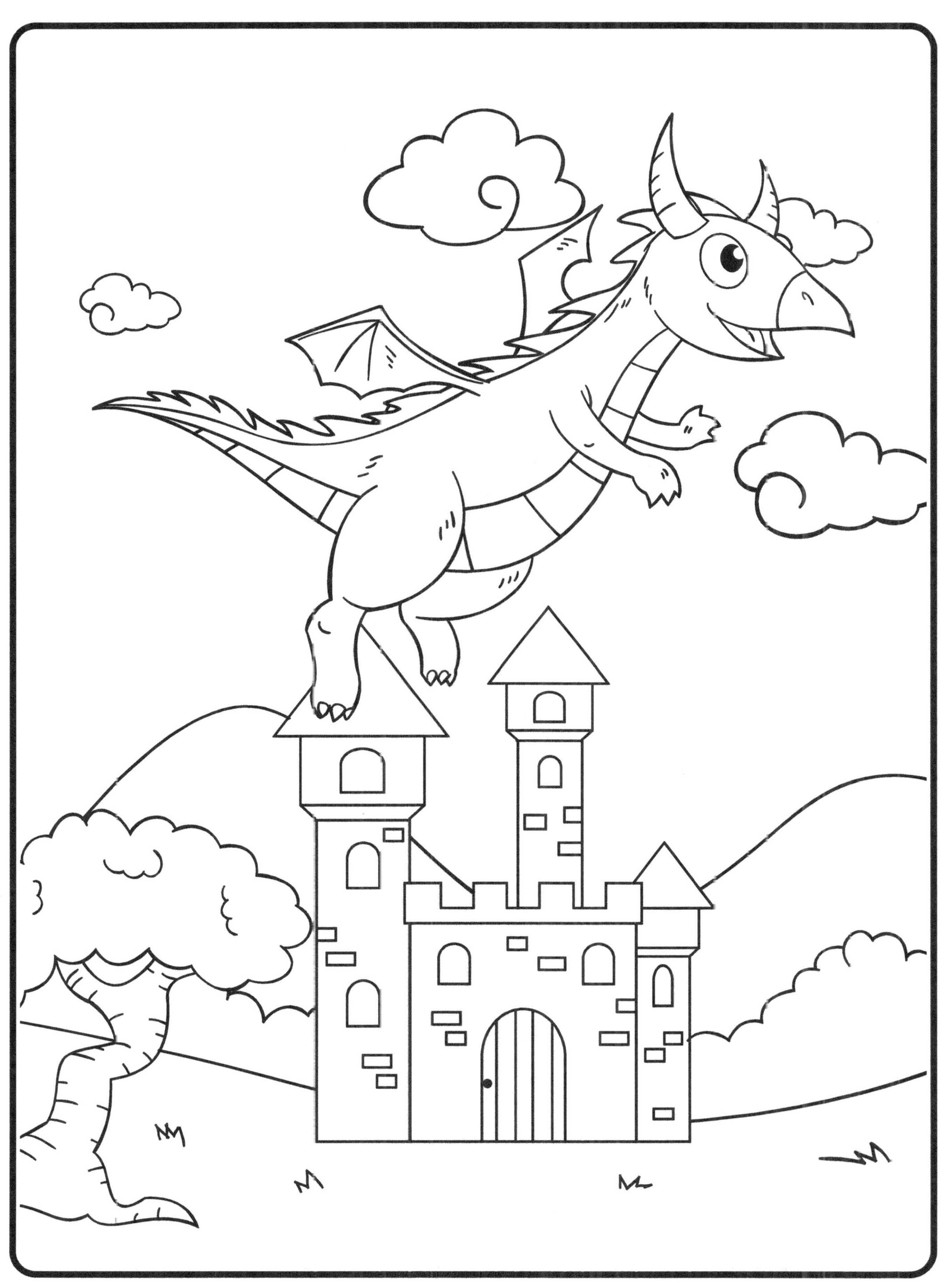

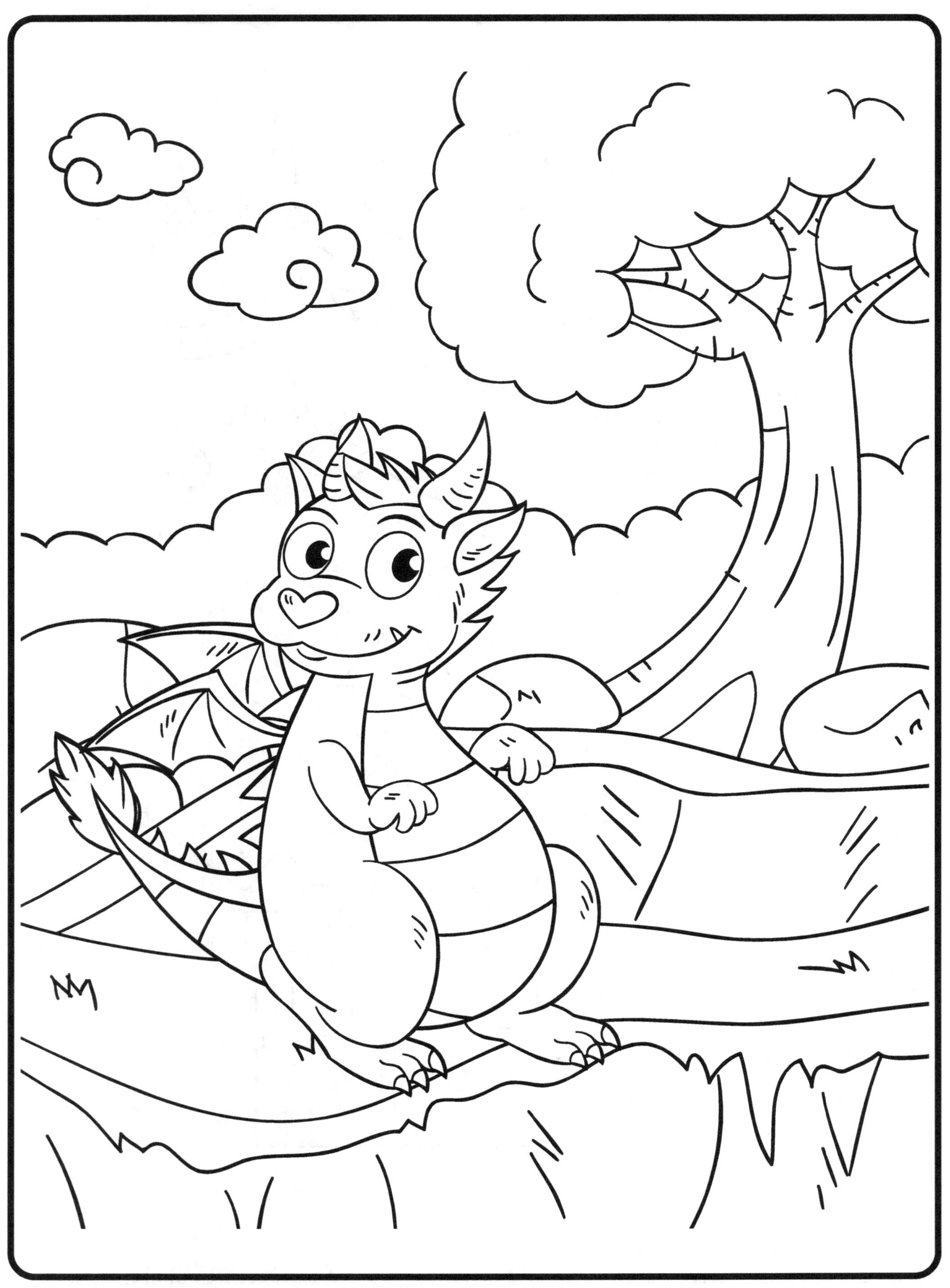

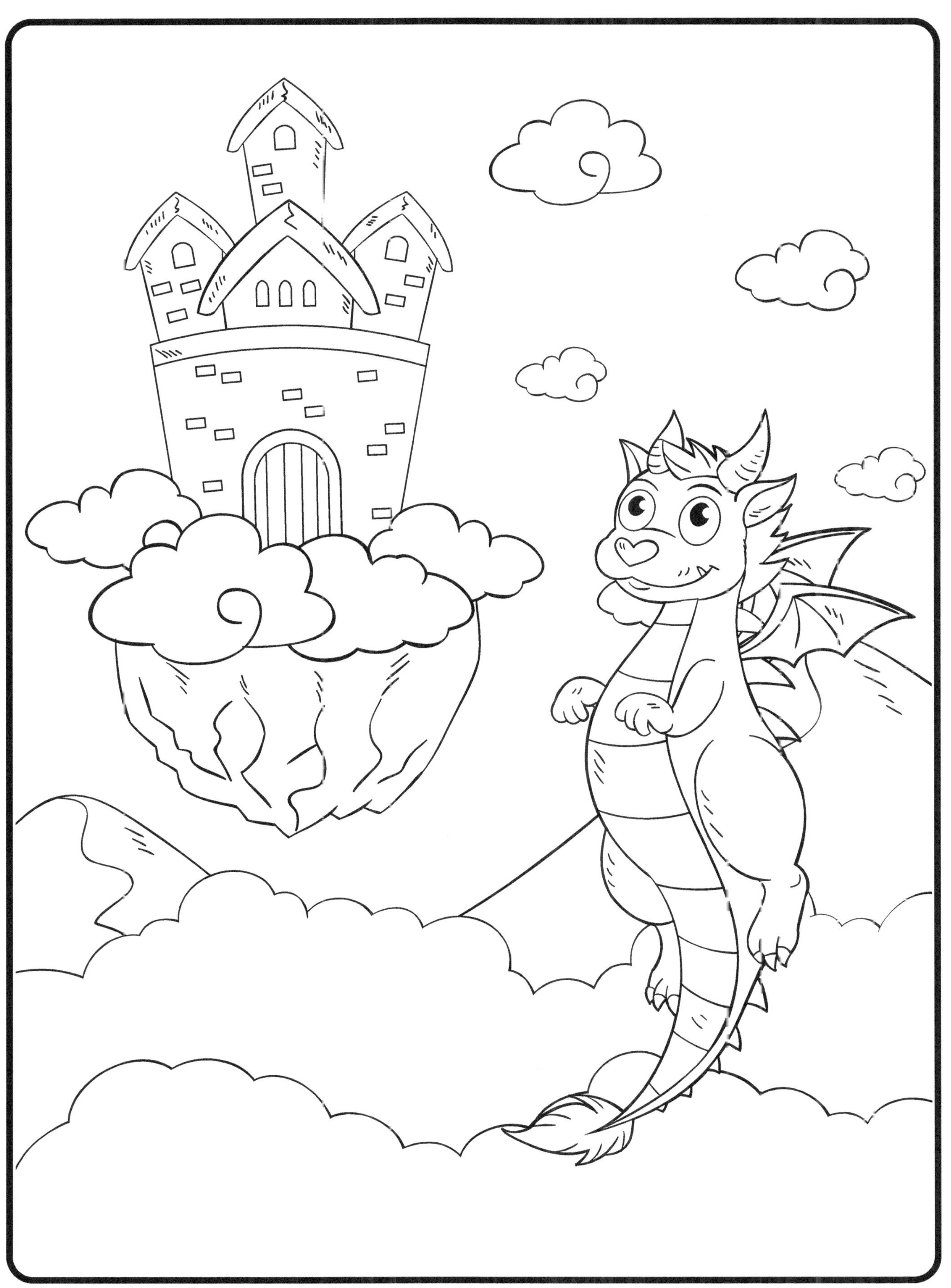

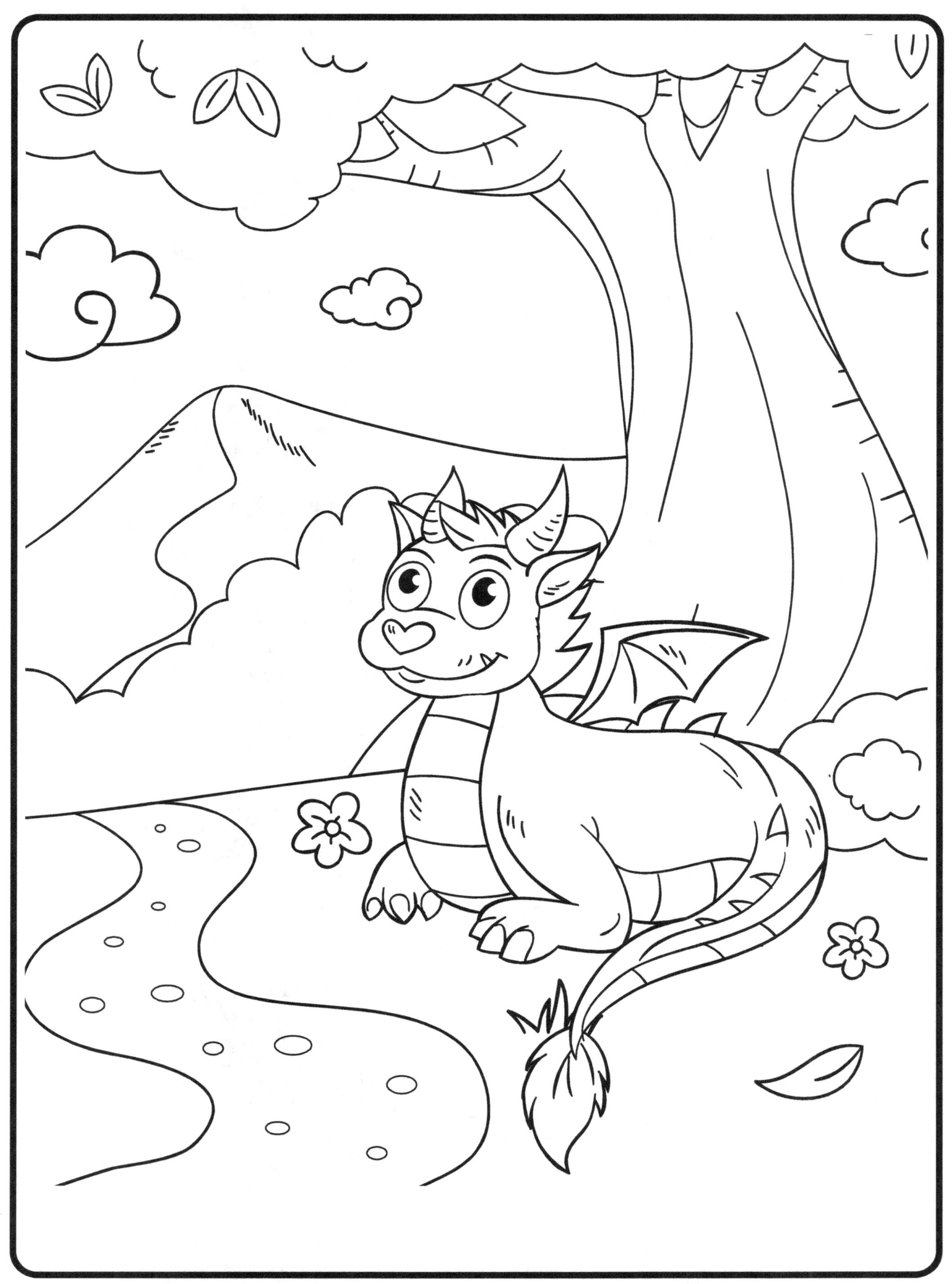

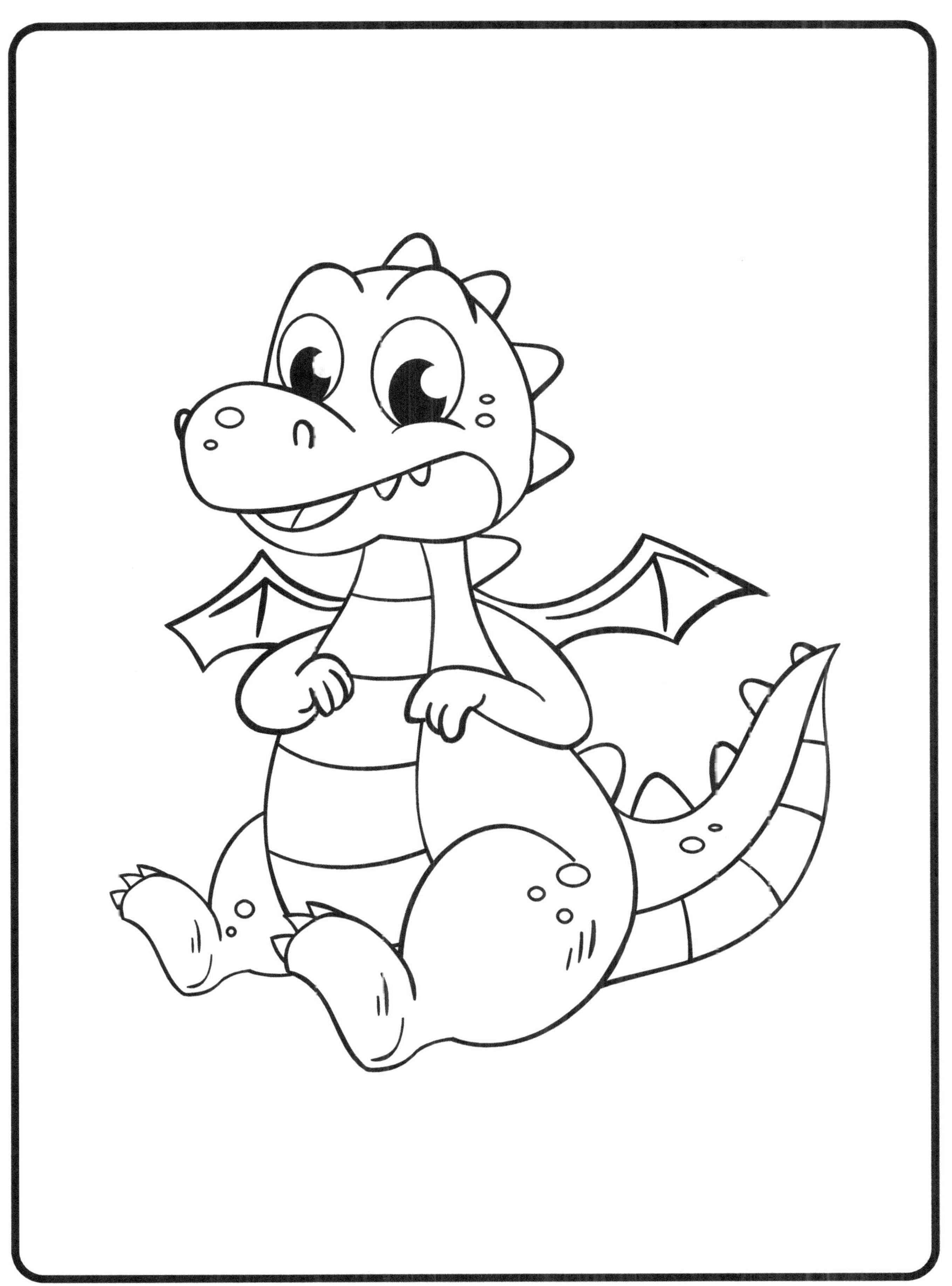

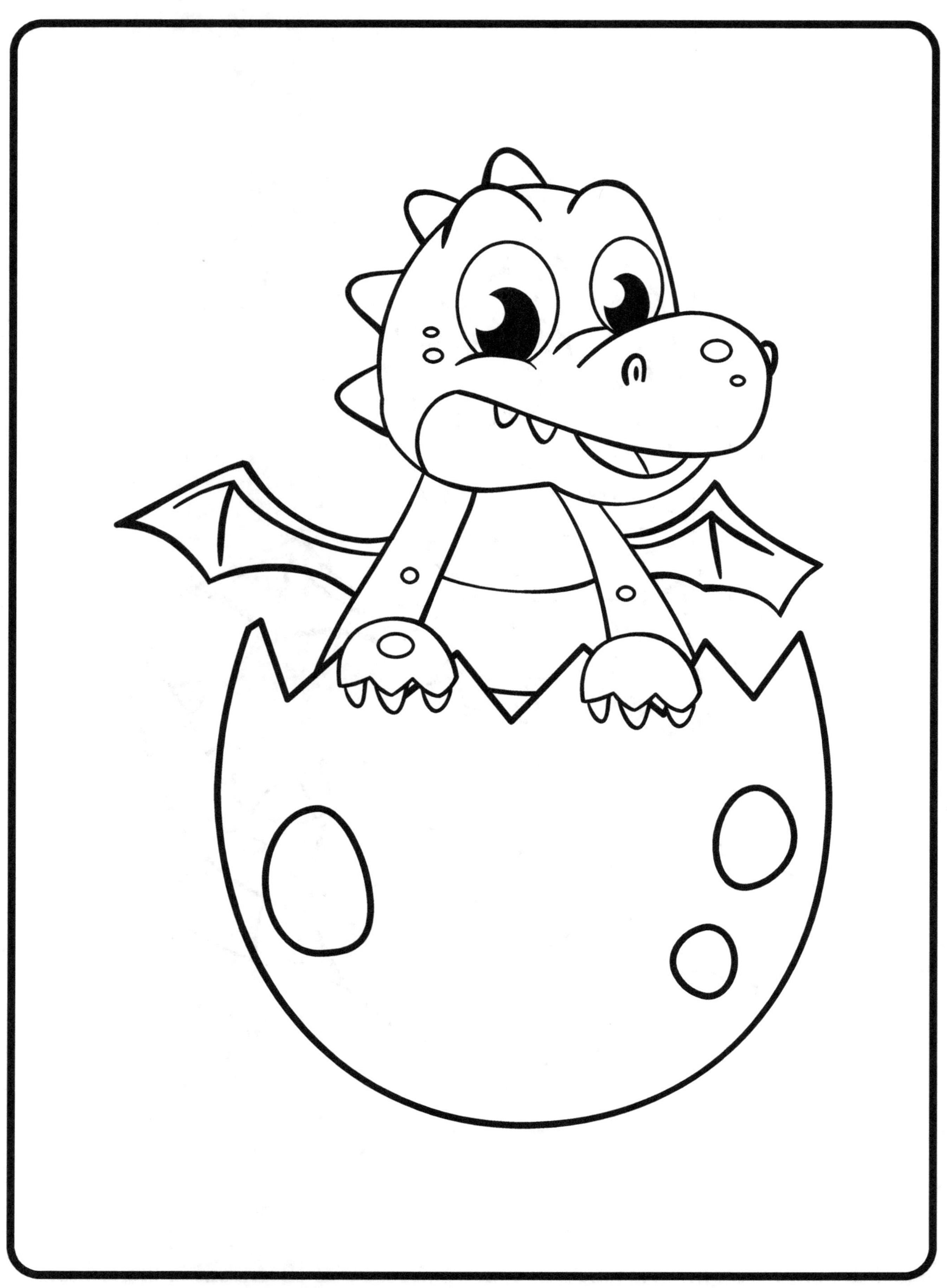

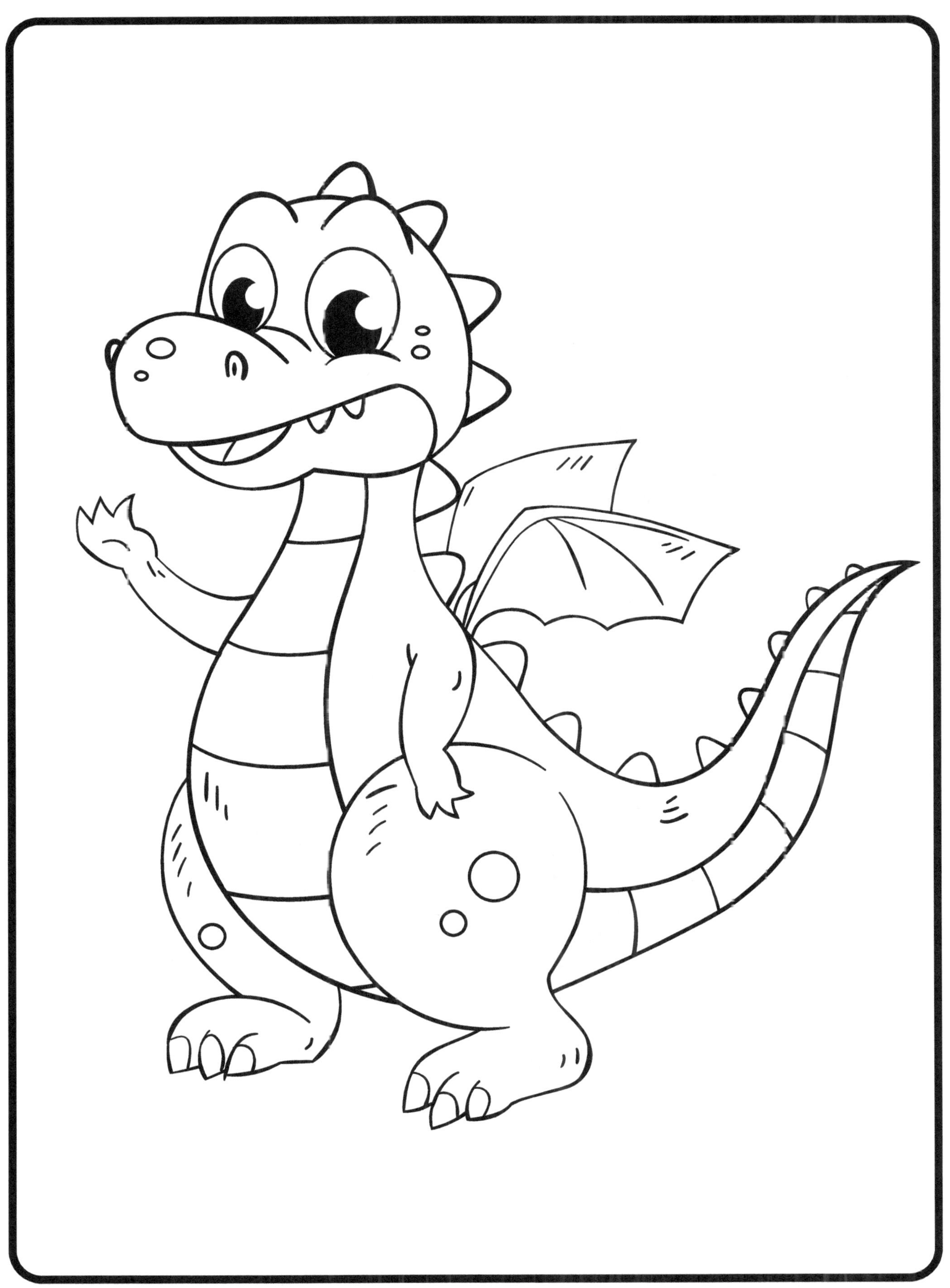

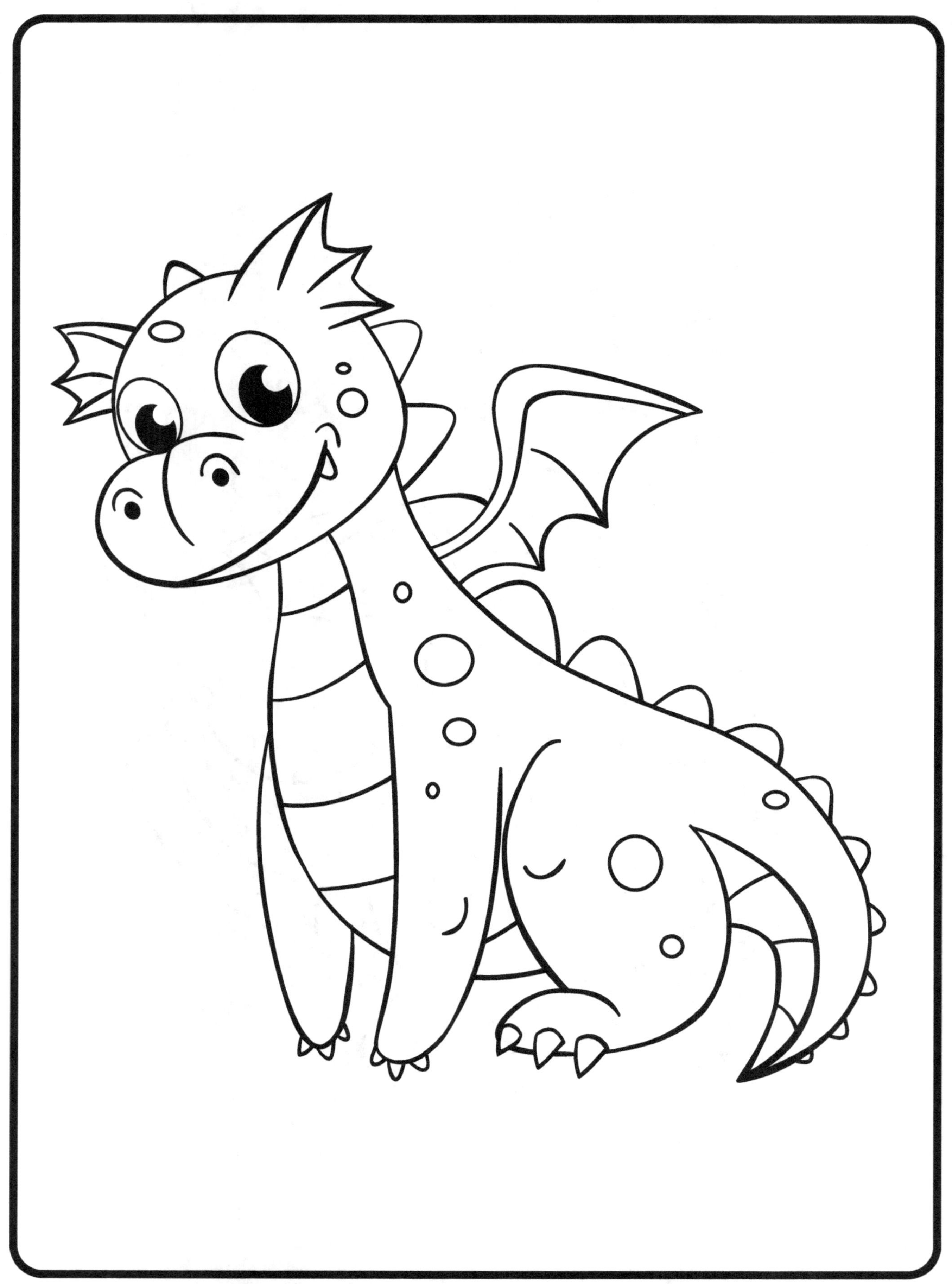

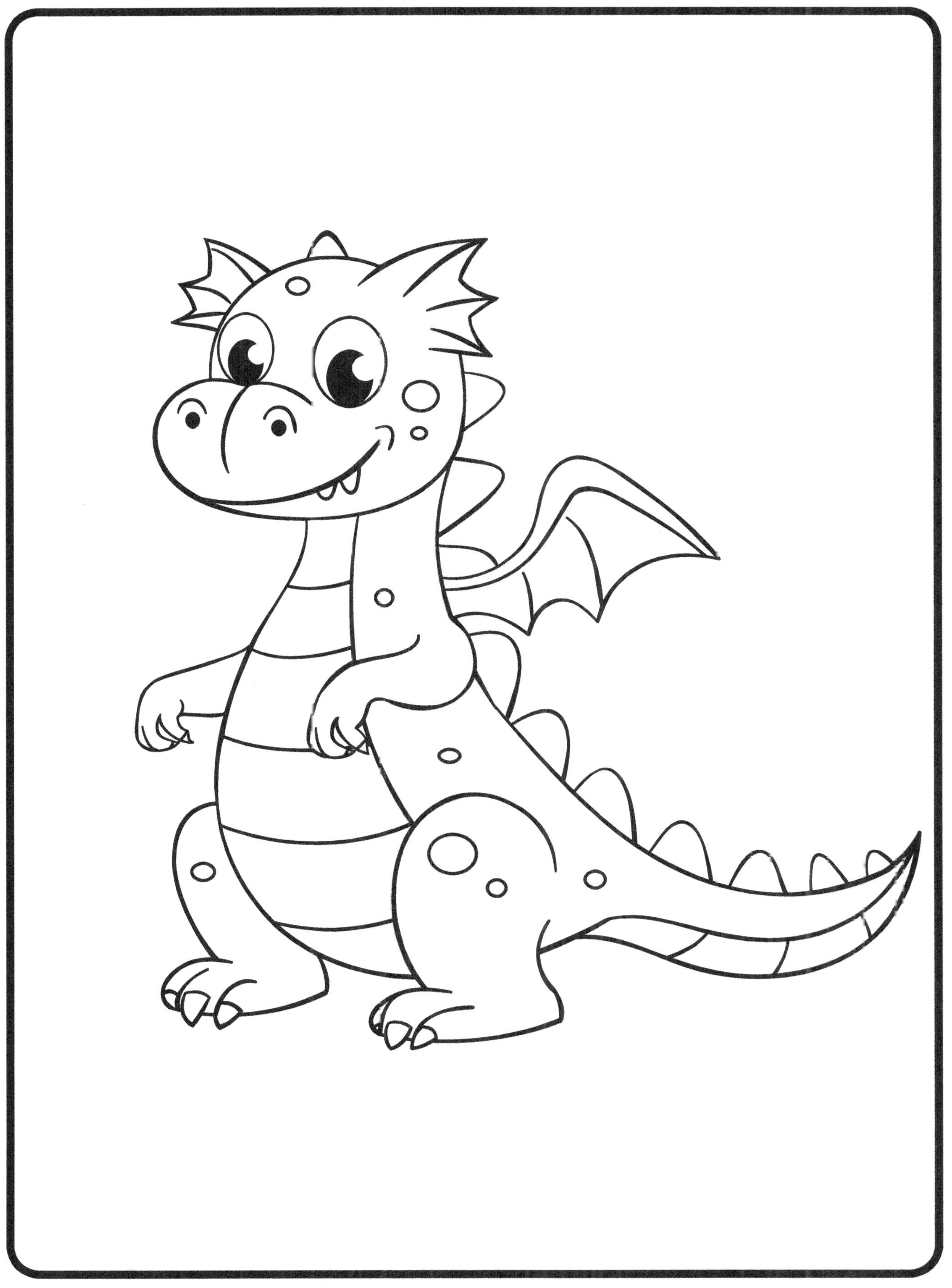

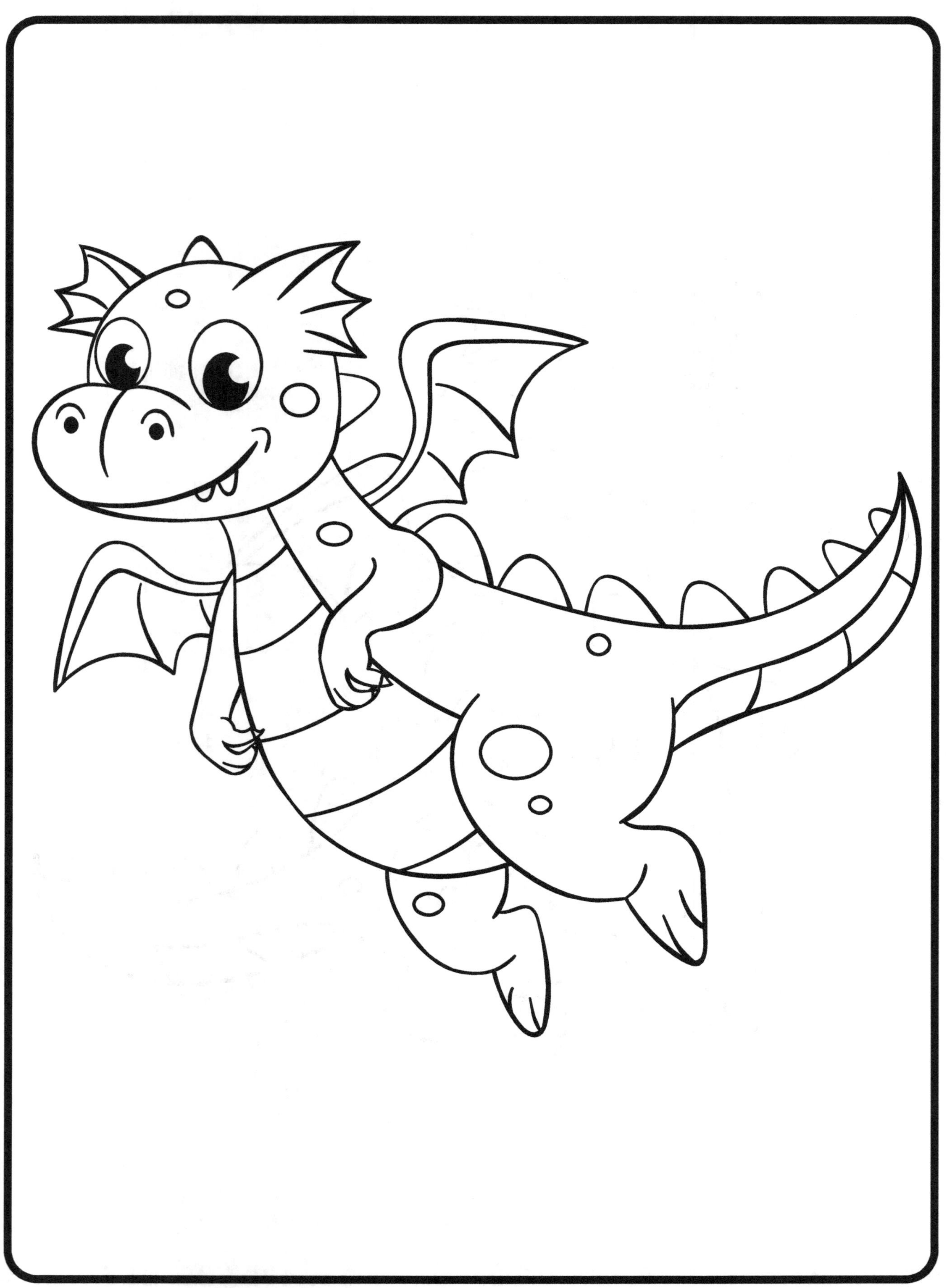

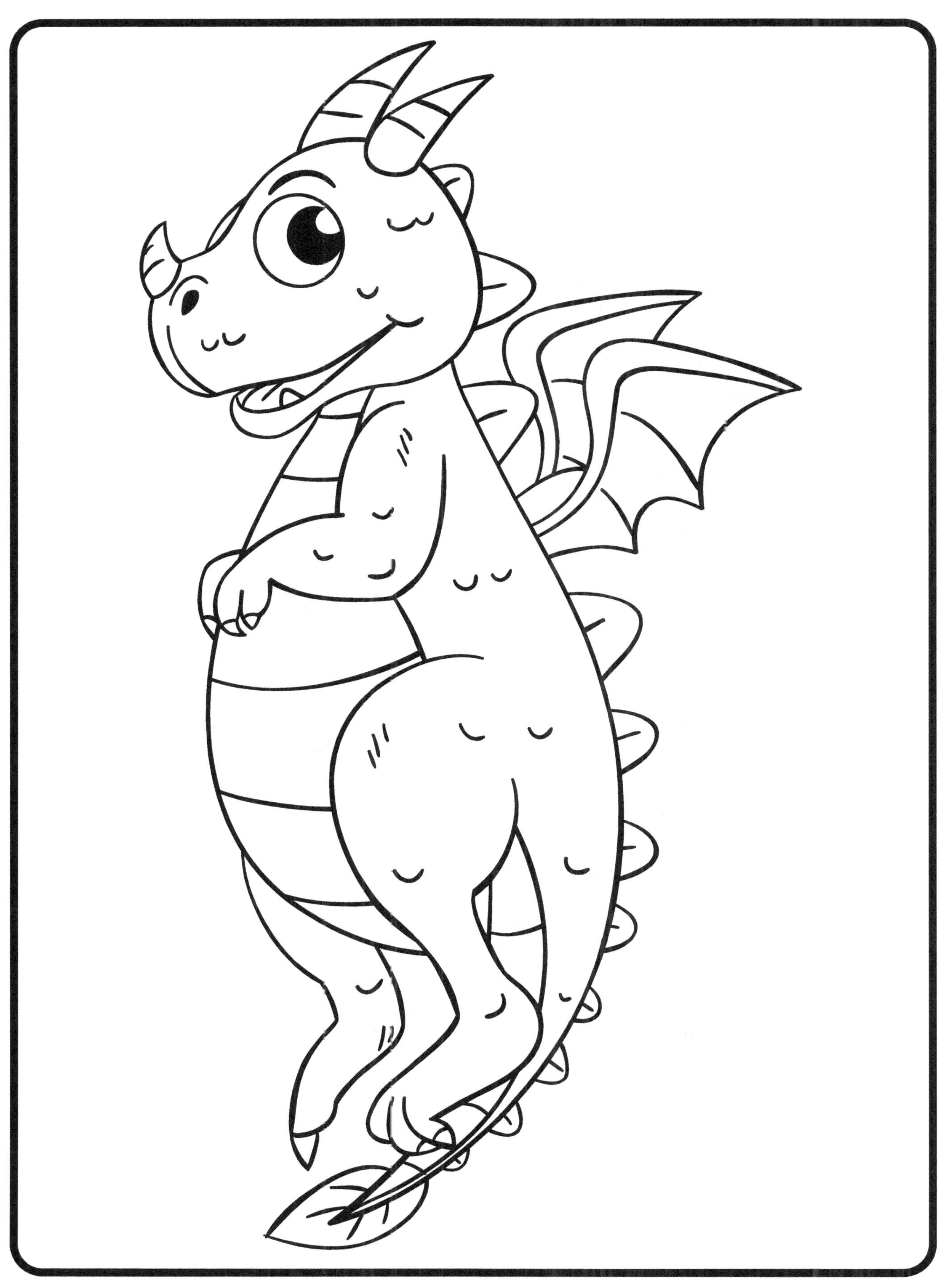

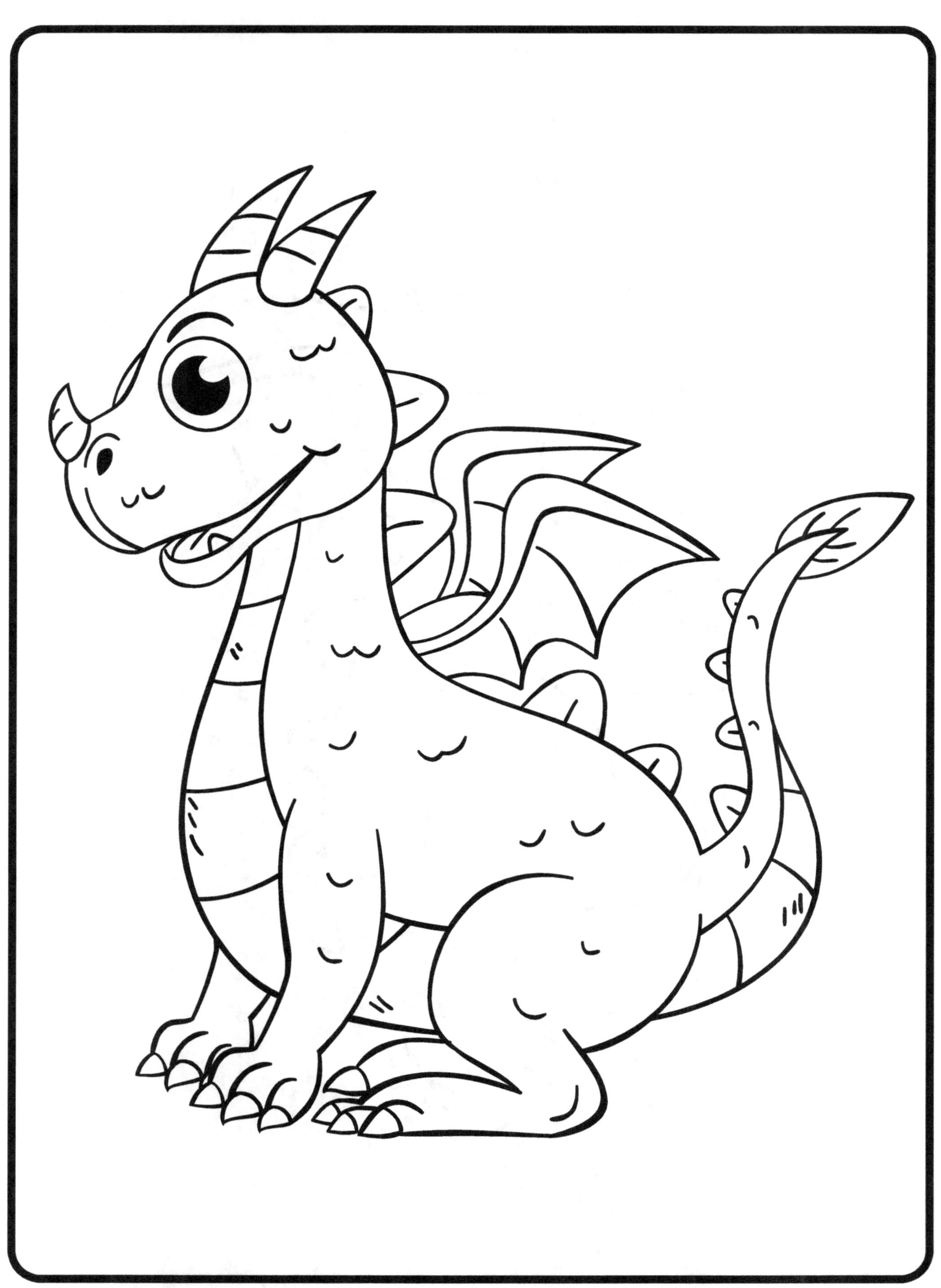

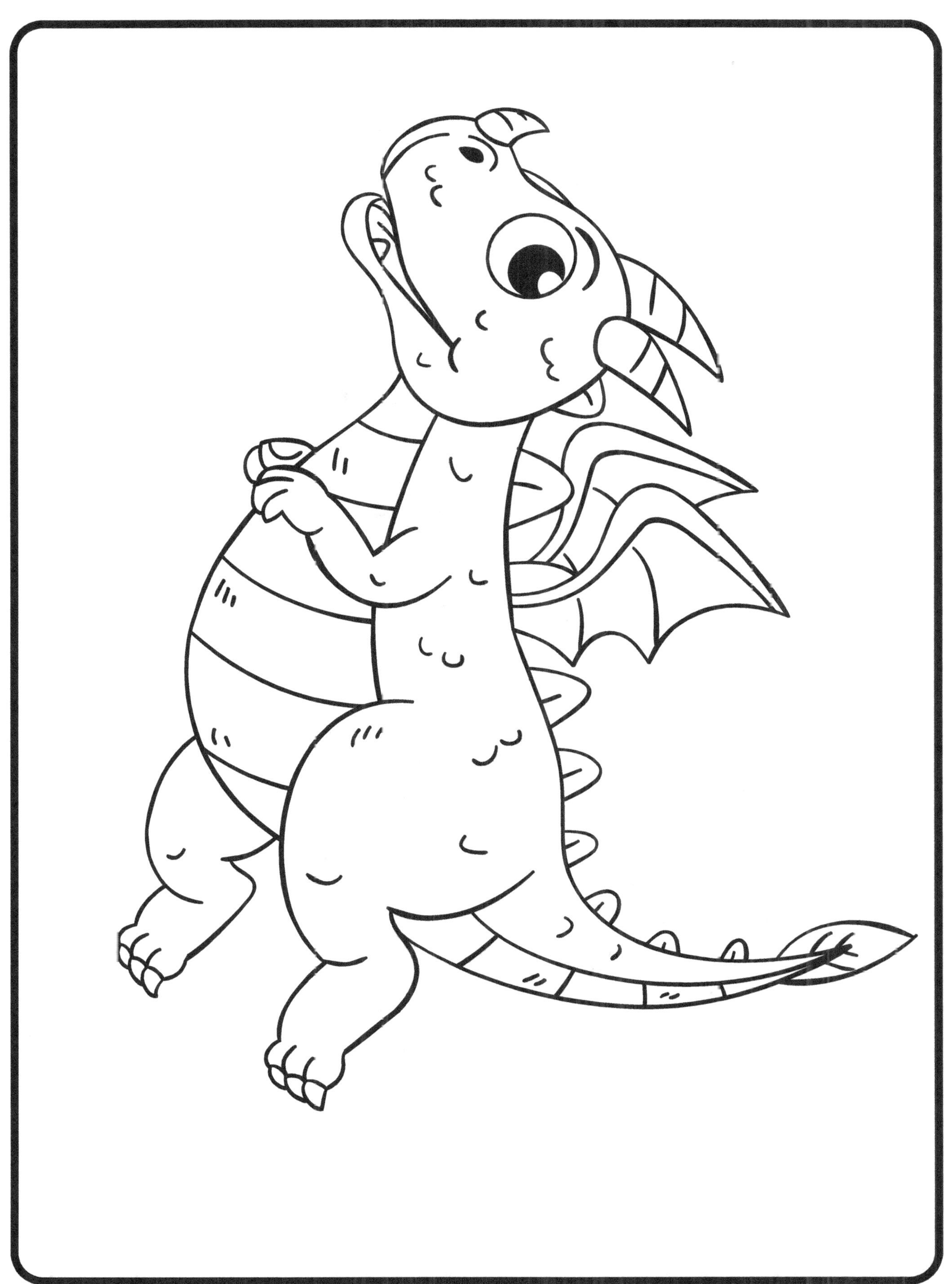

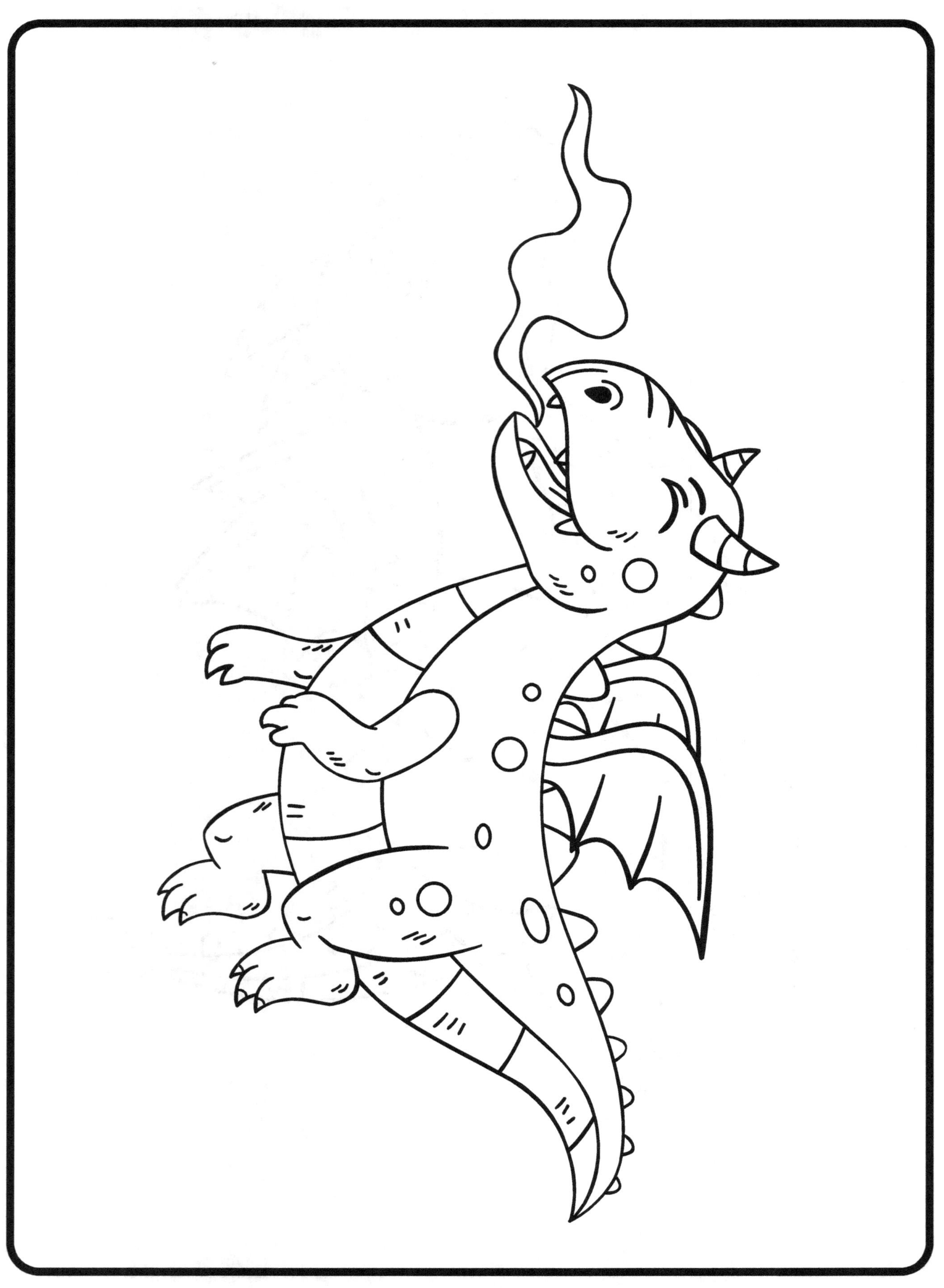

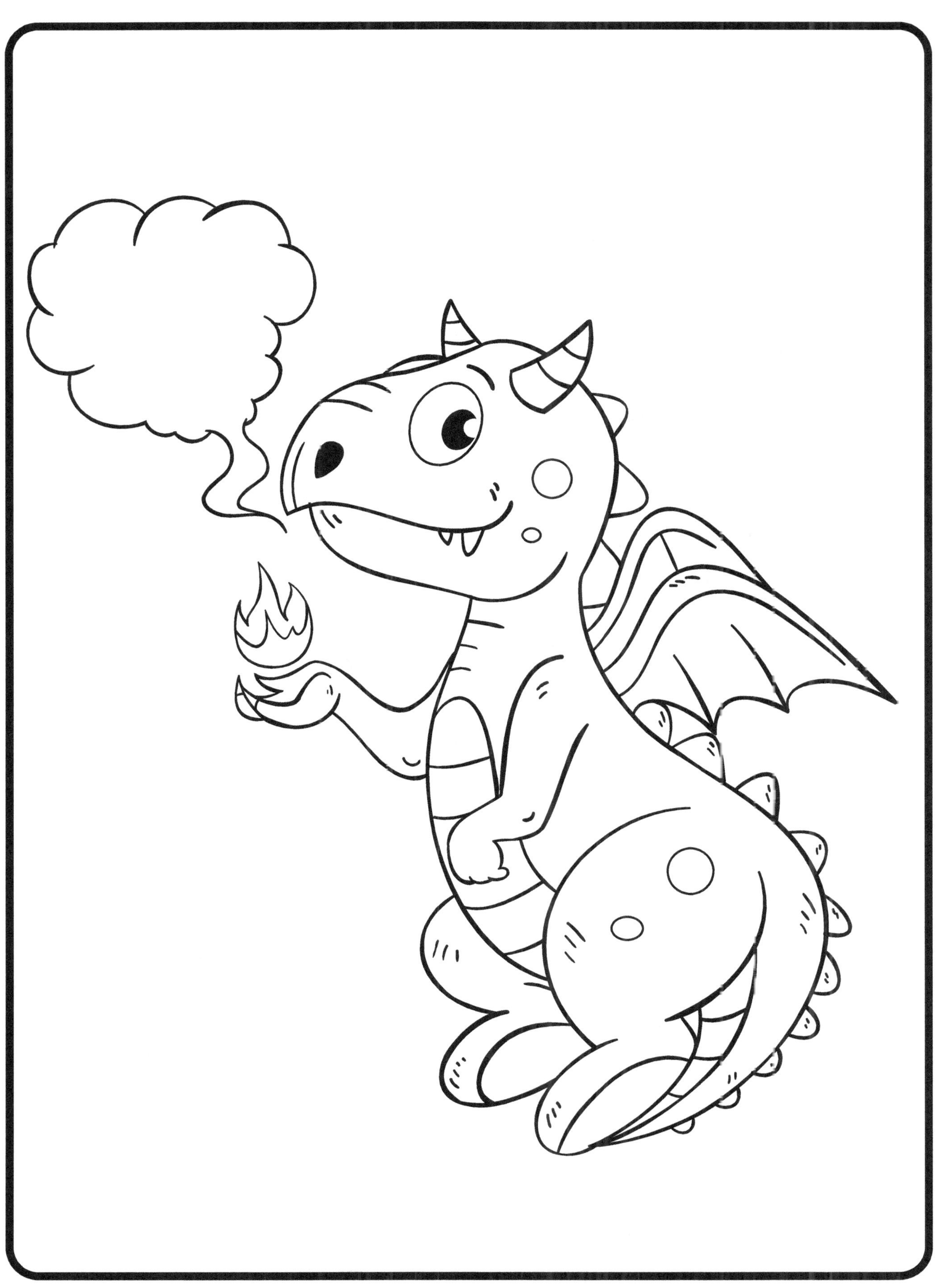

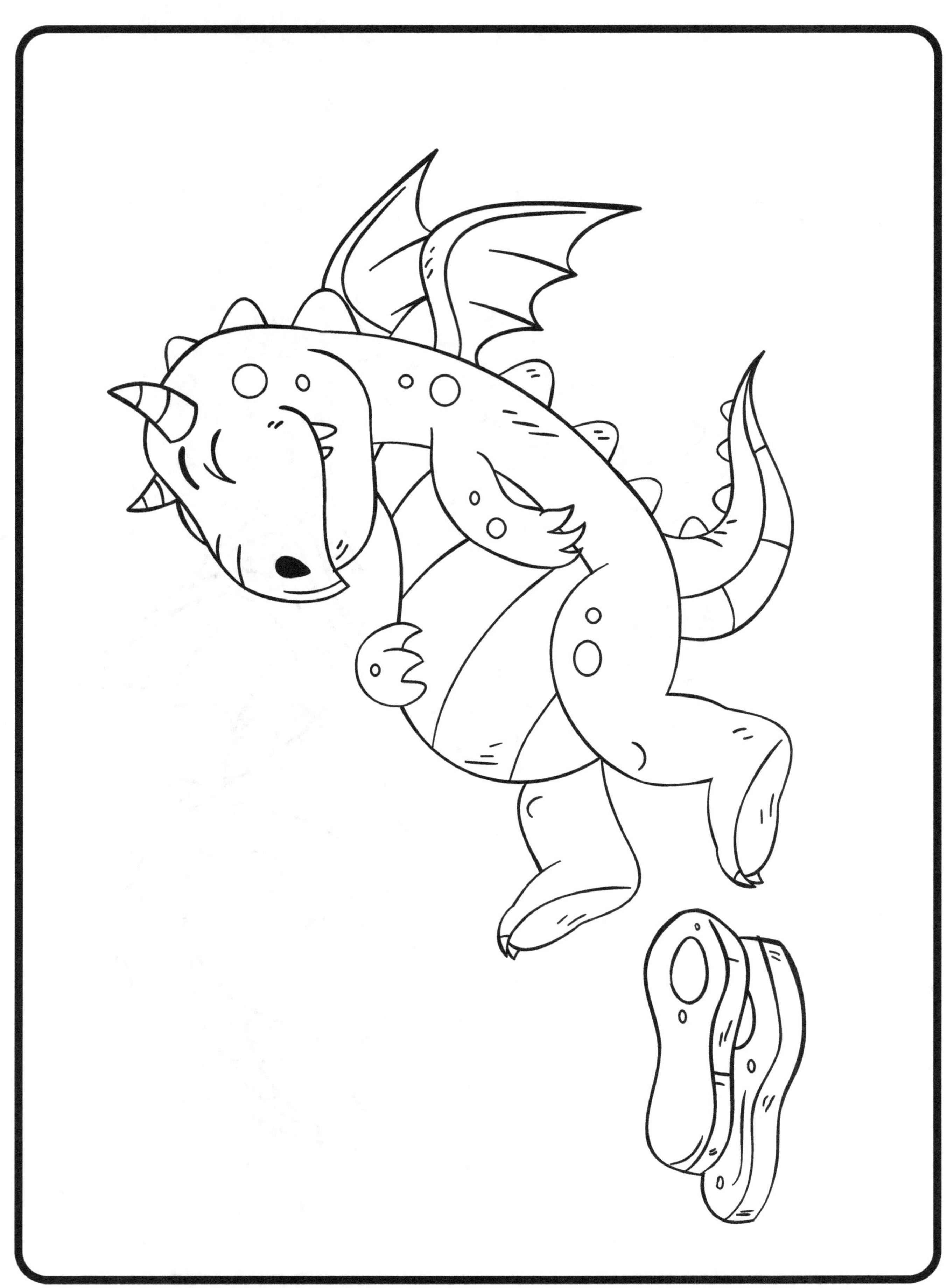

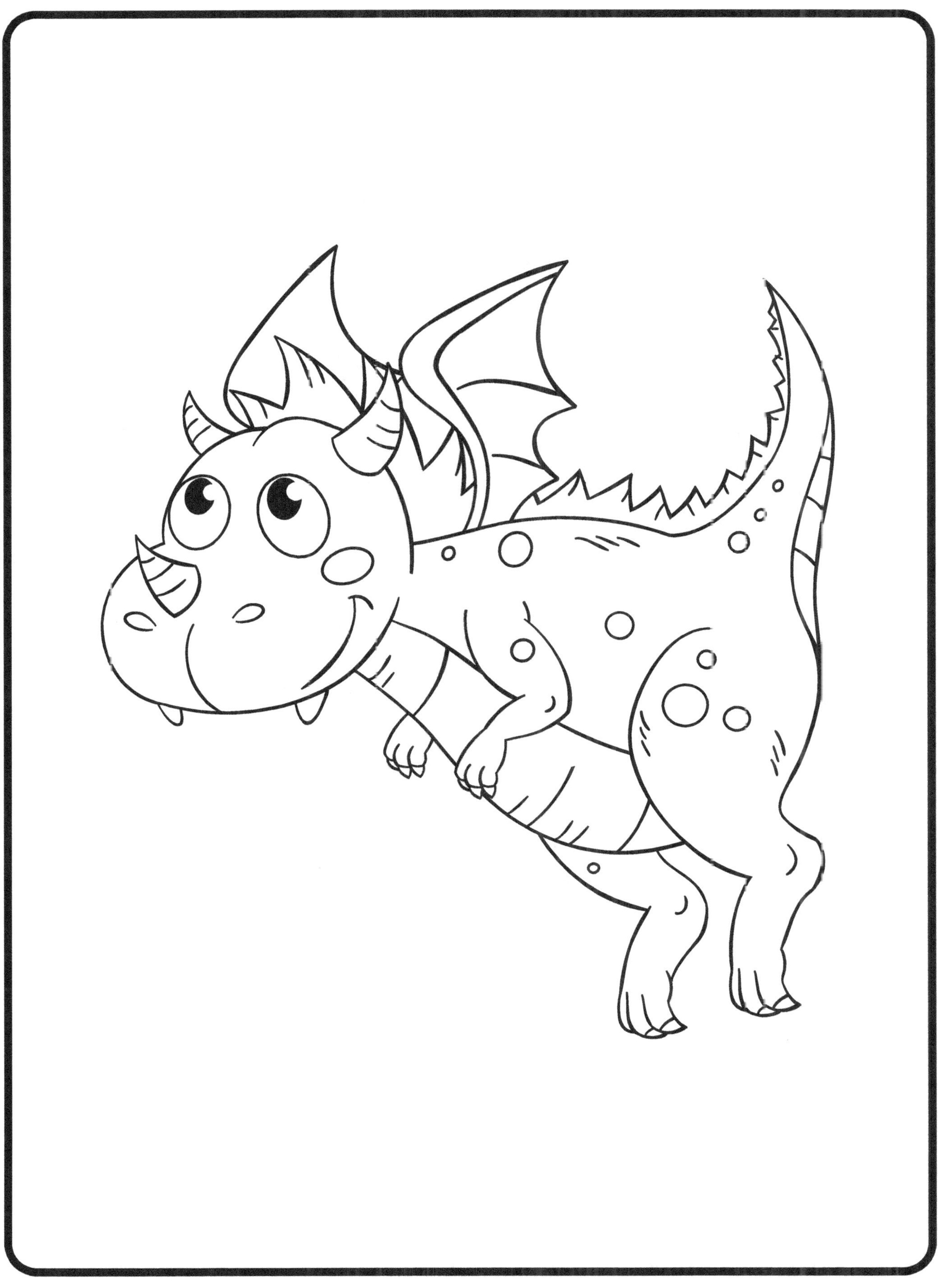

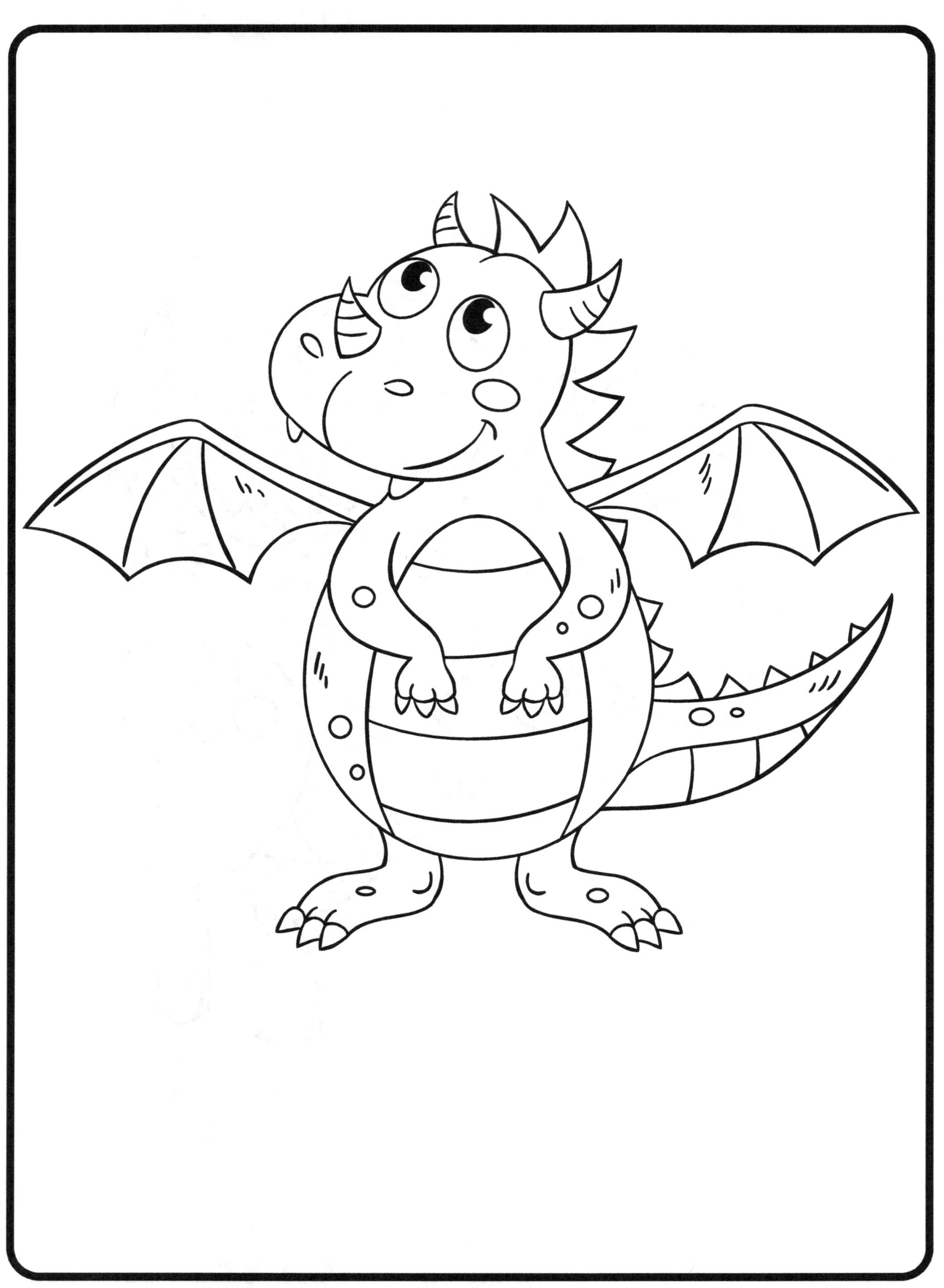

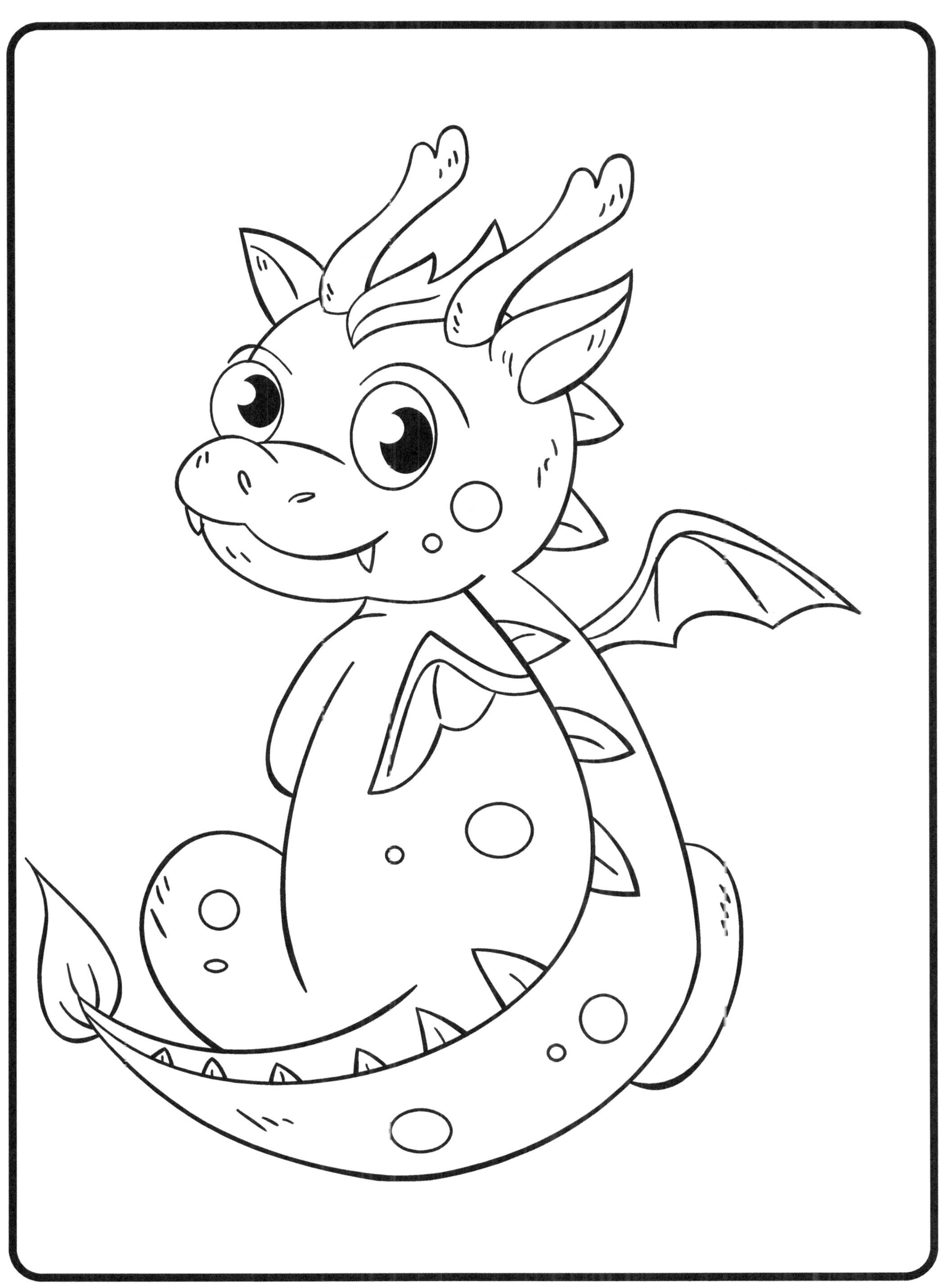

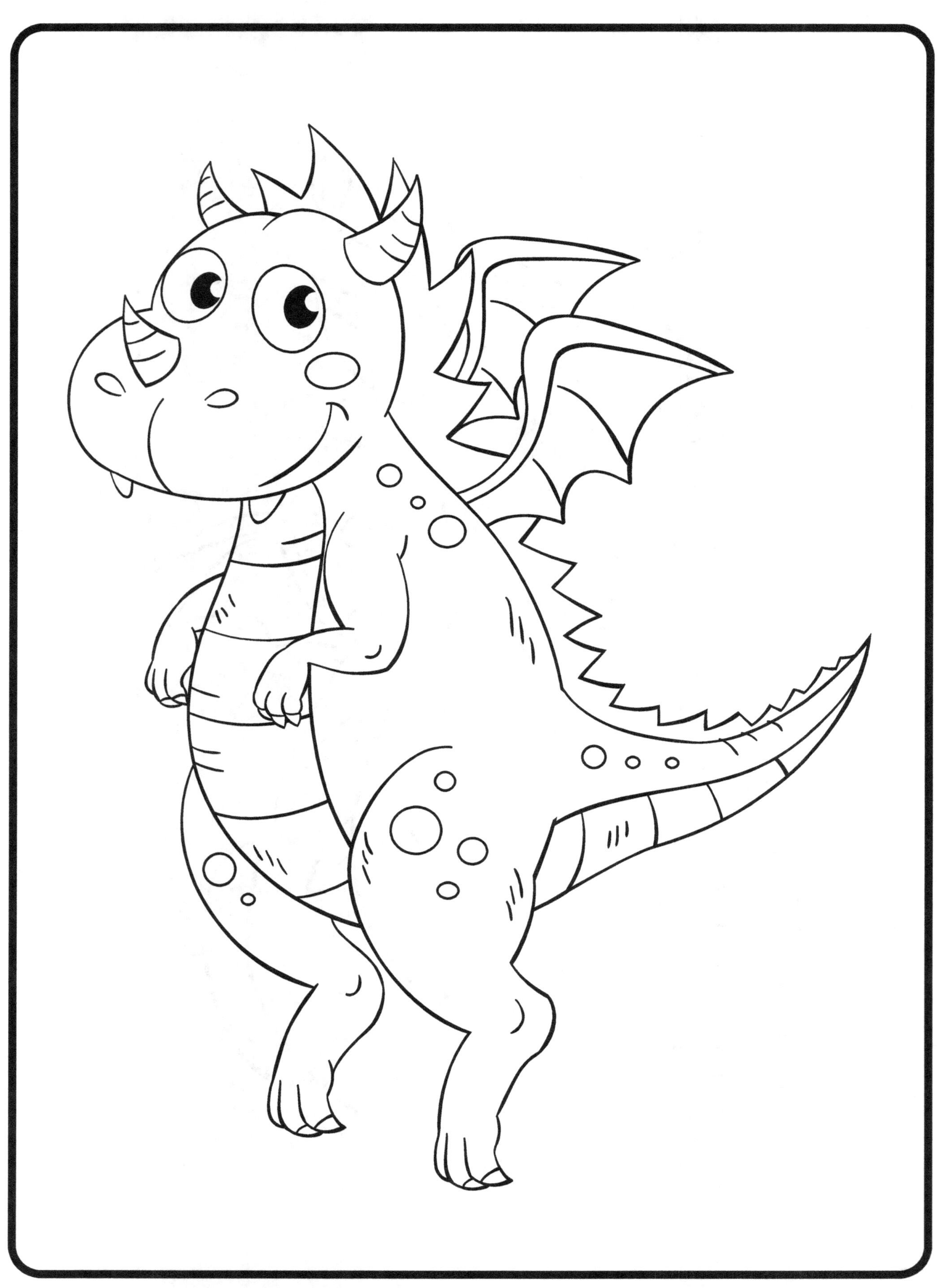

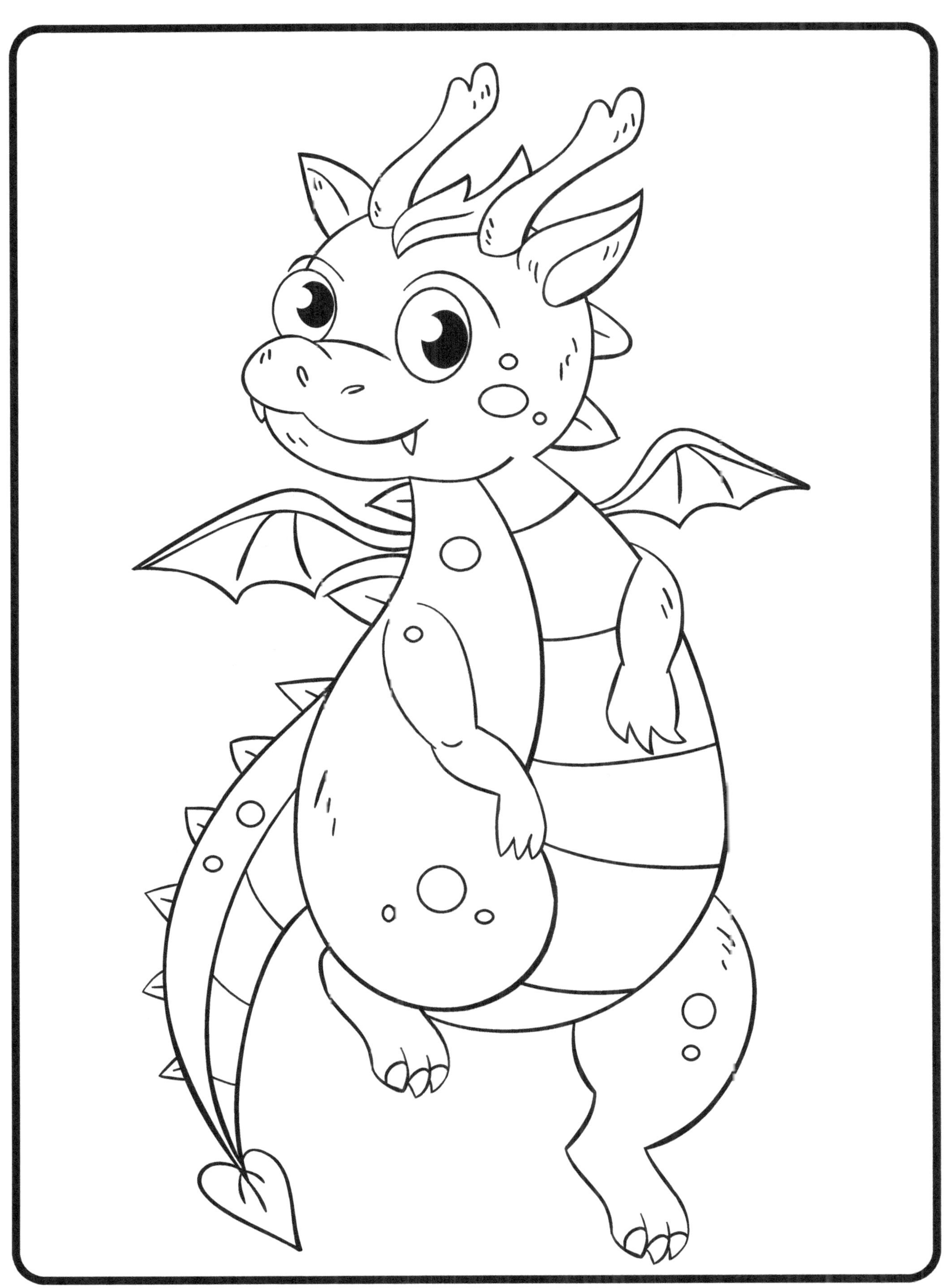

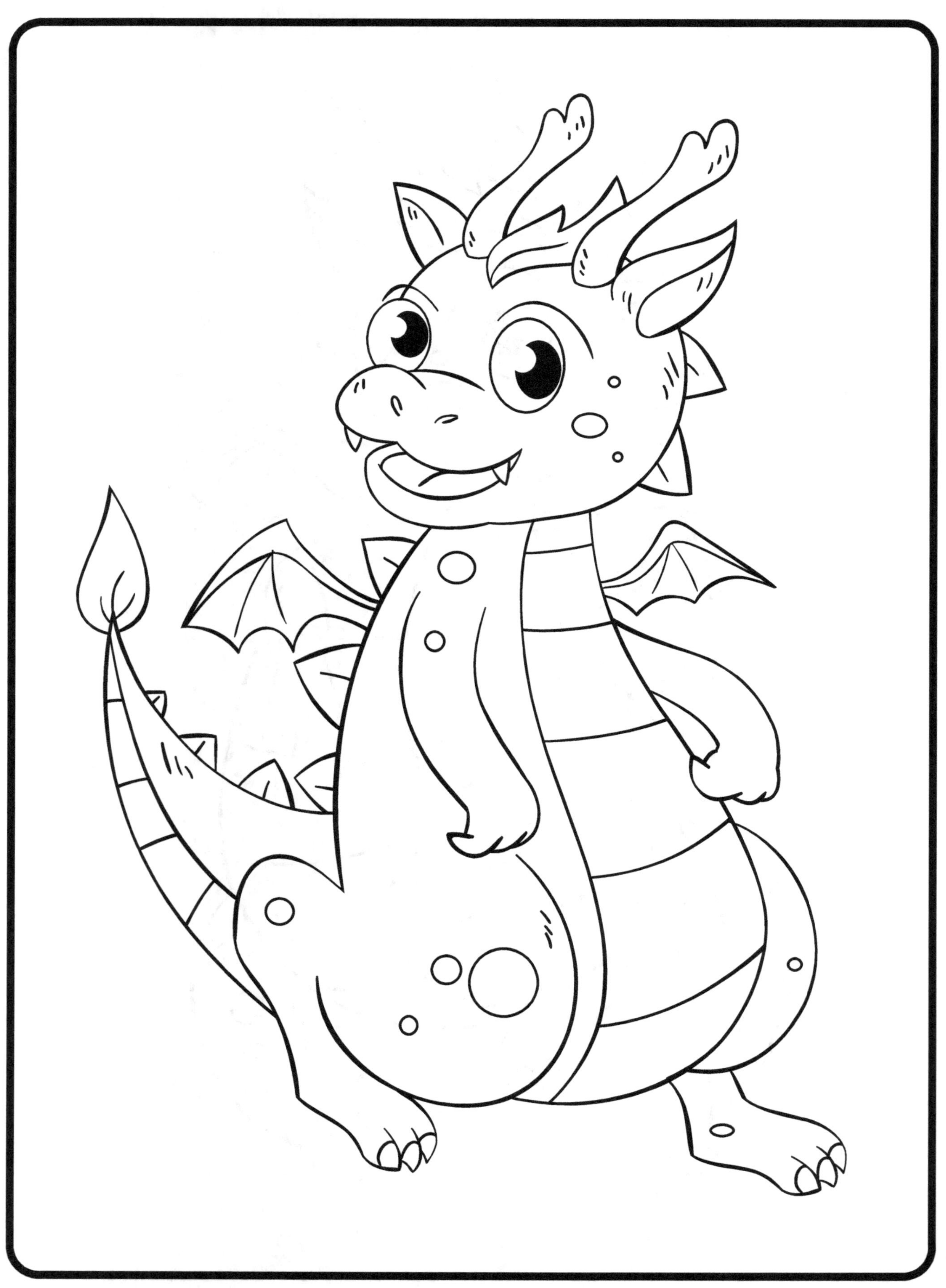

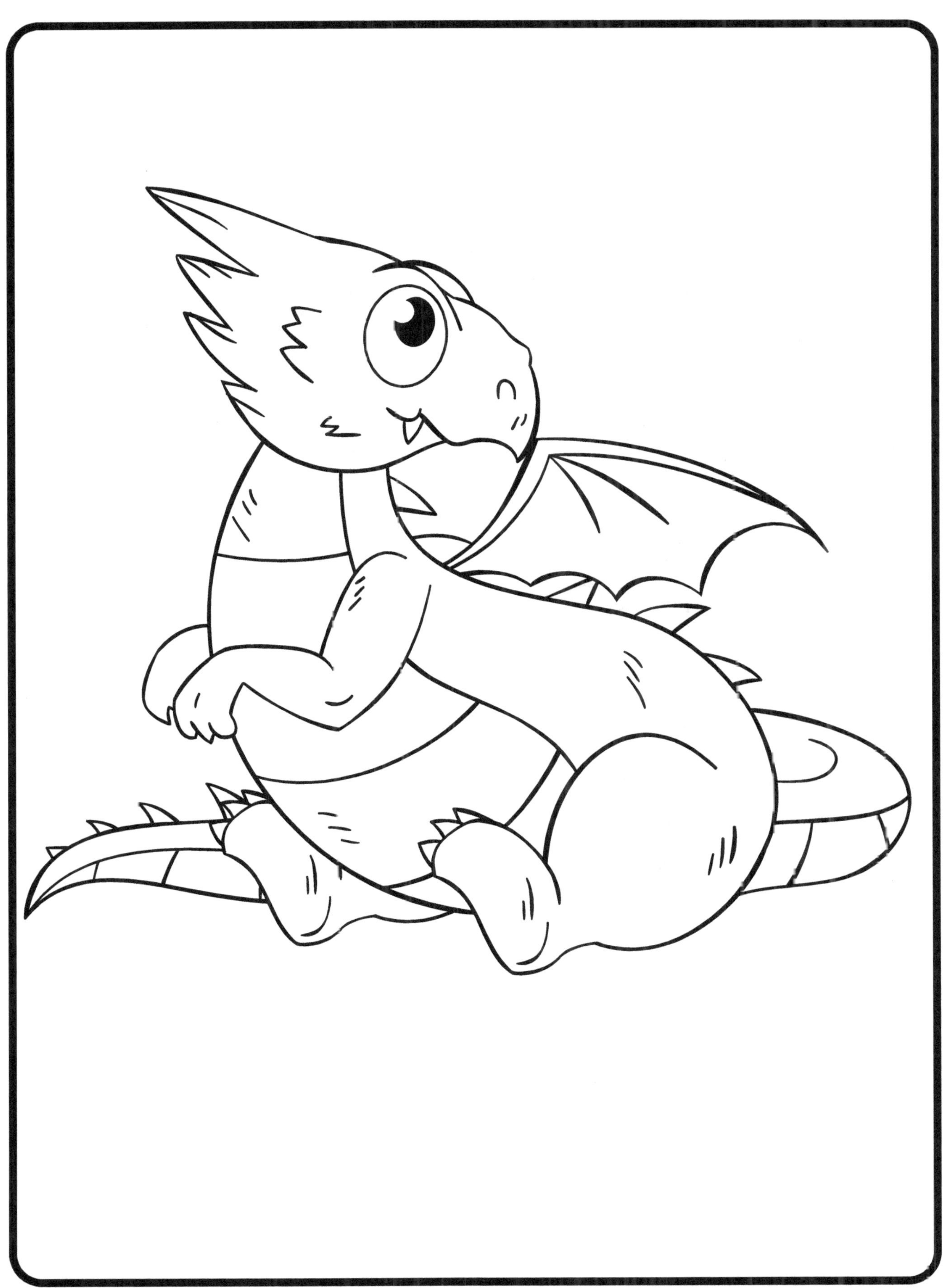

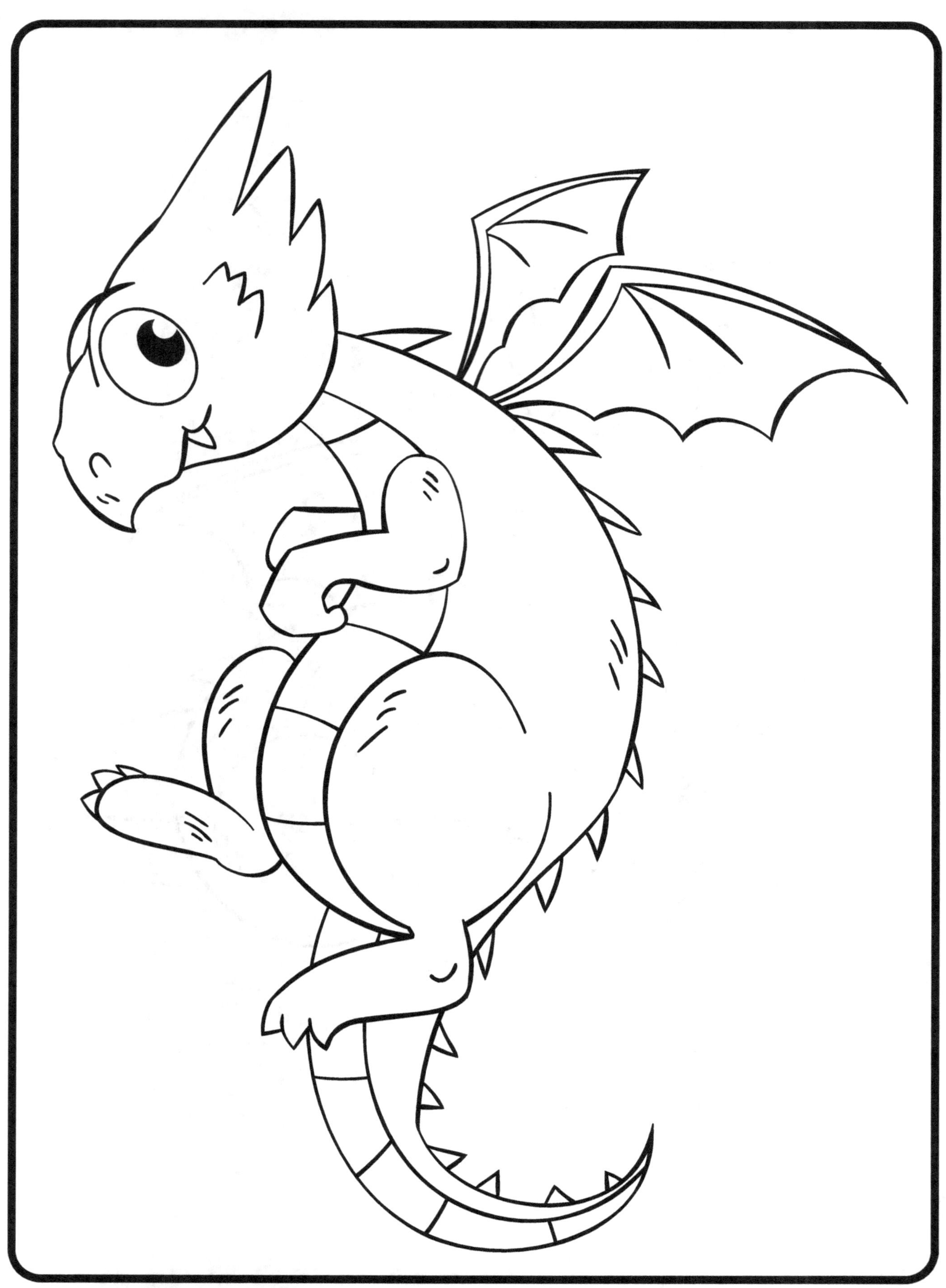

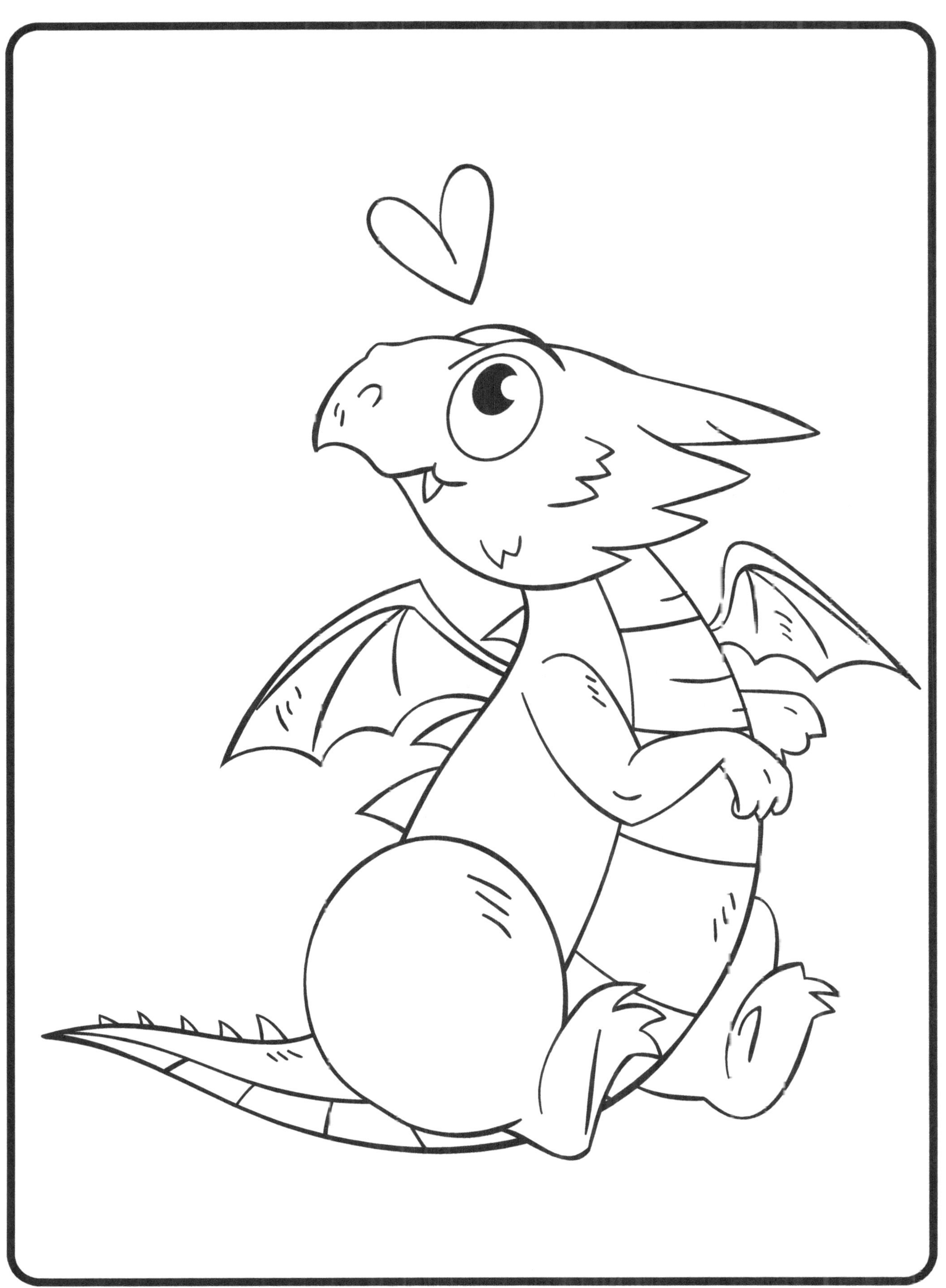

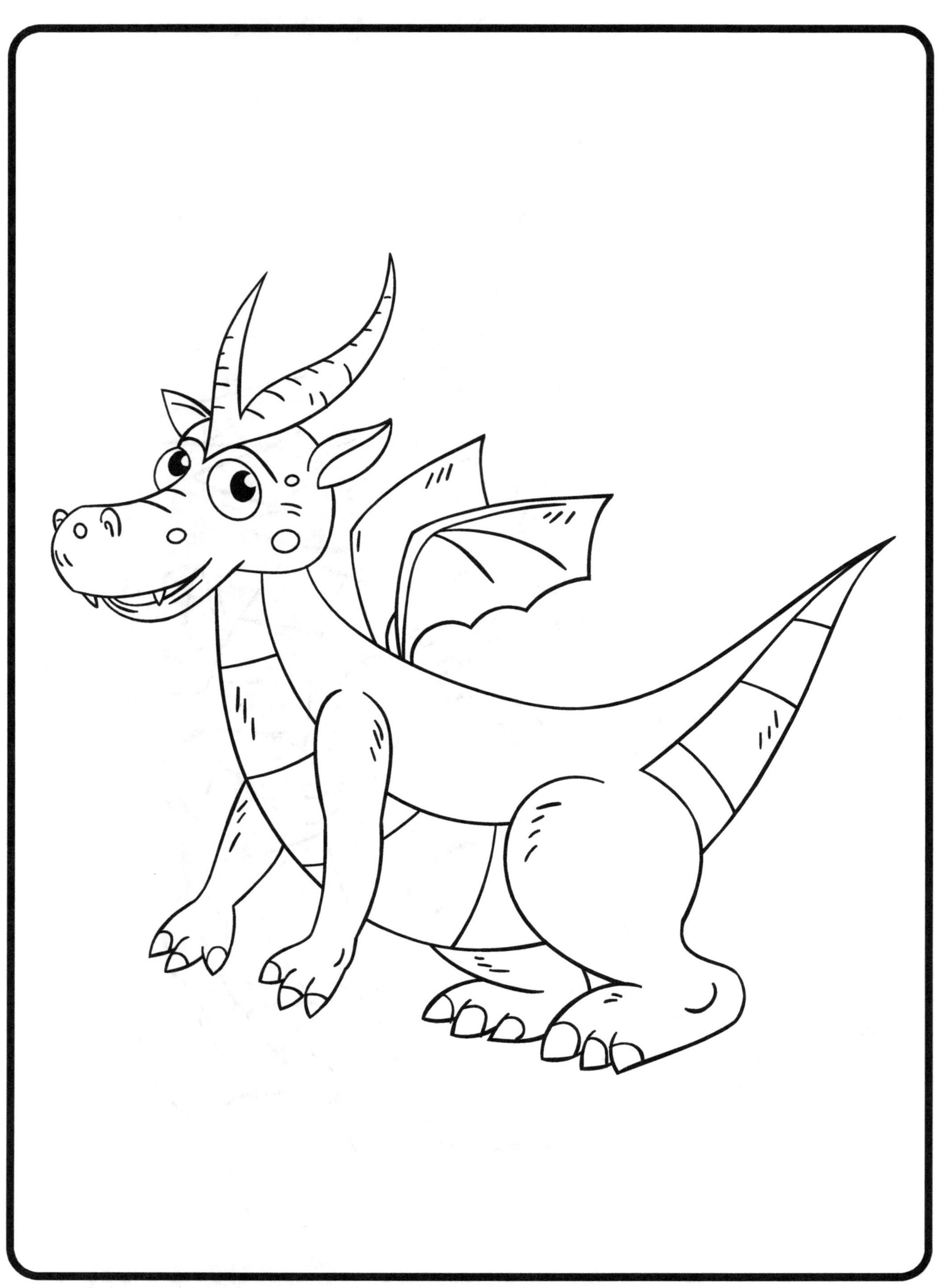

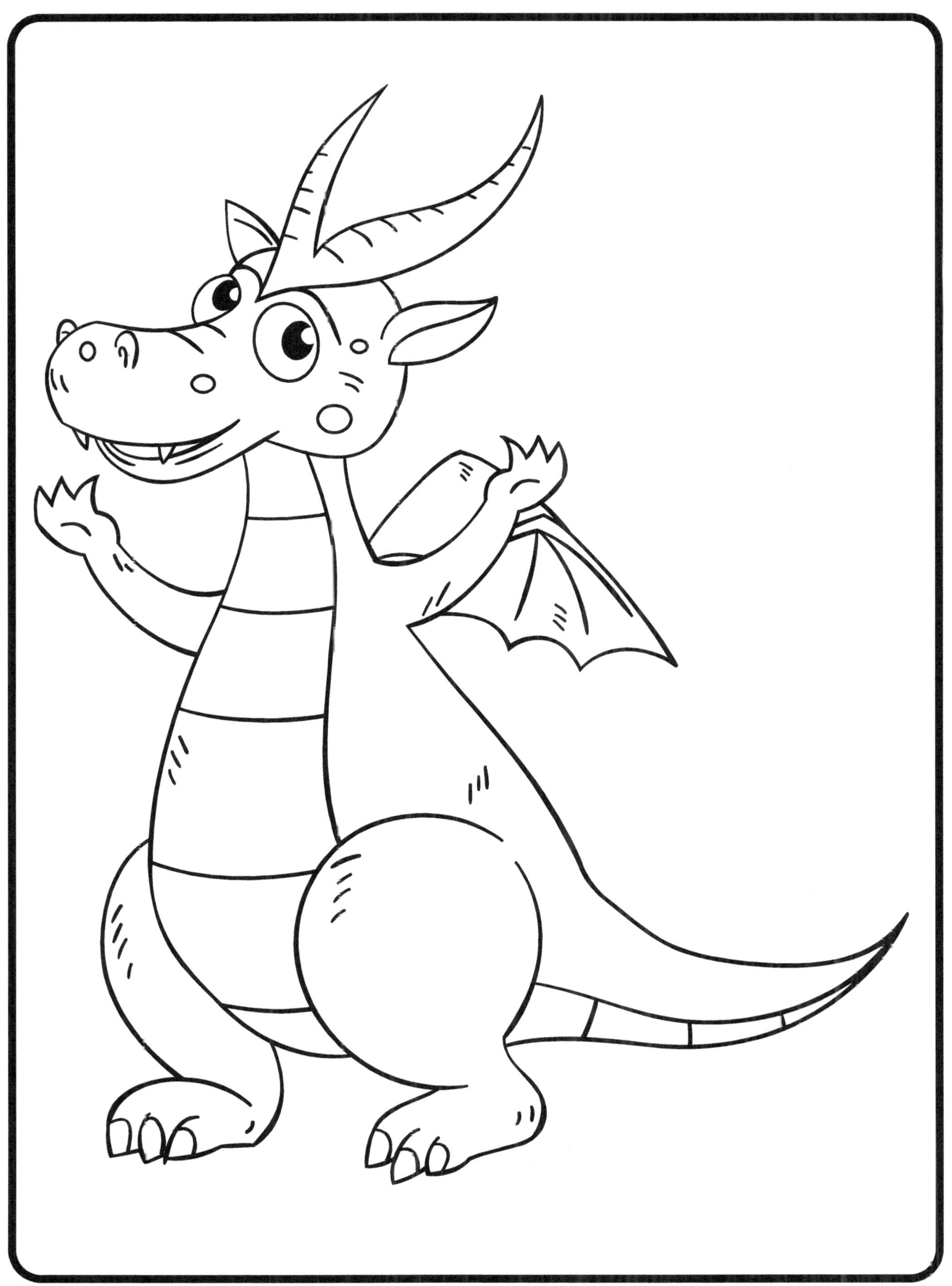

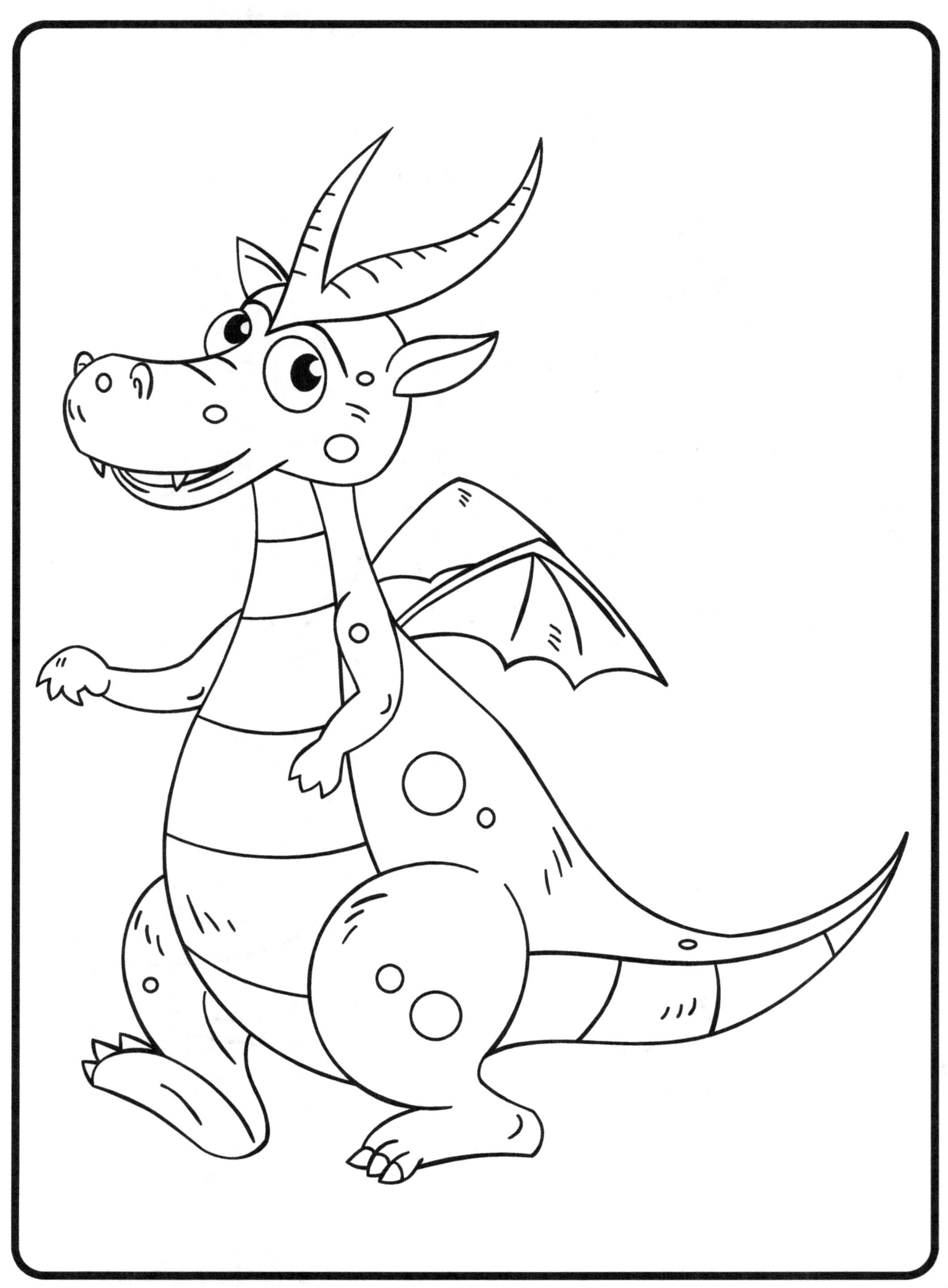

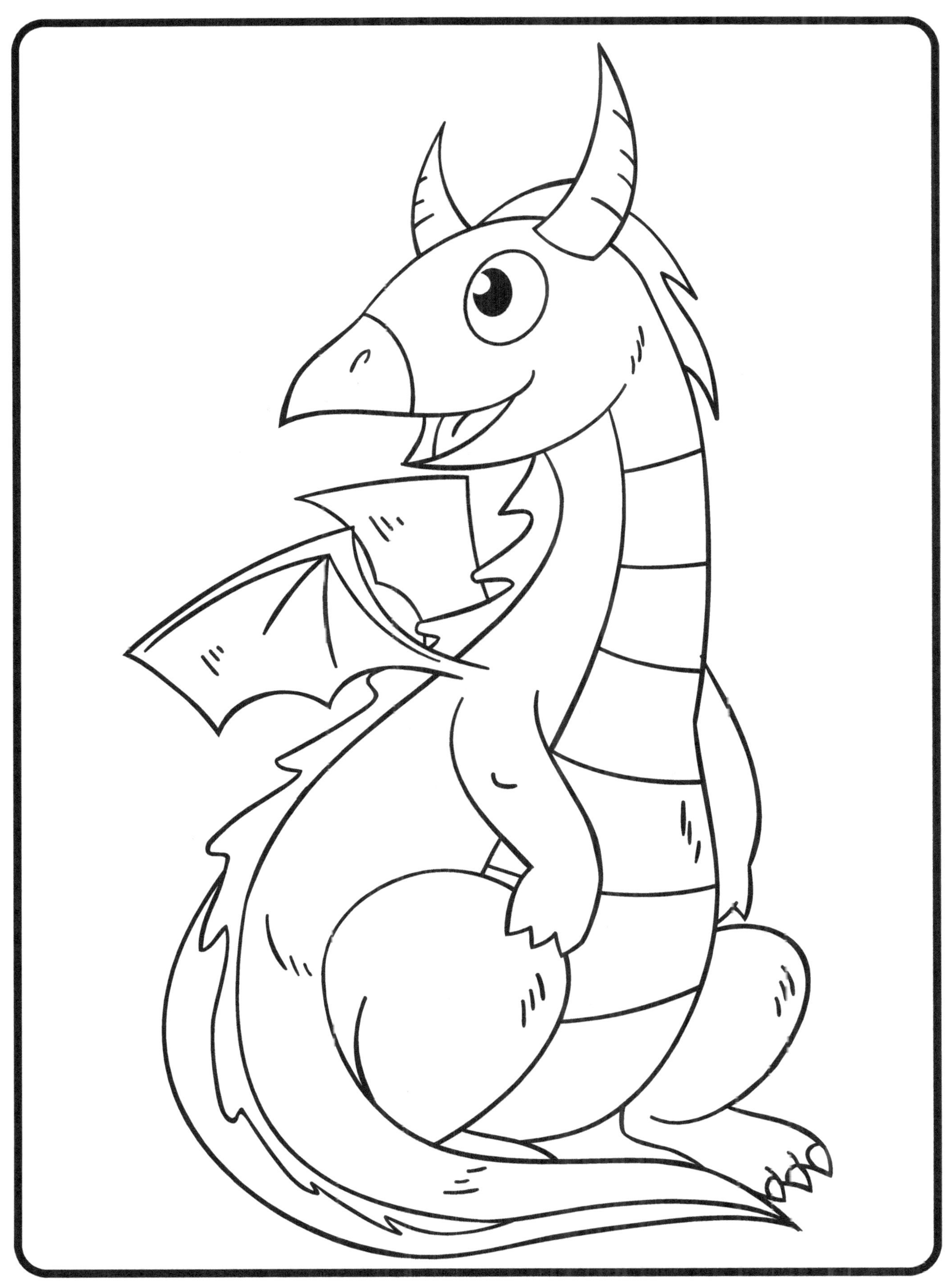

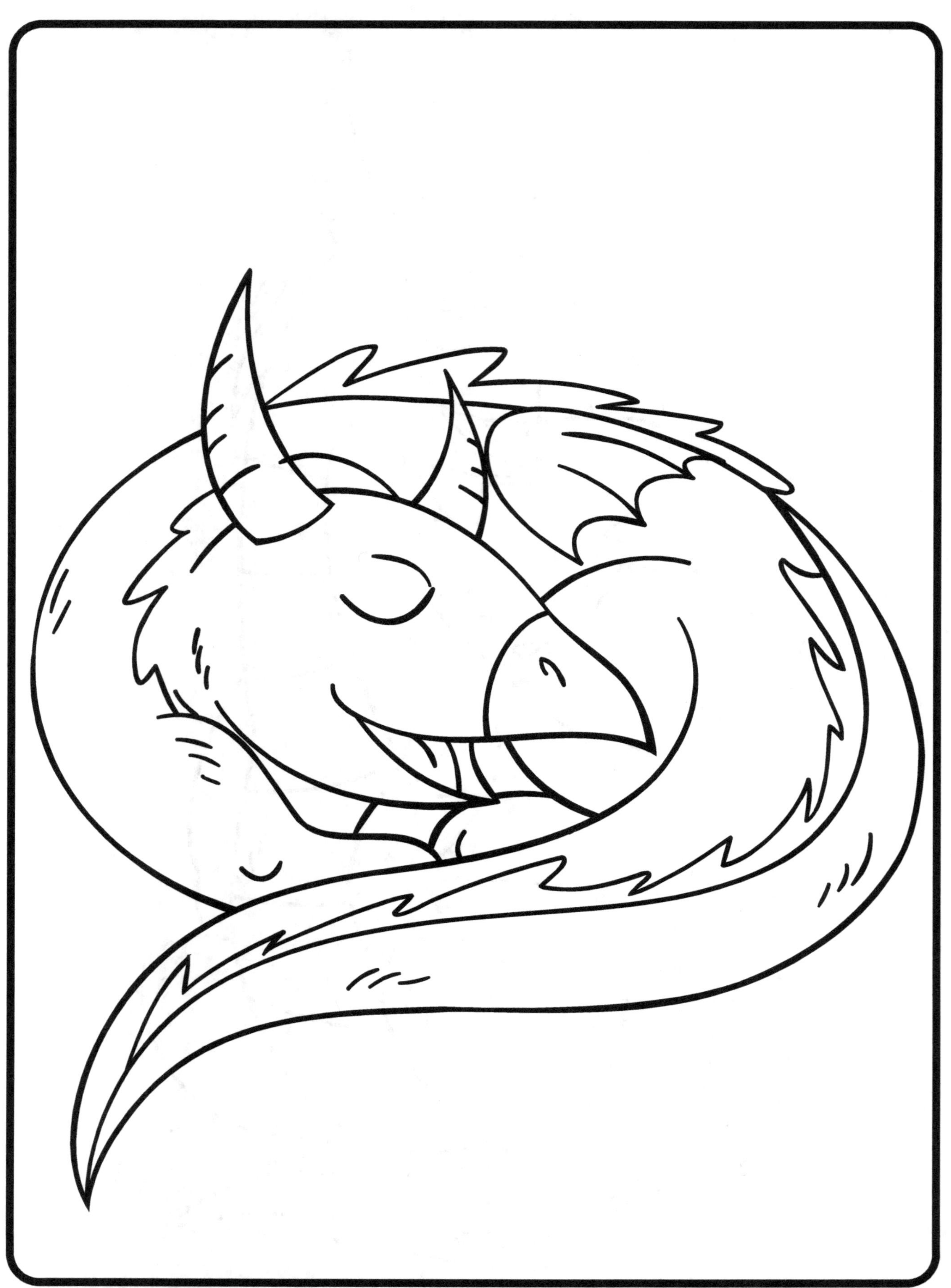

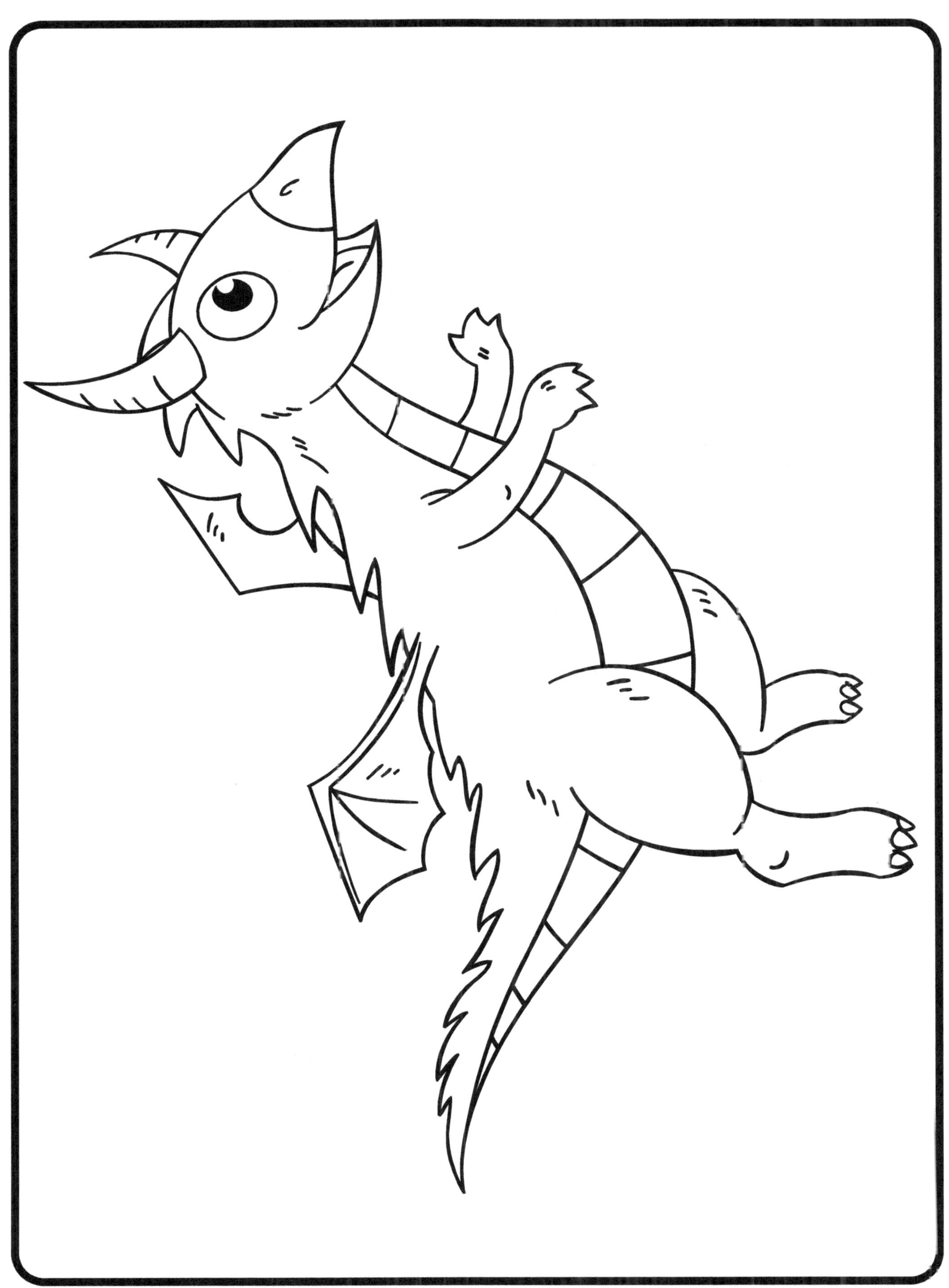

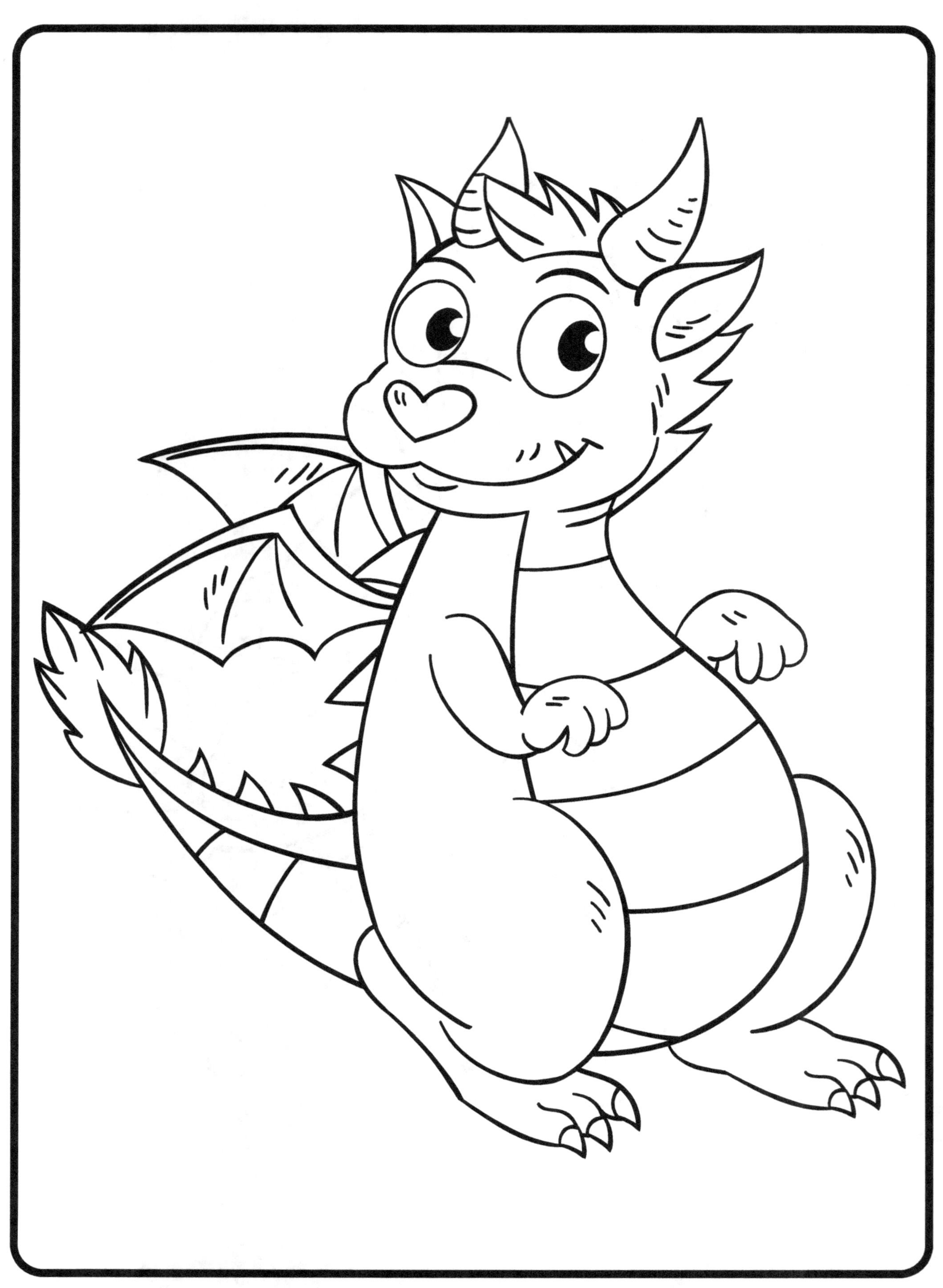

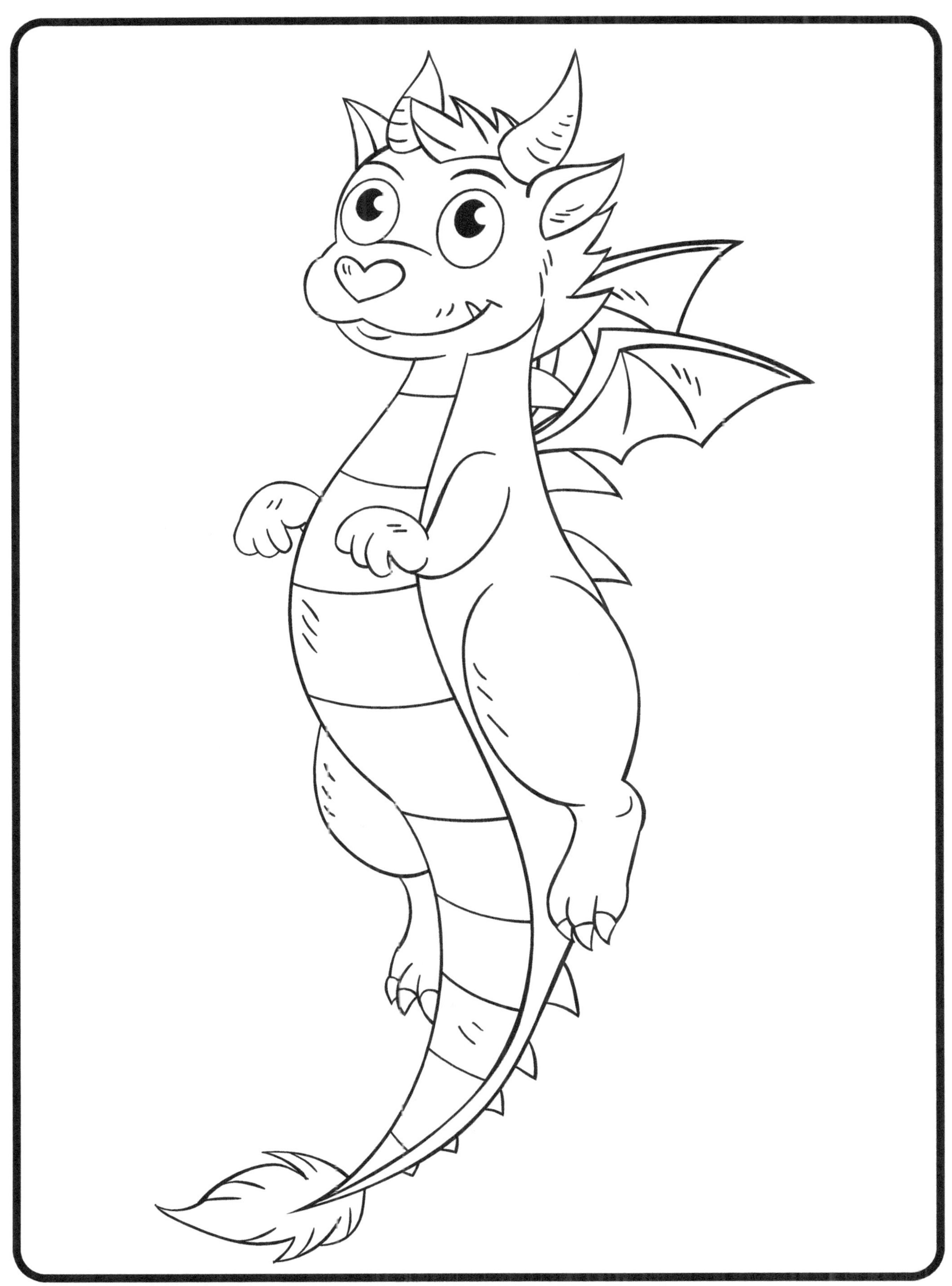

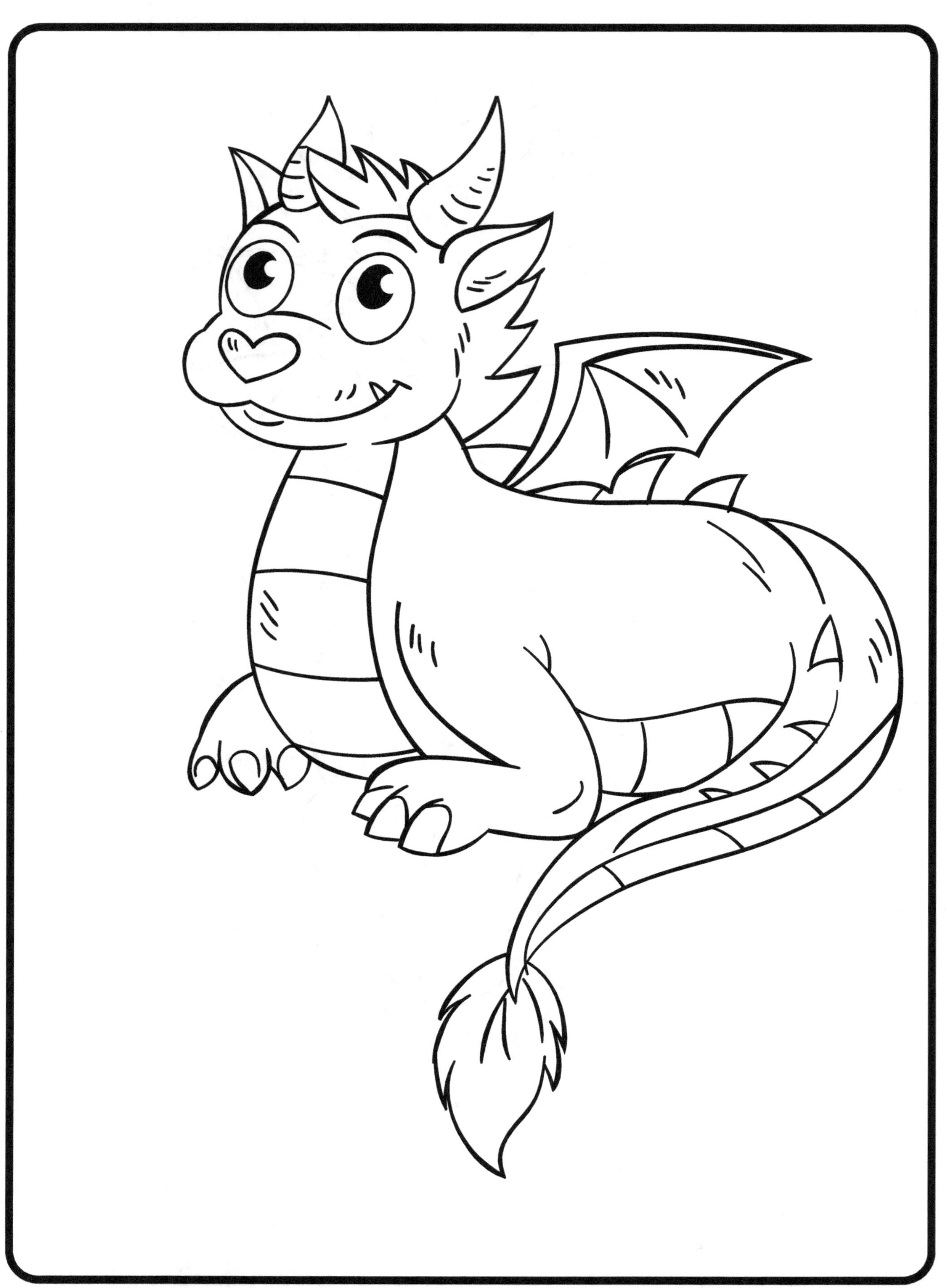

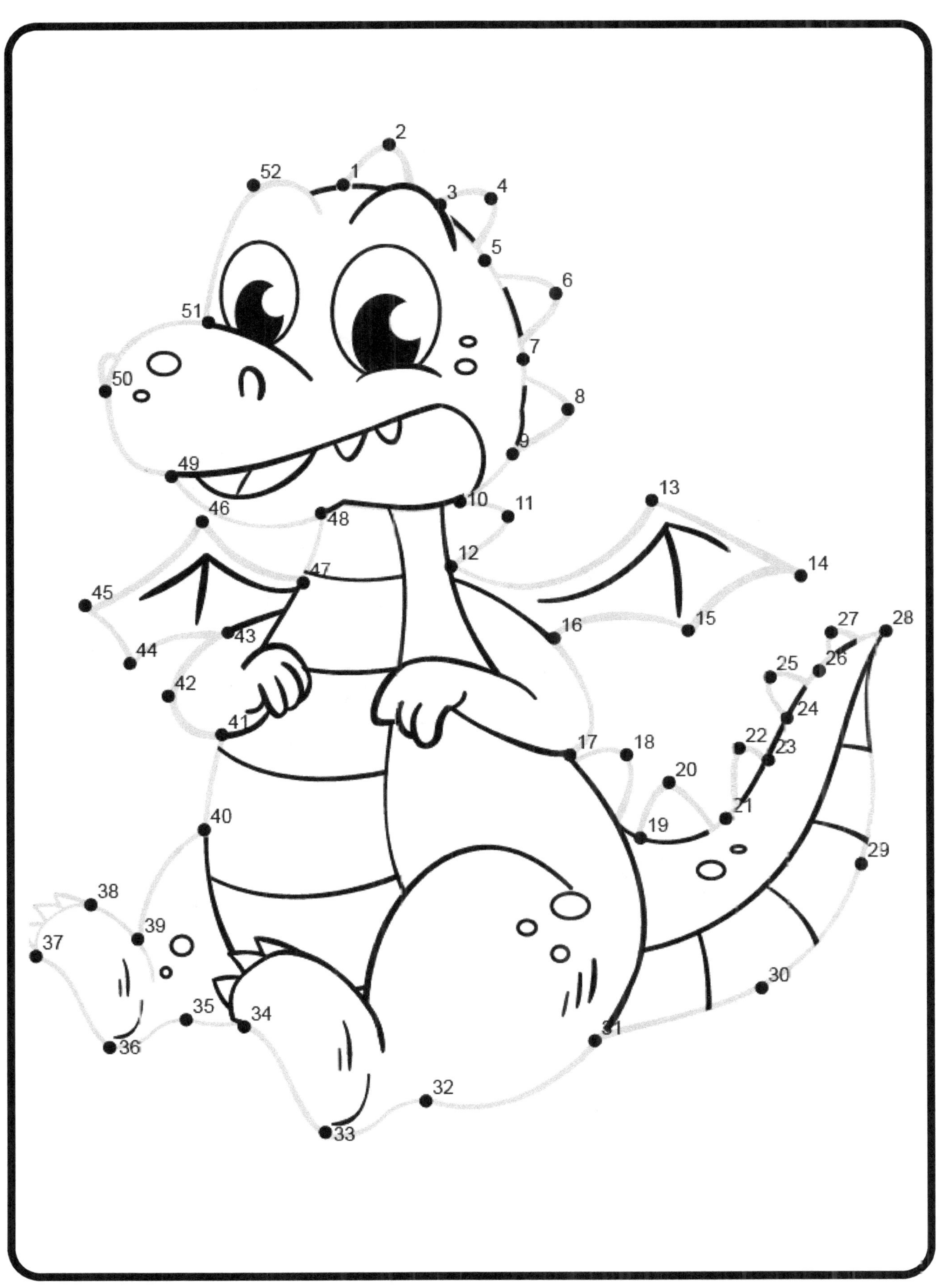

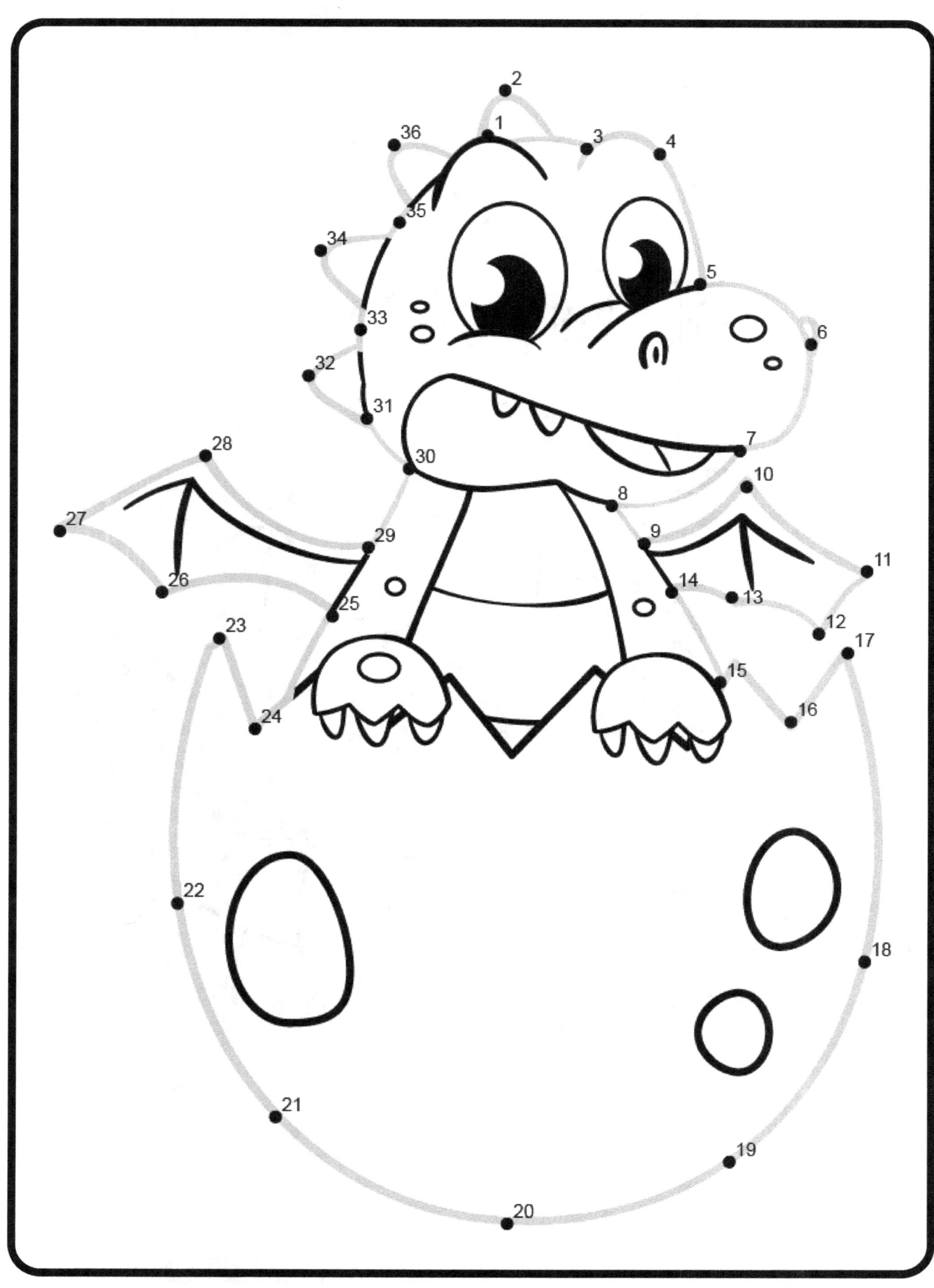

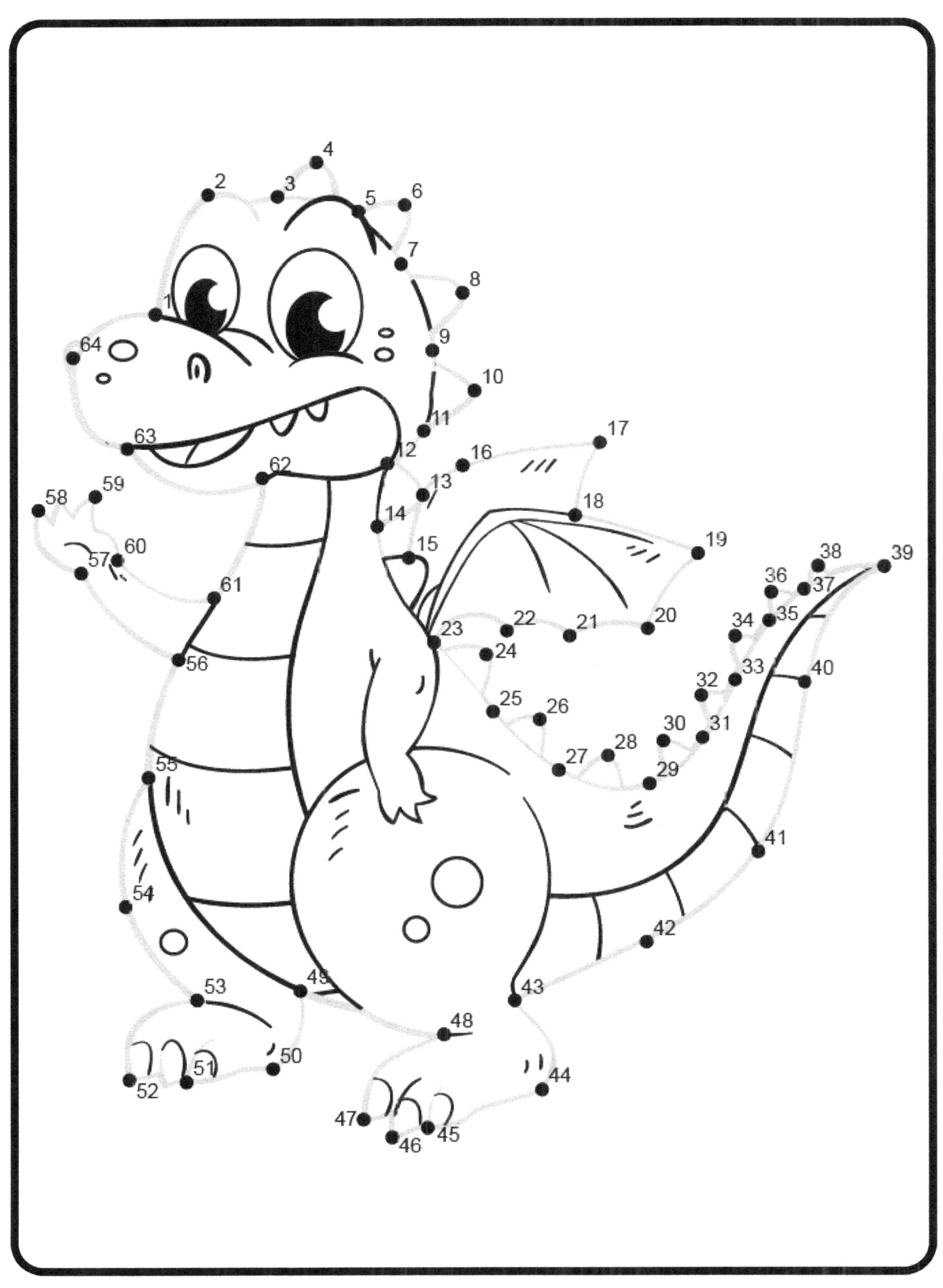

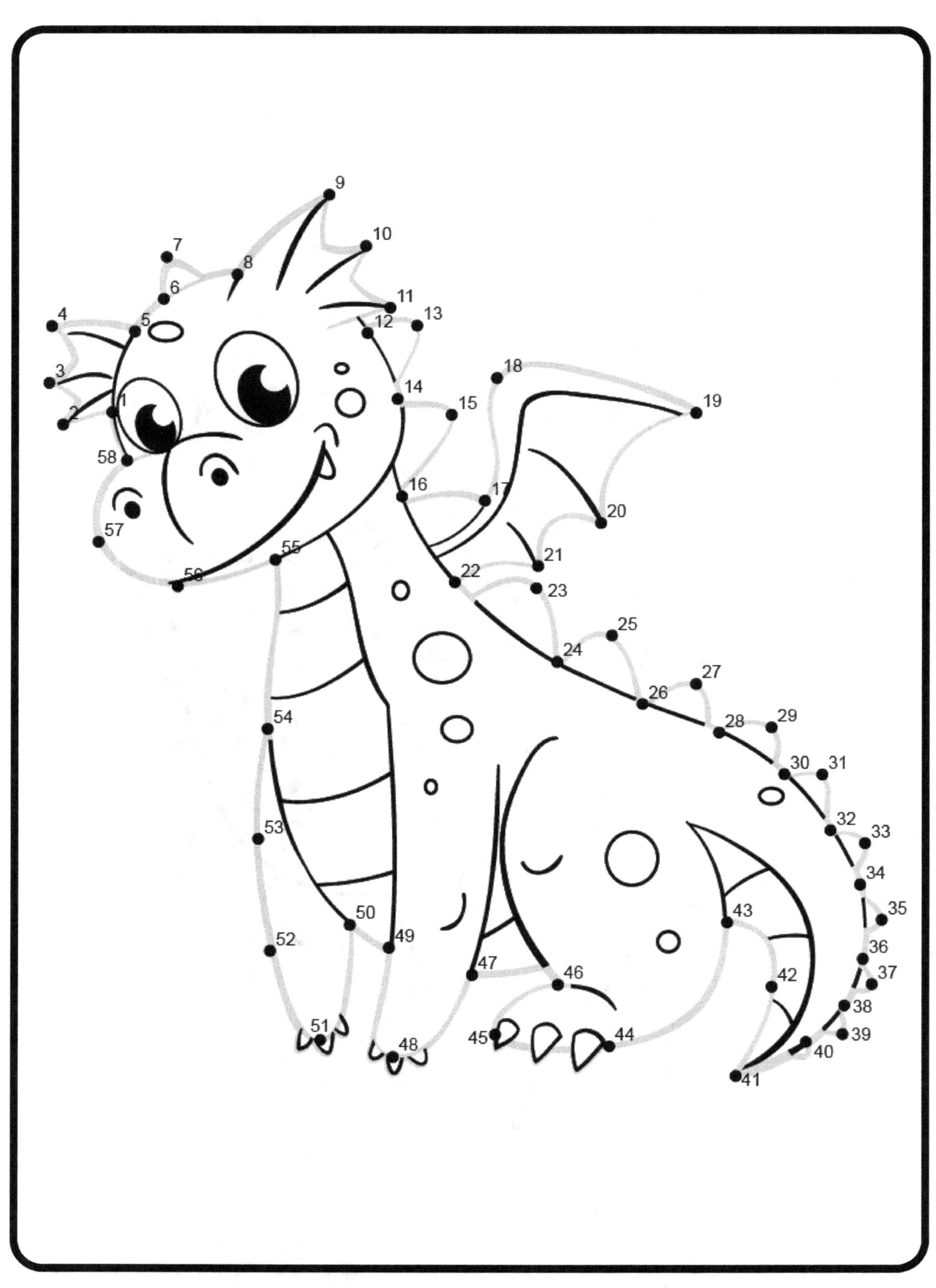

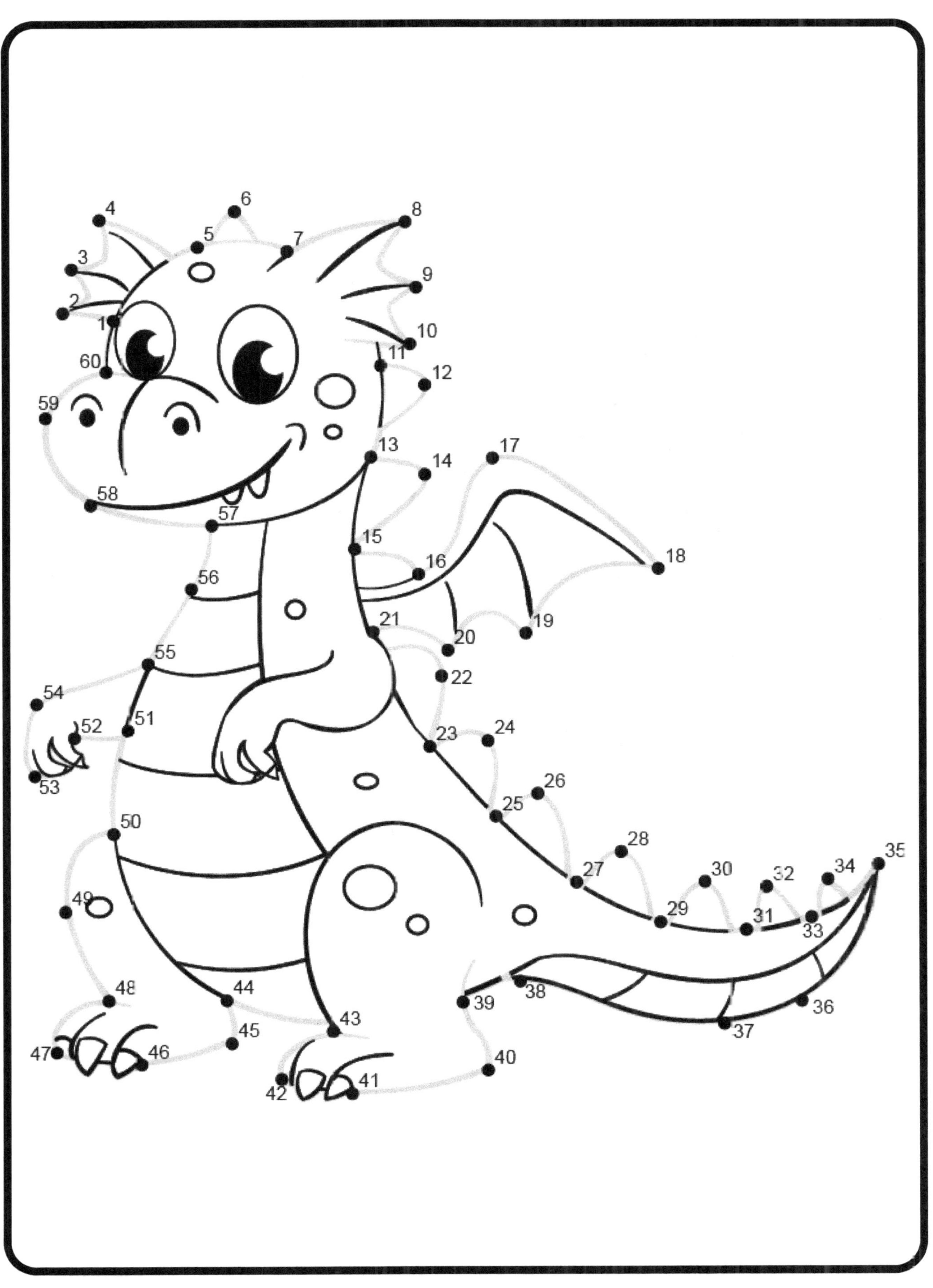

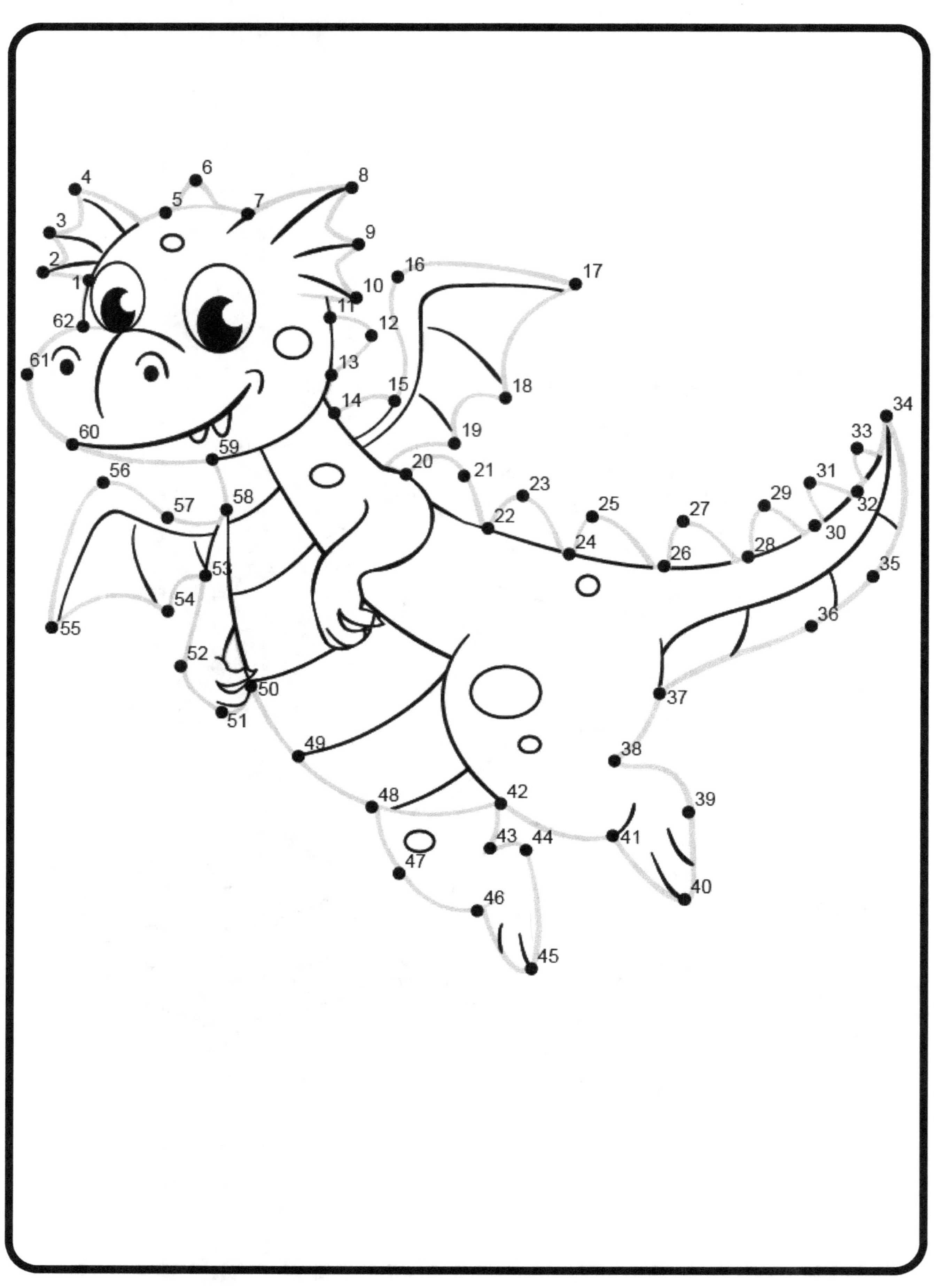

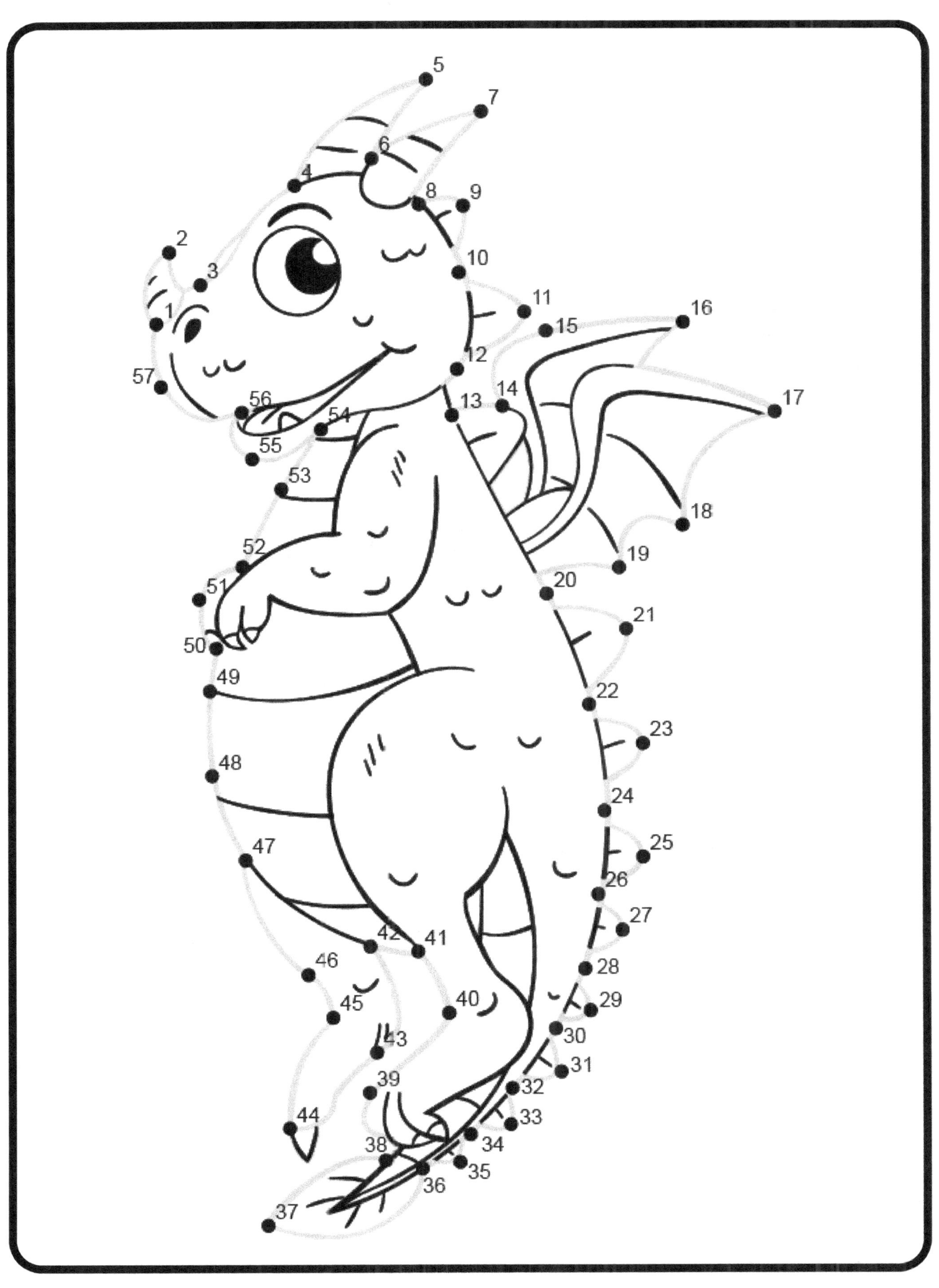

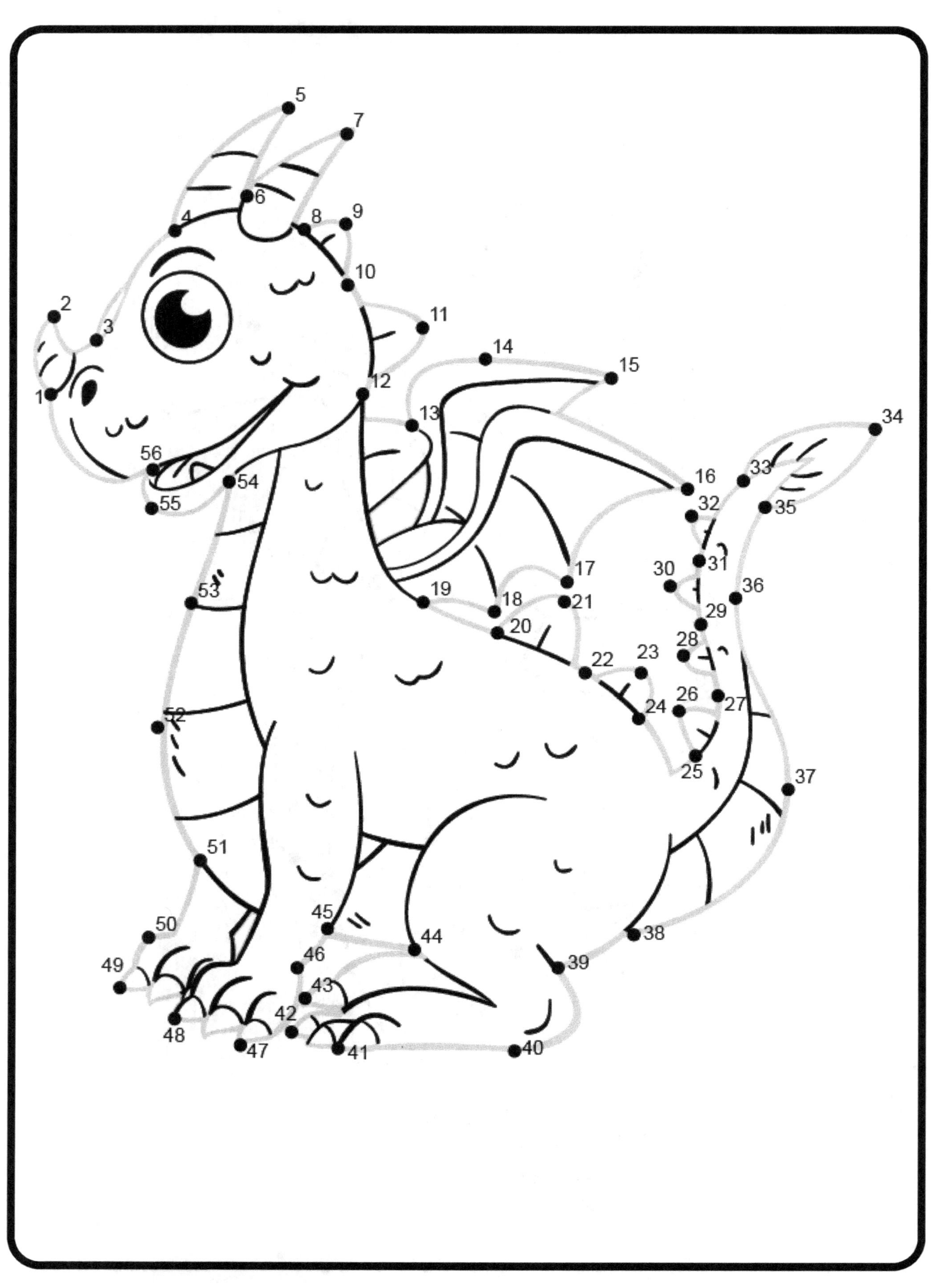

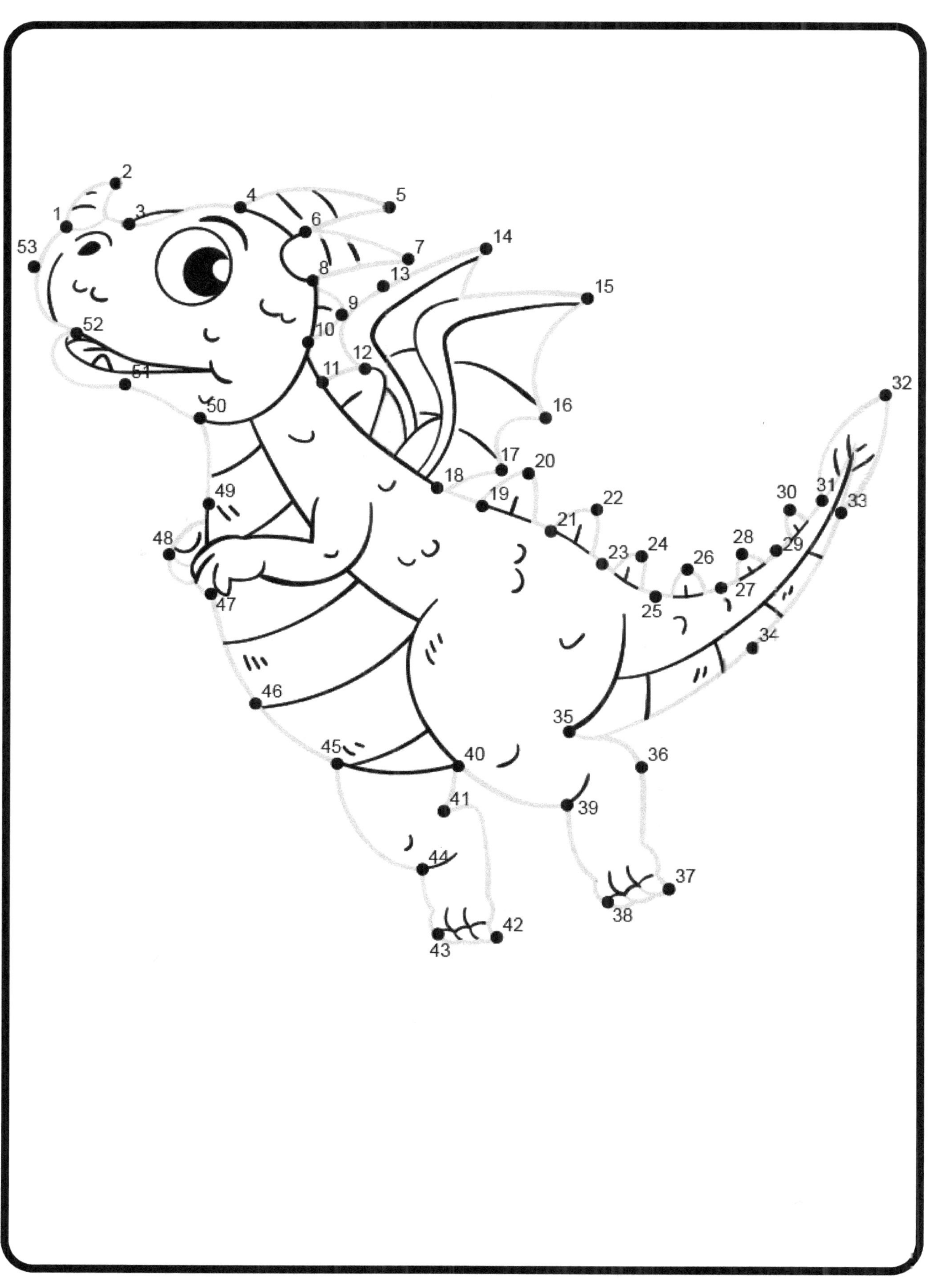

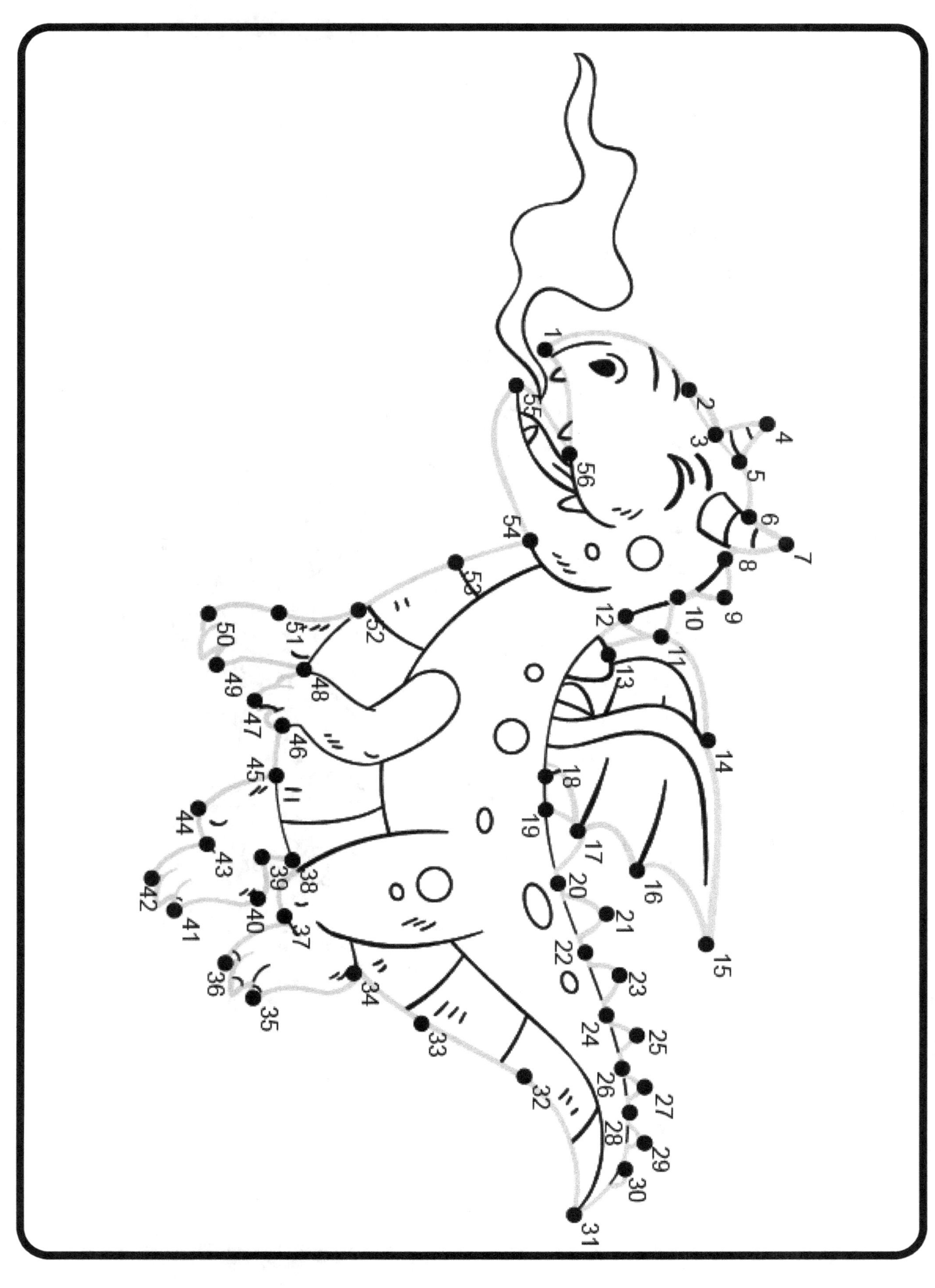

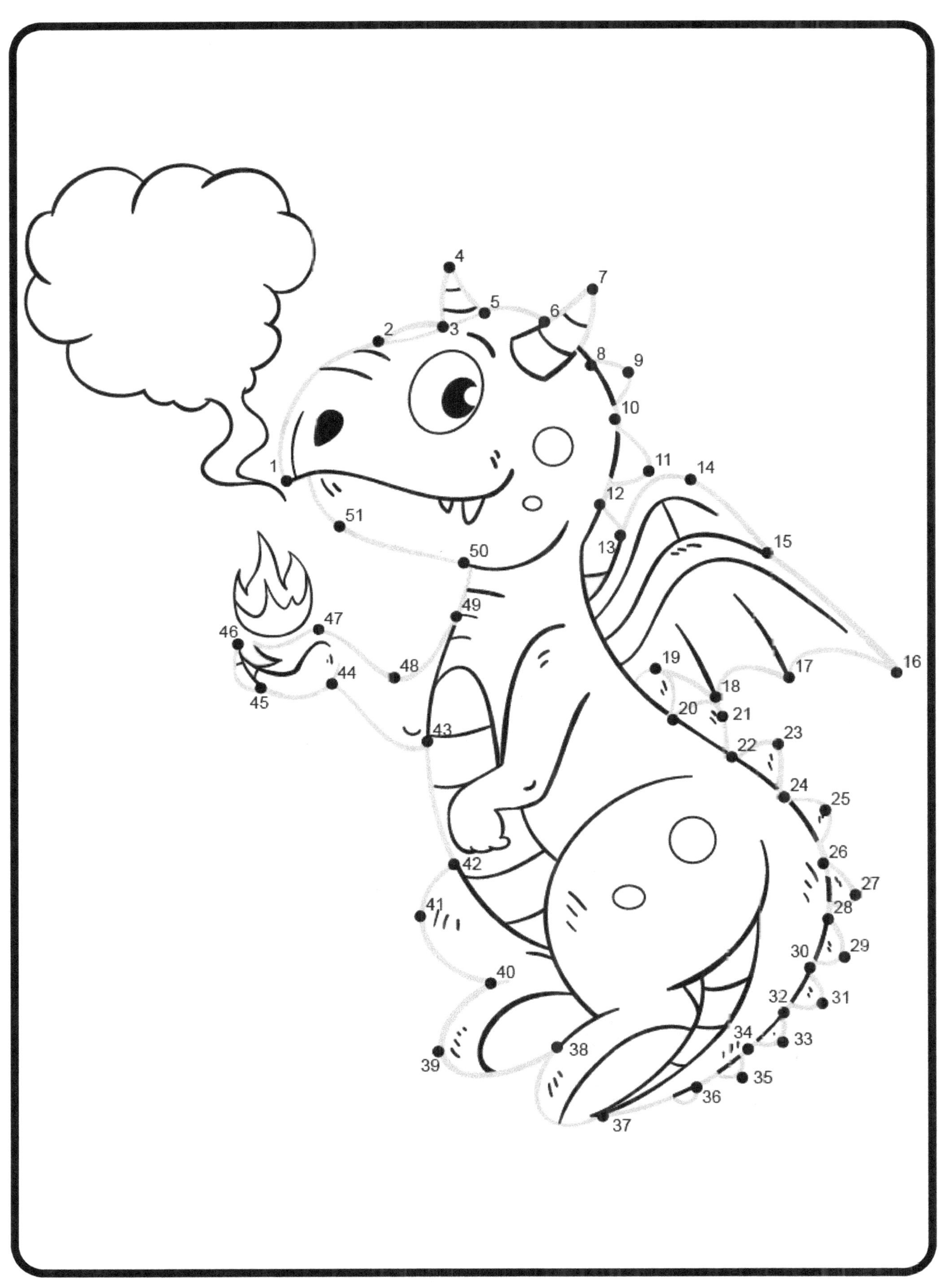

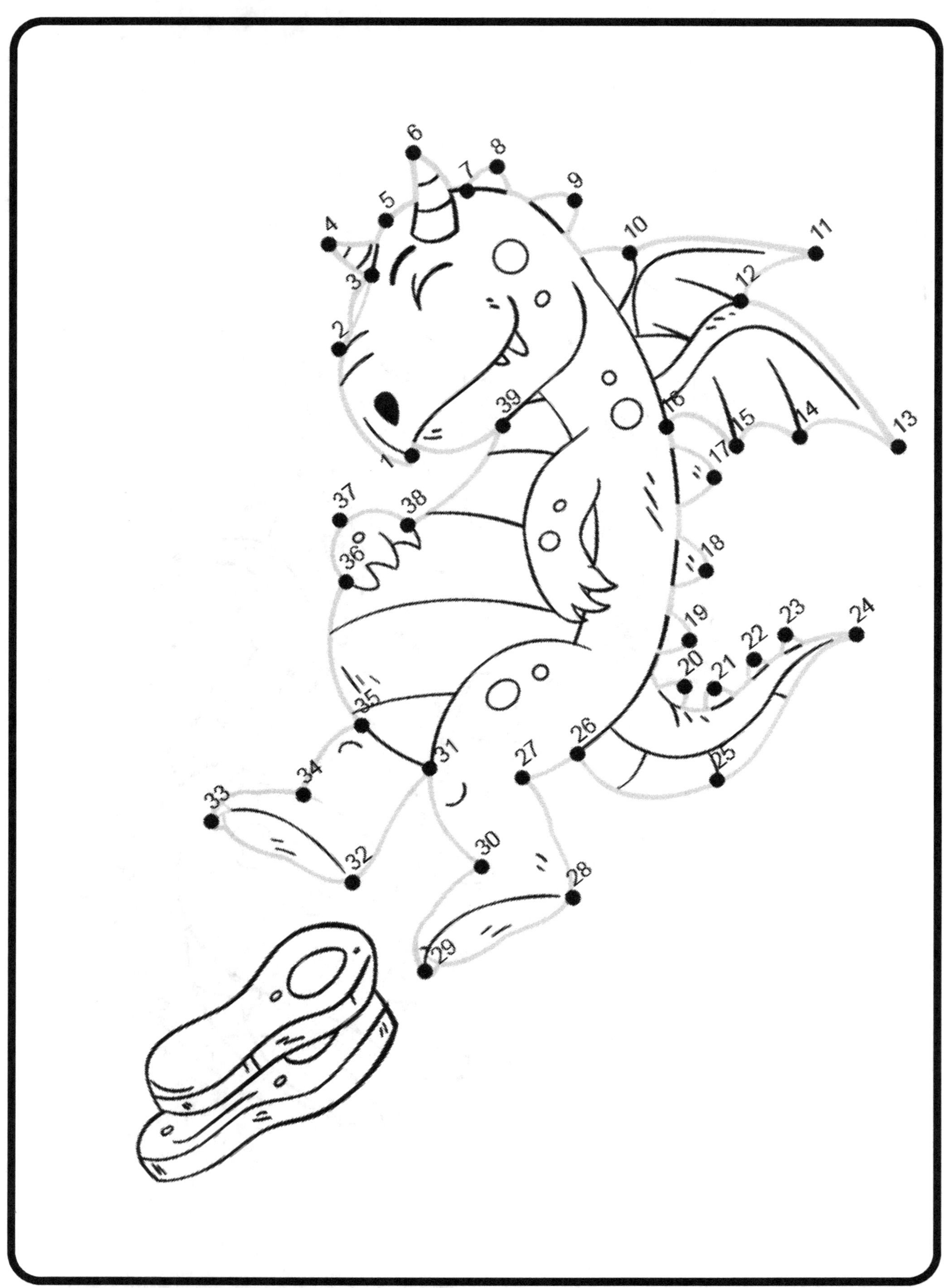

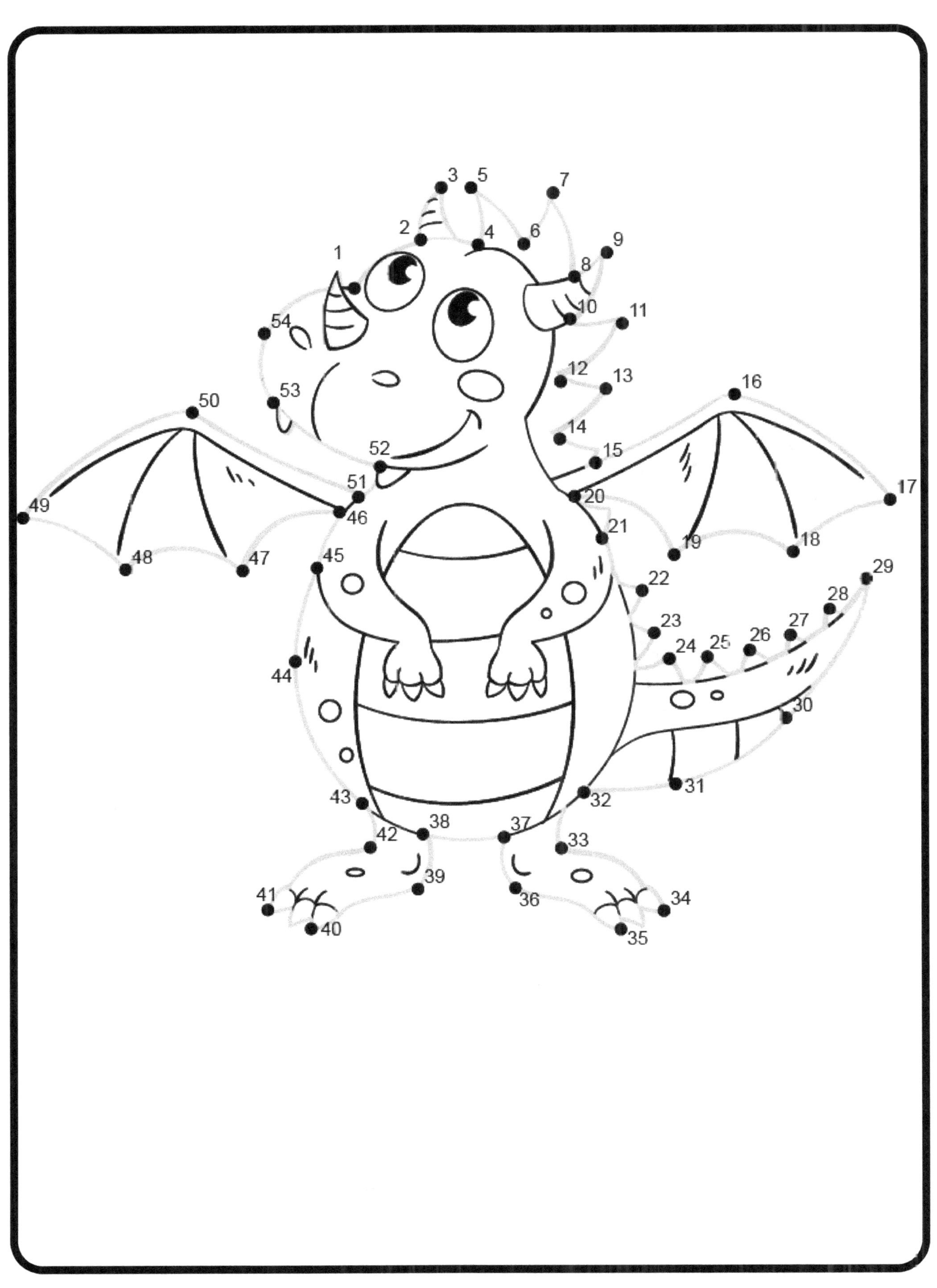

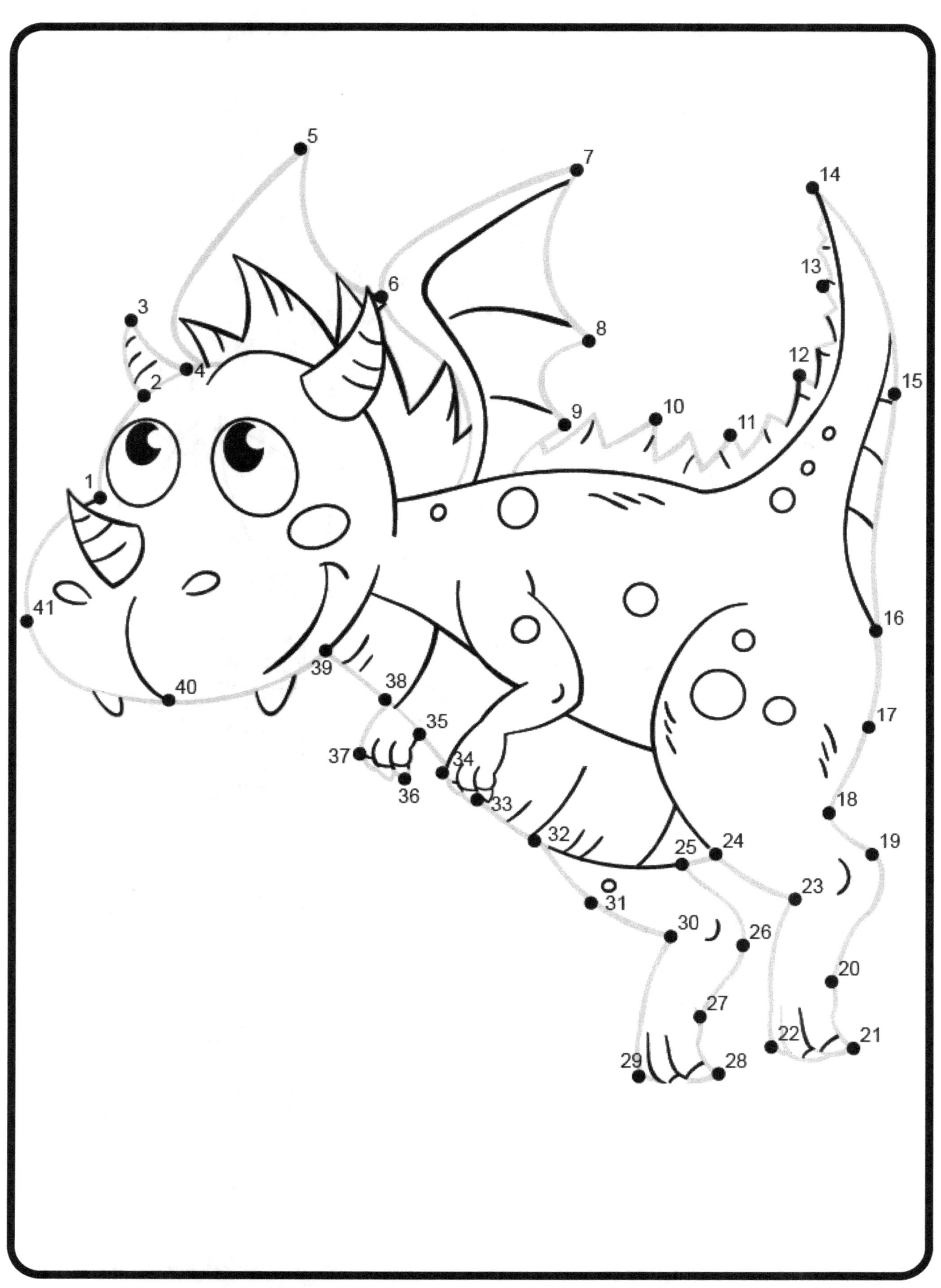

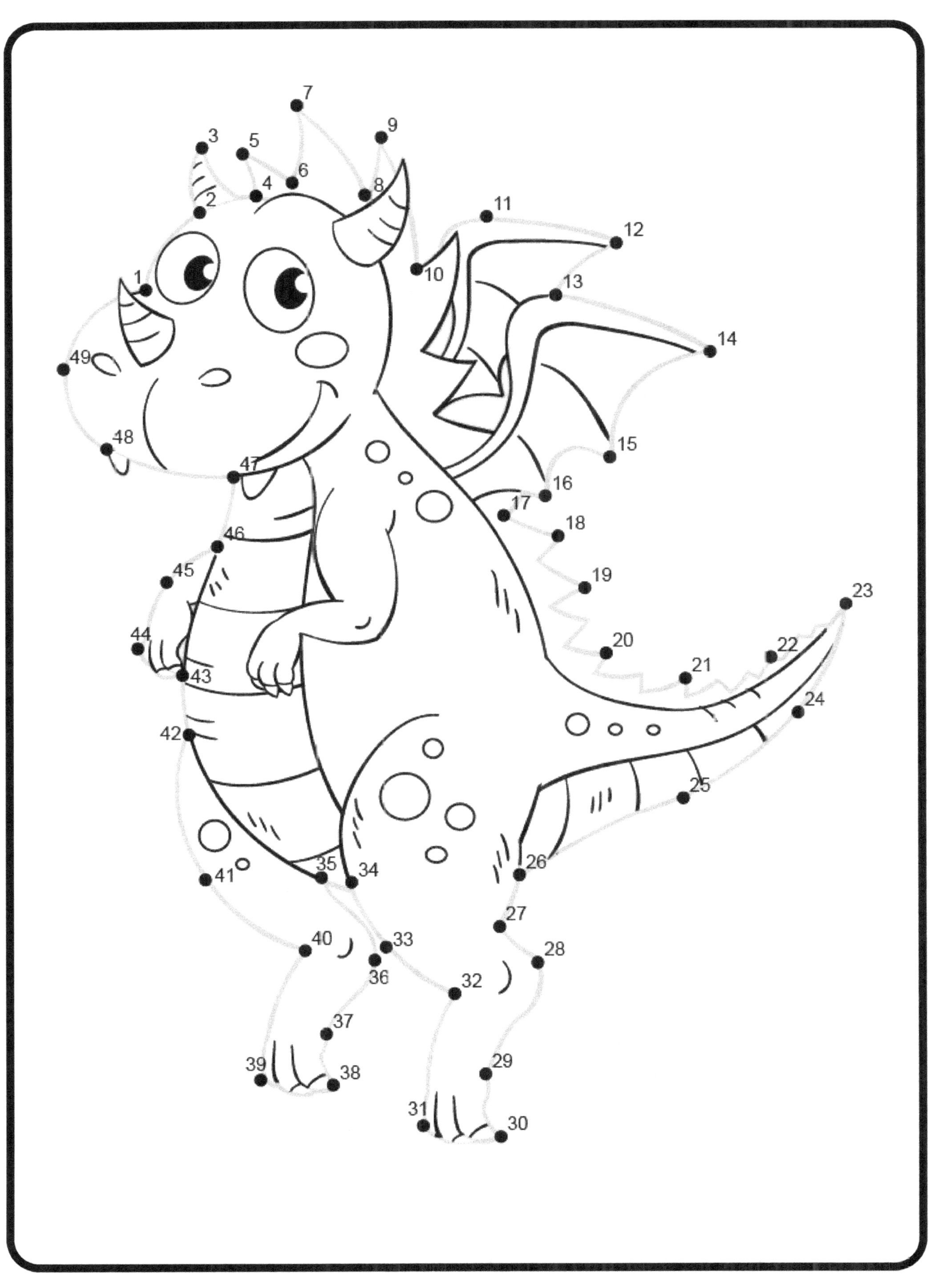

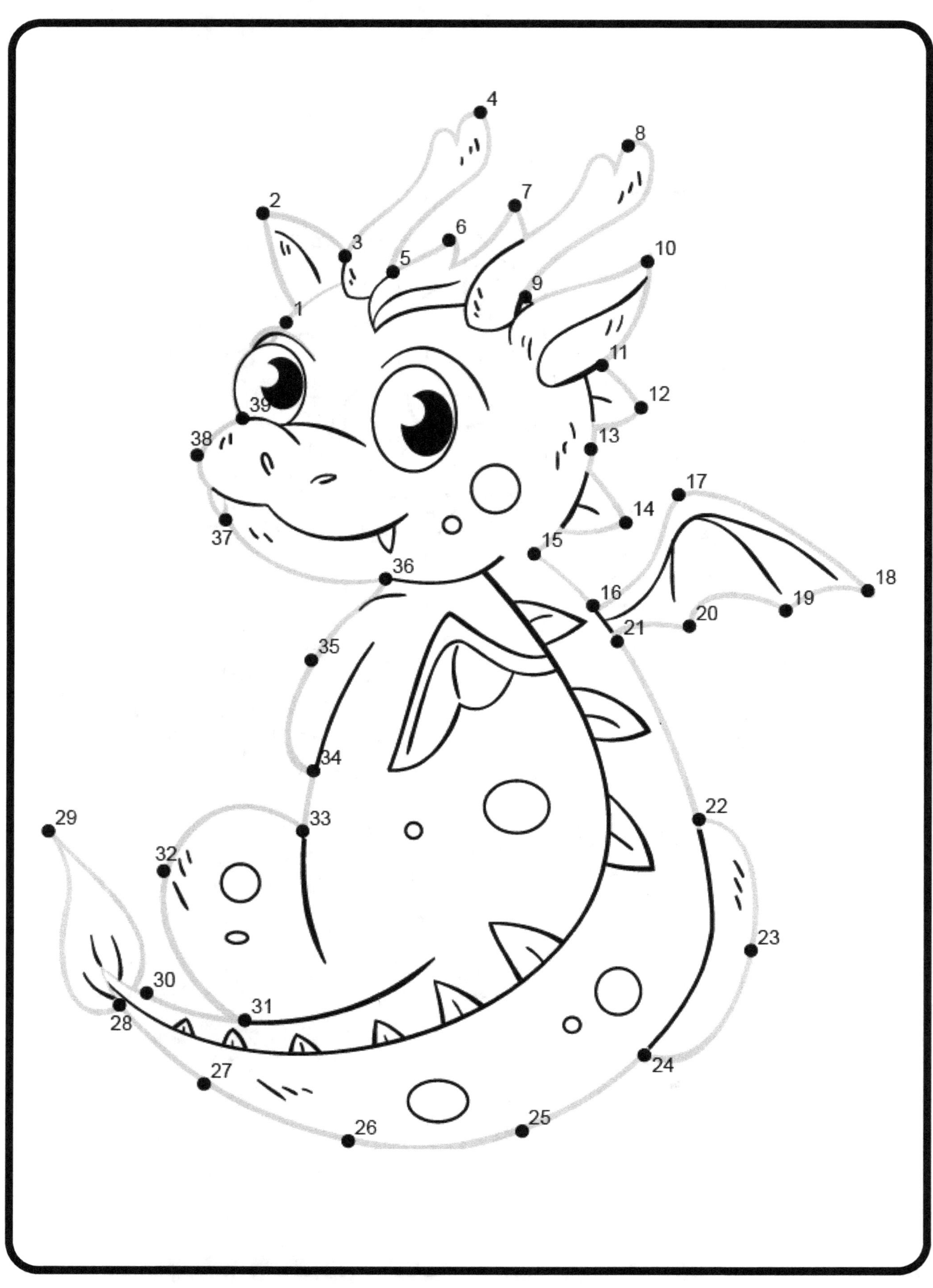

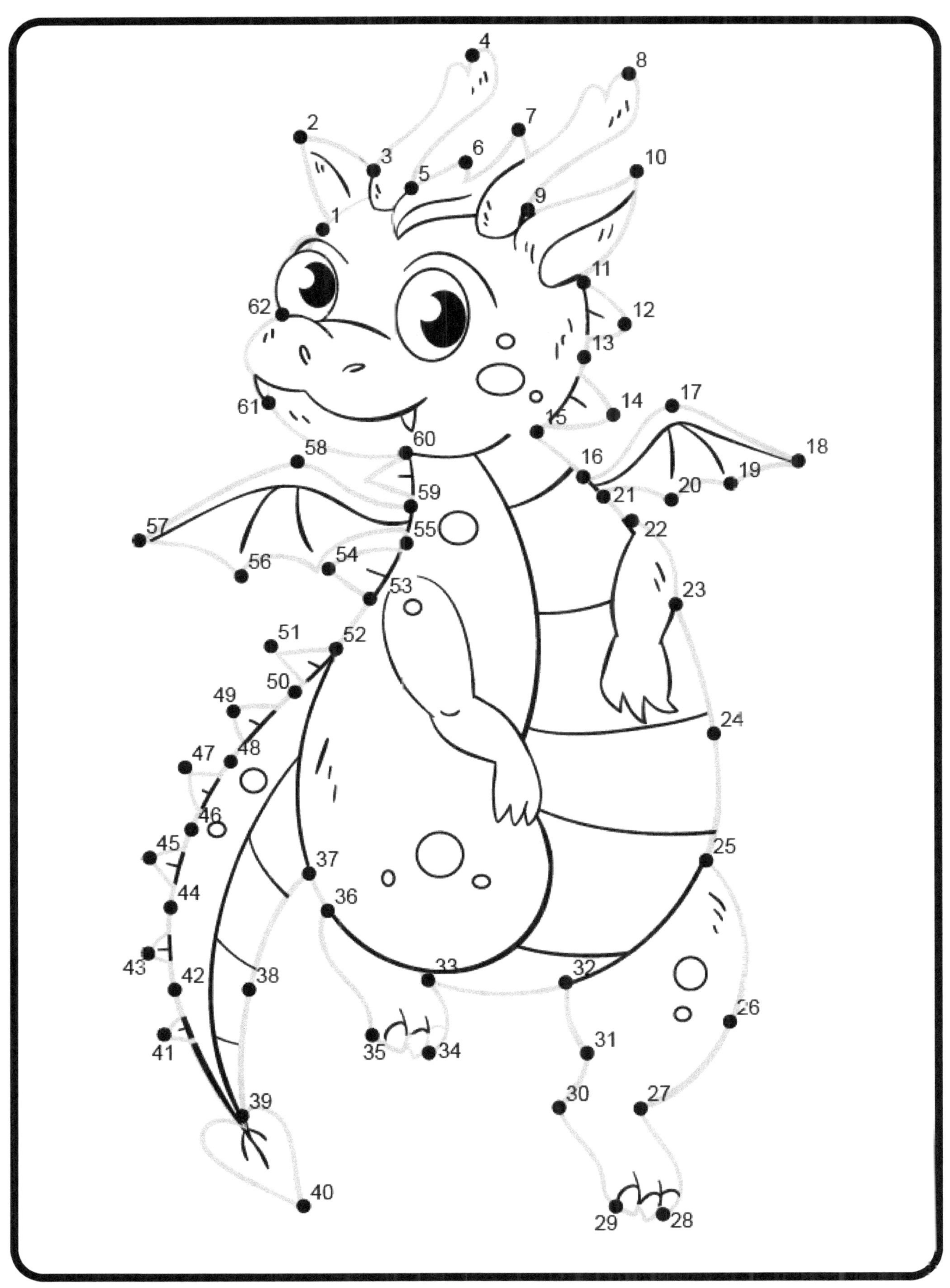

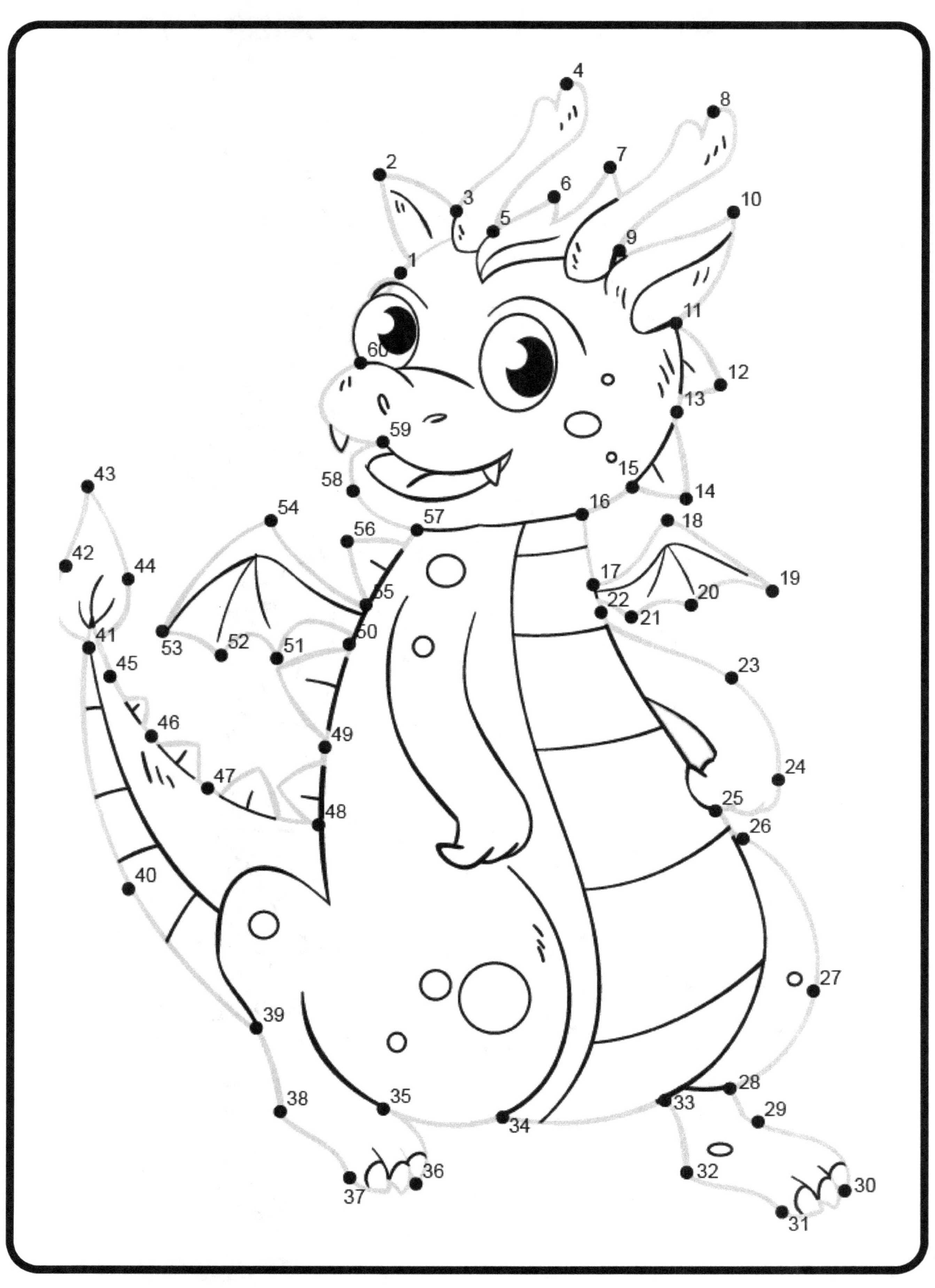

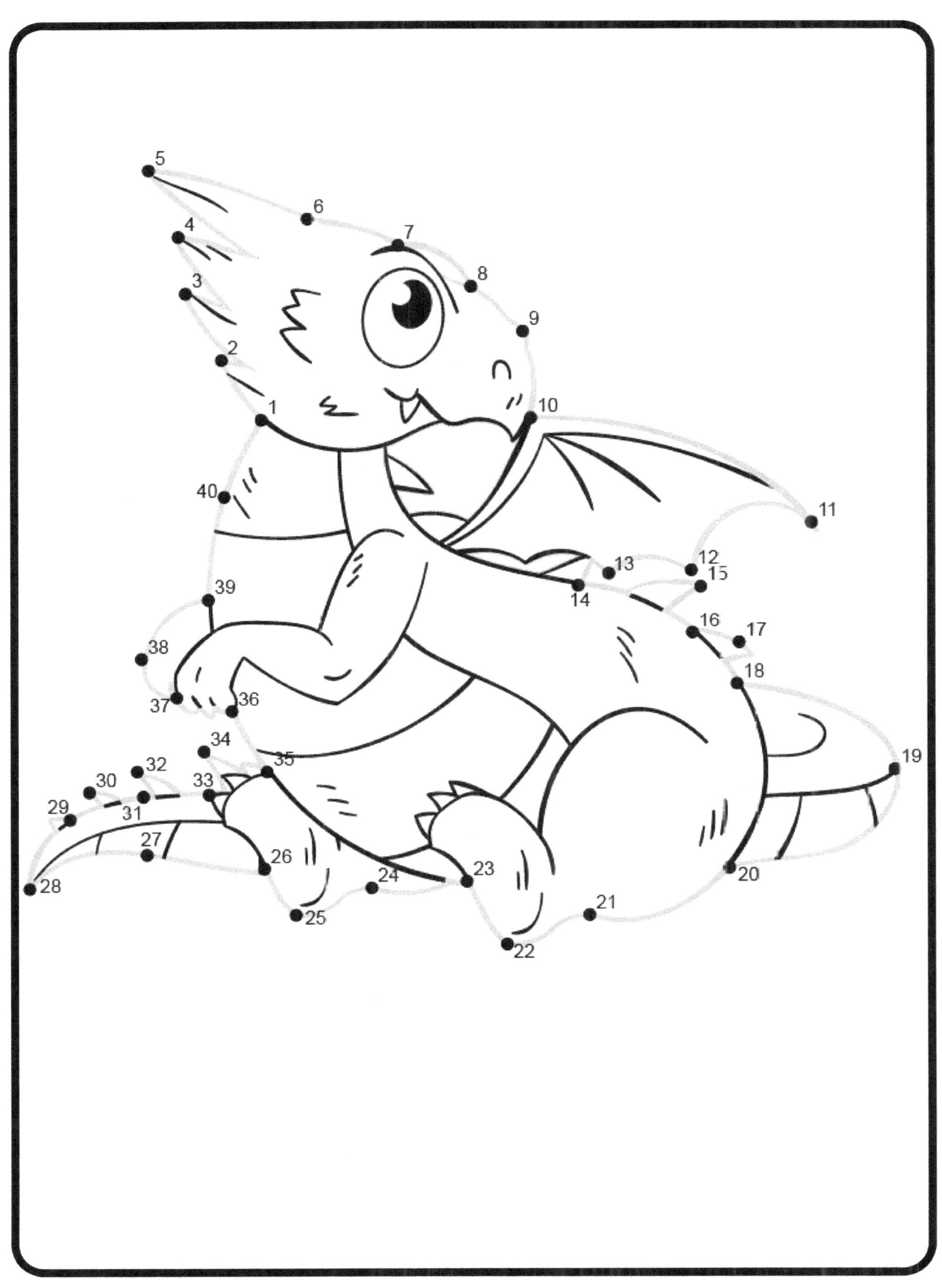

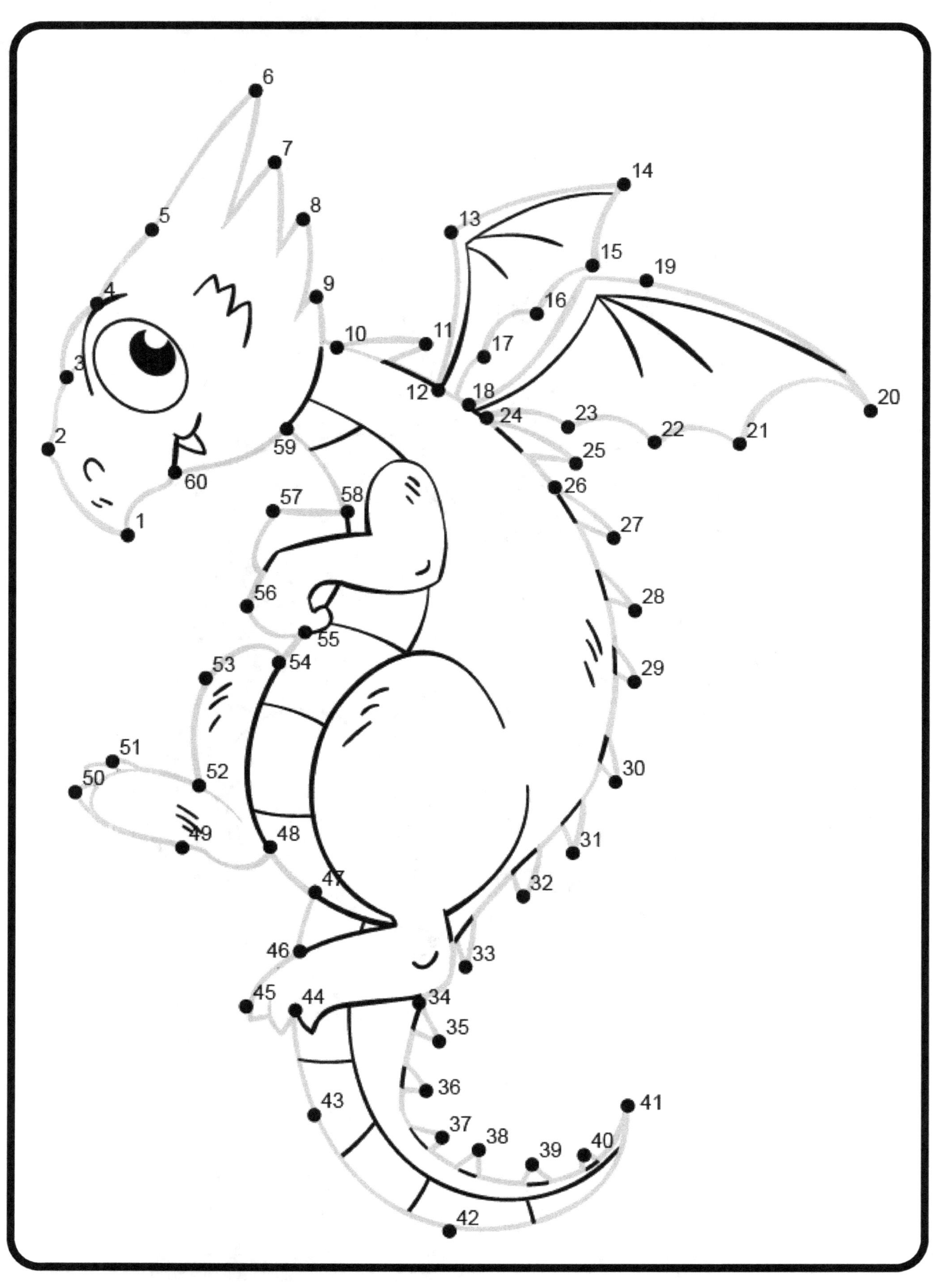

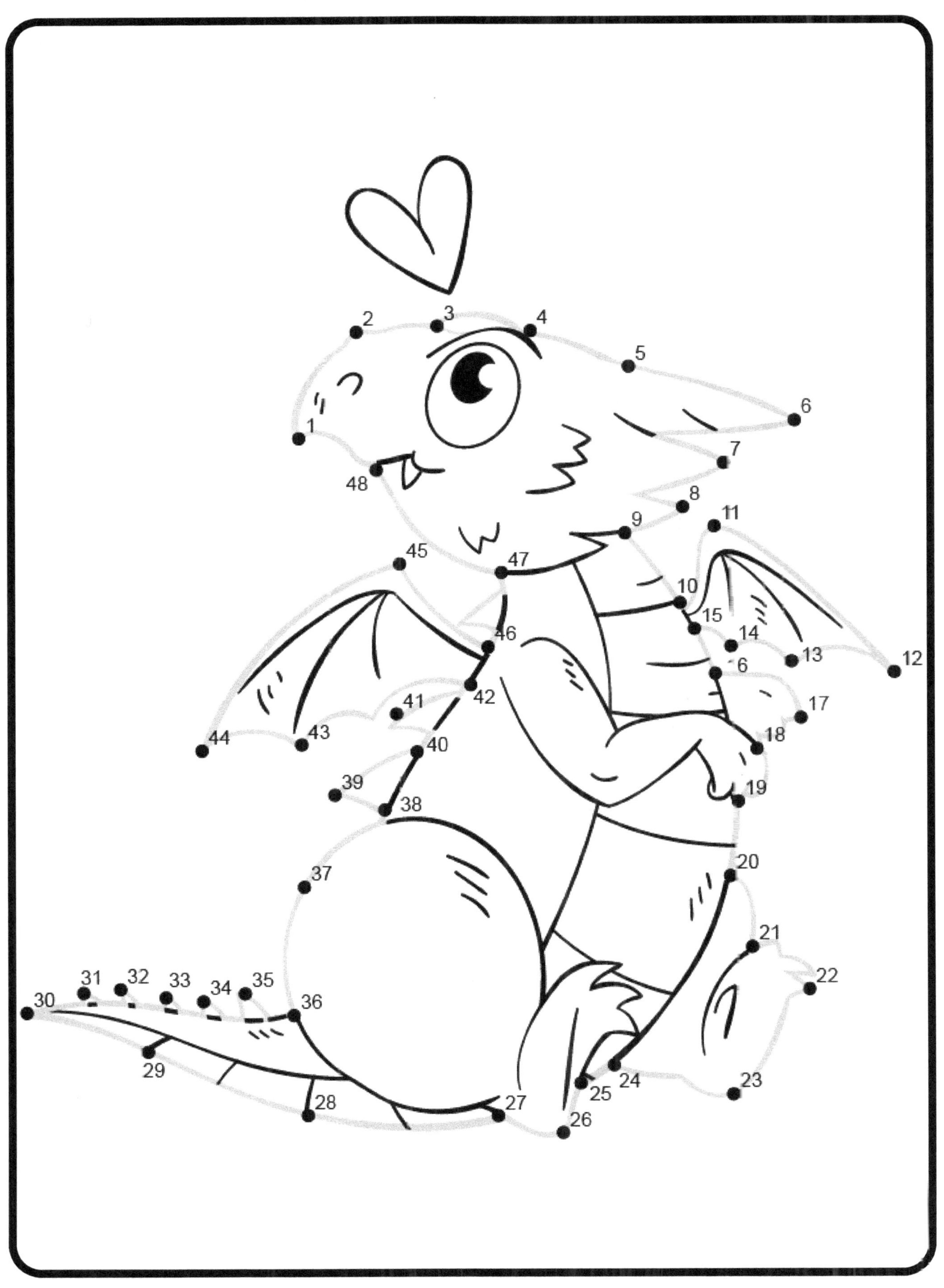

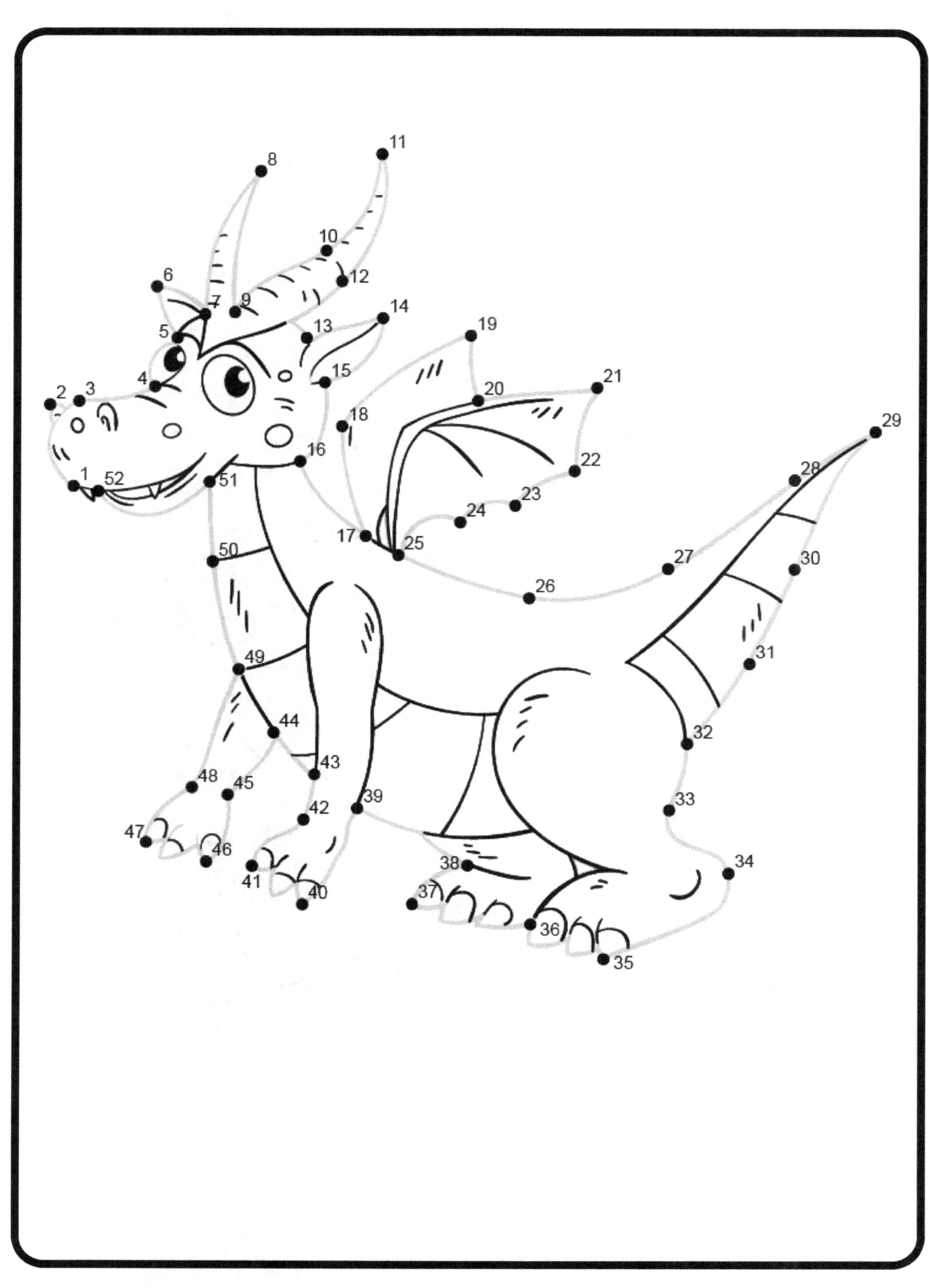

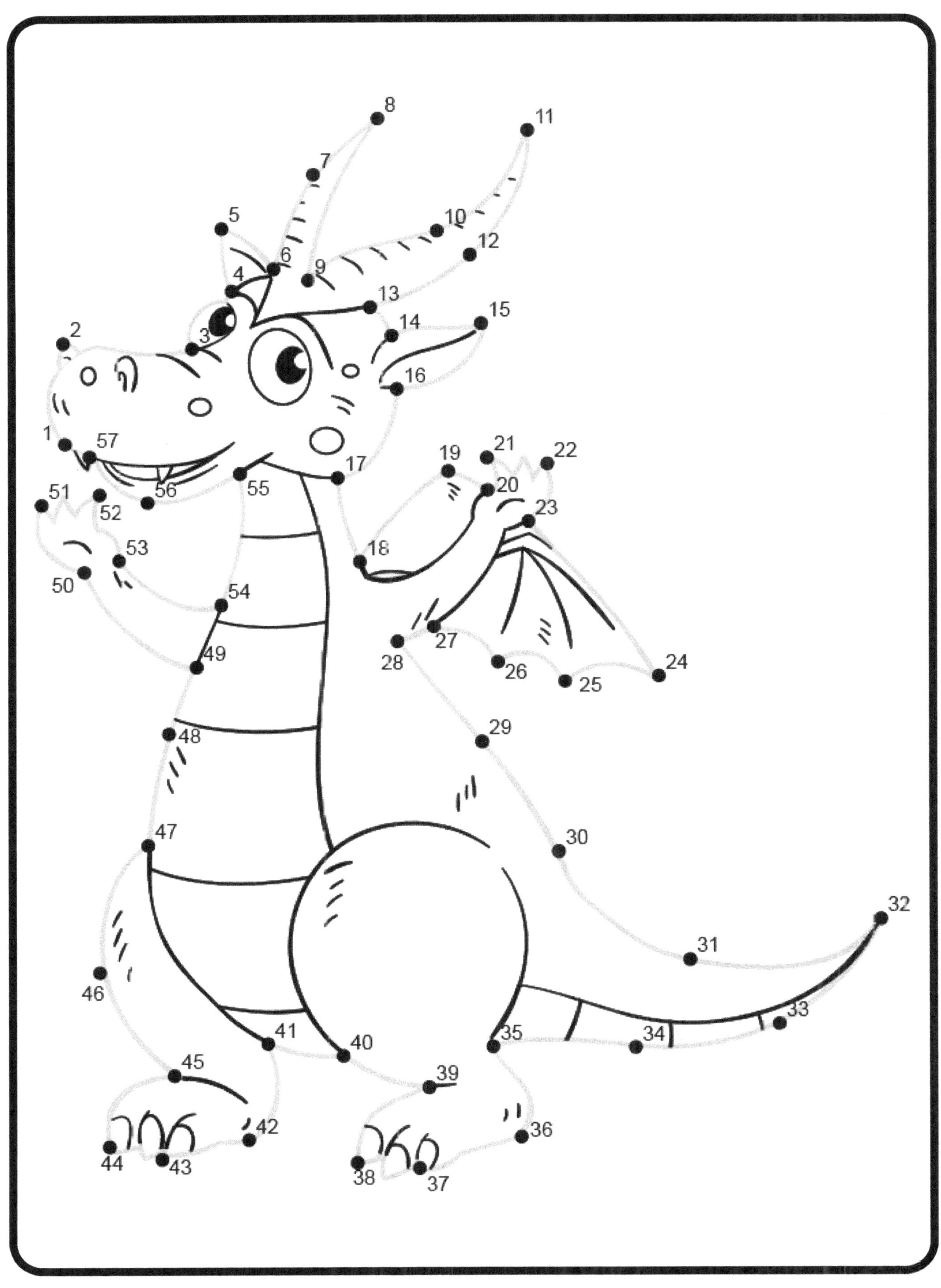

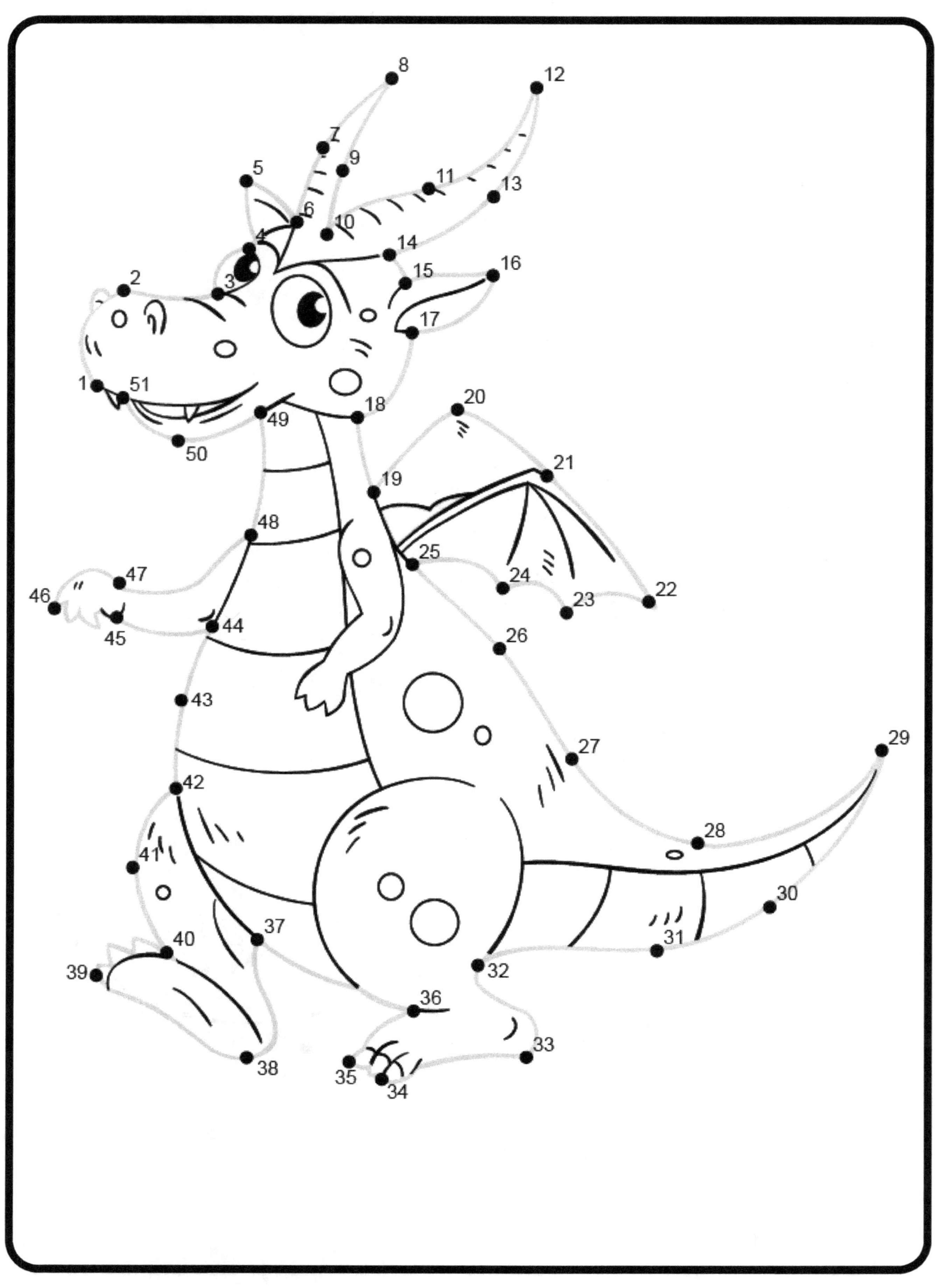

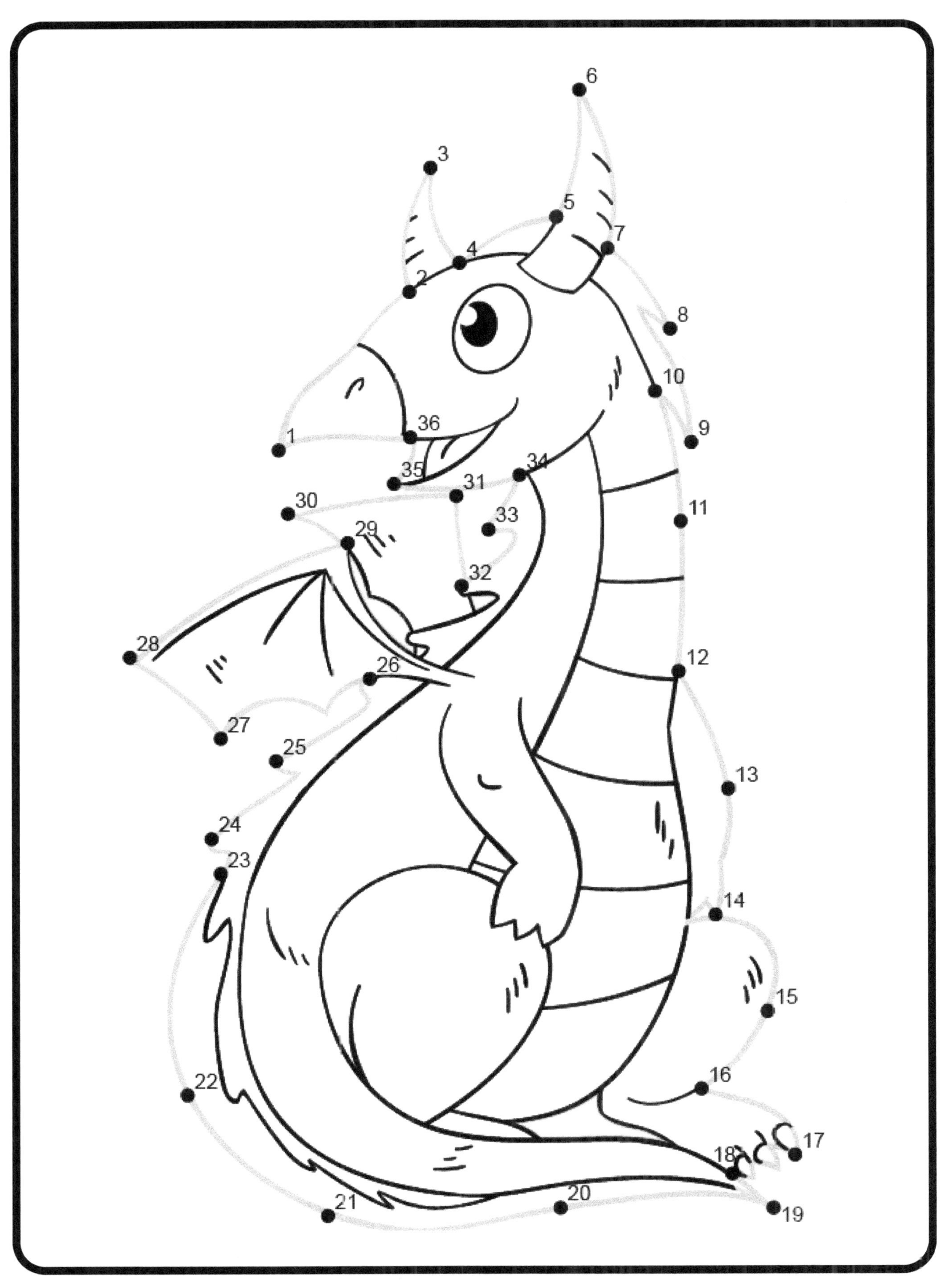

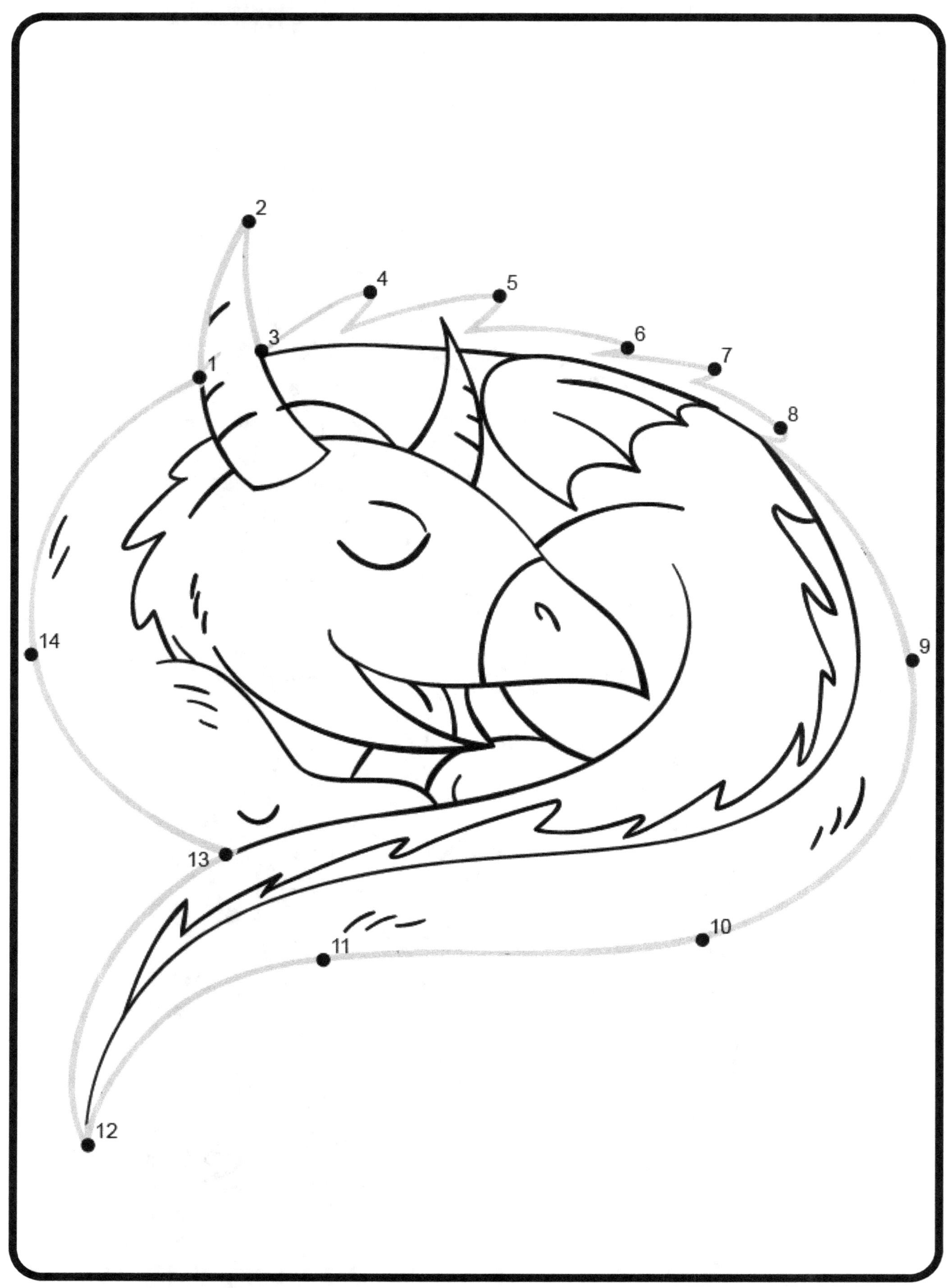

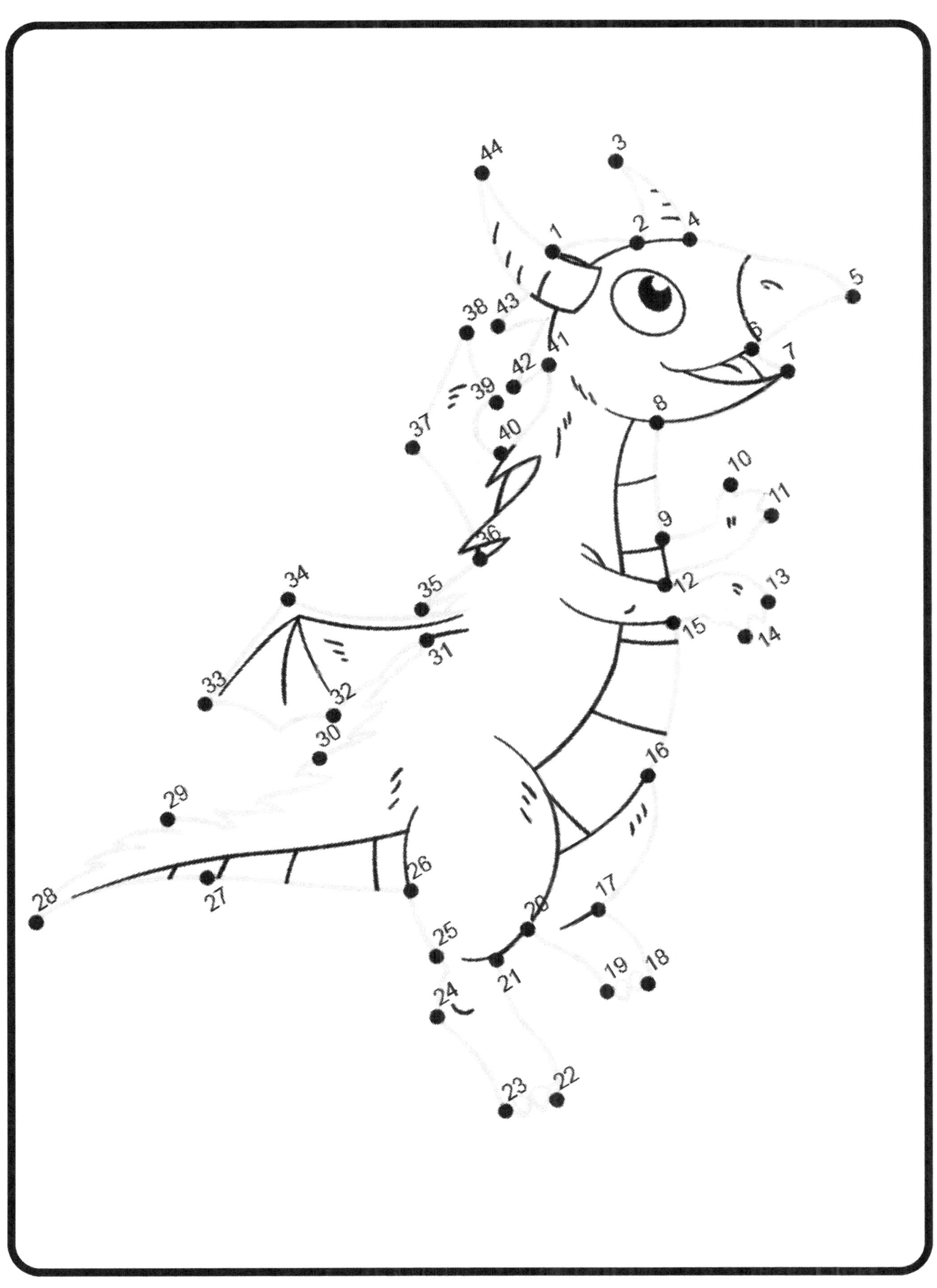

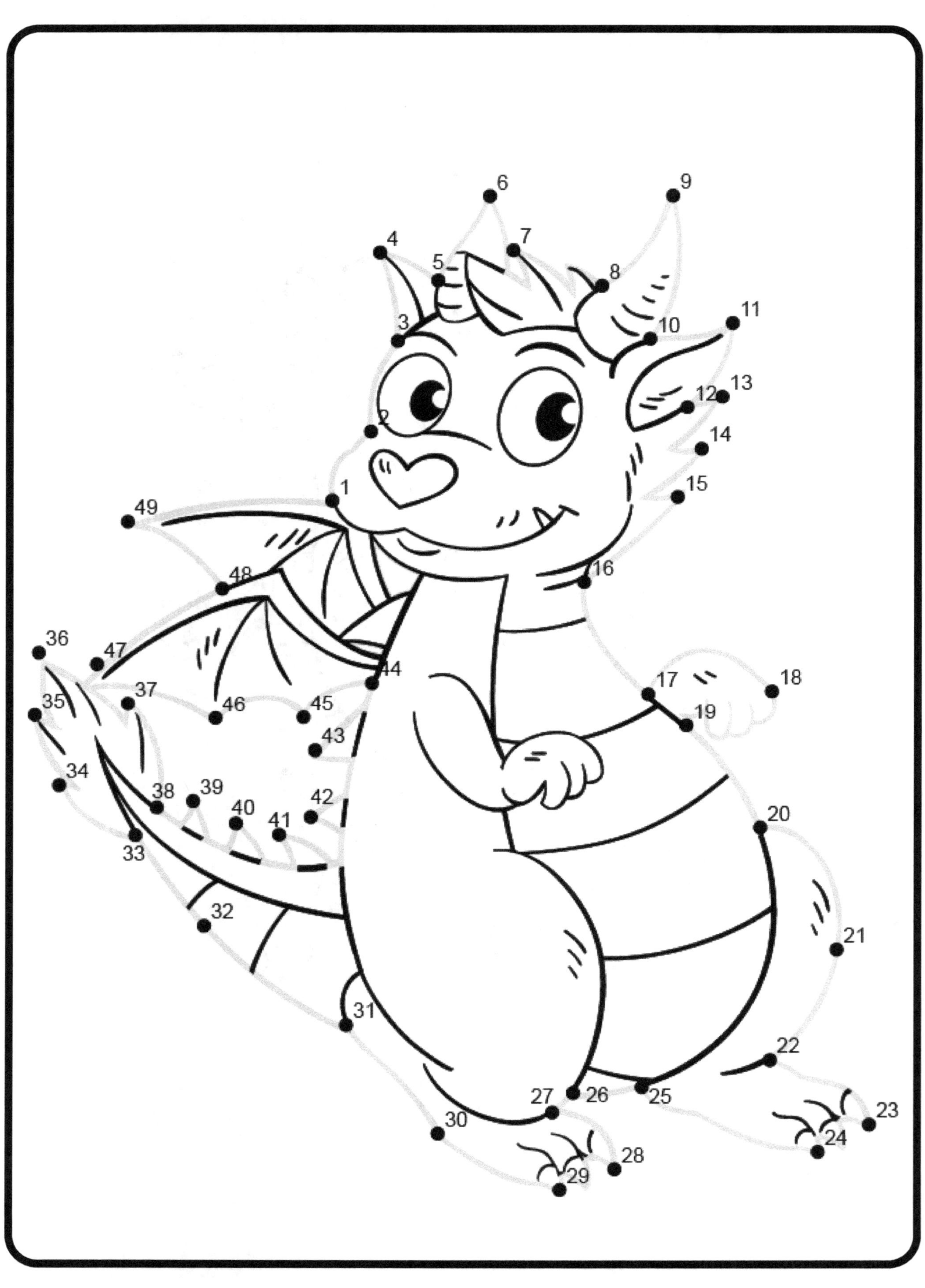

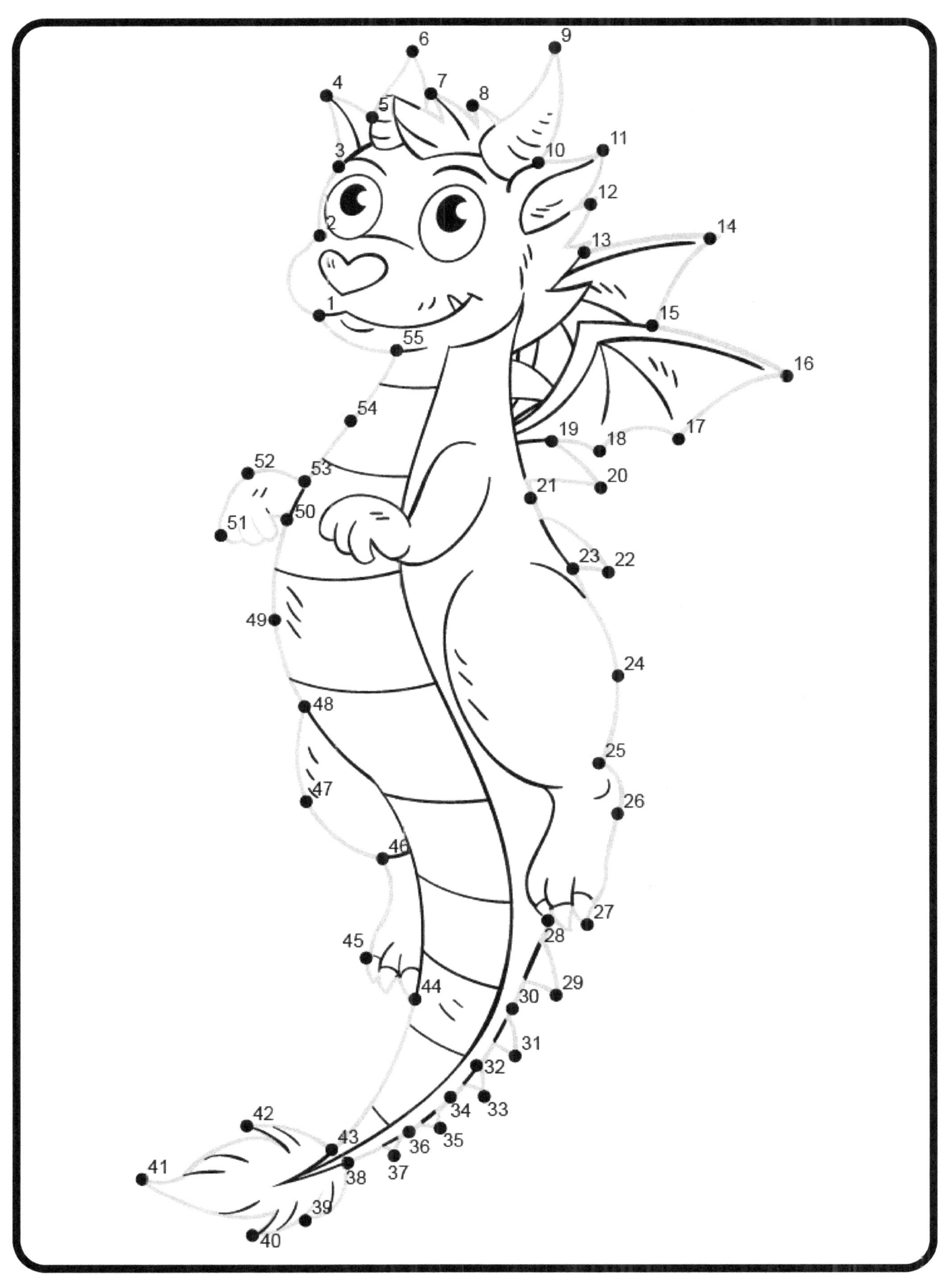

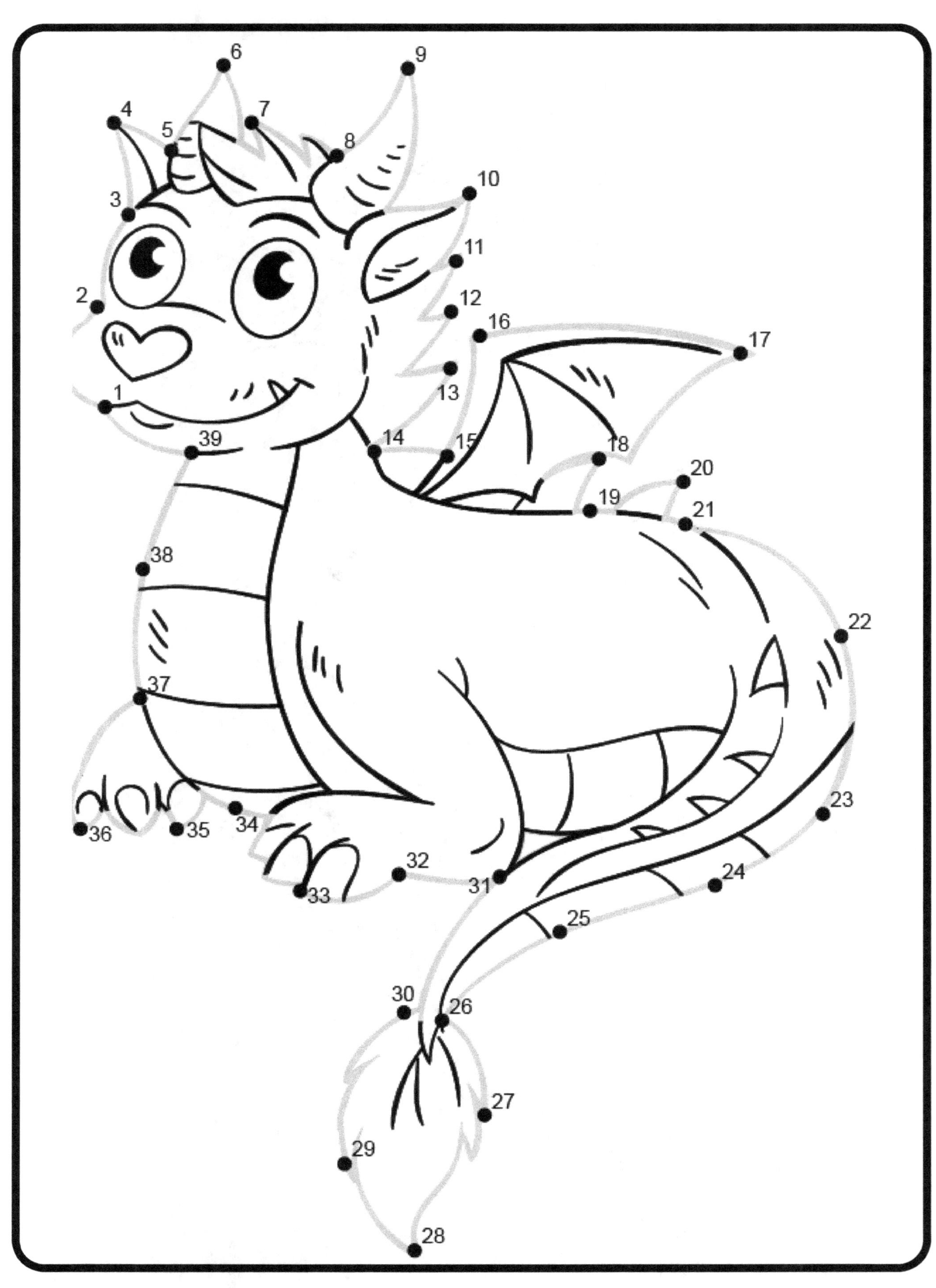

WHALE
COLORING BOOK
FOR ADULTS

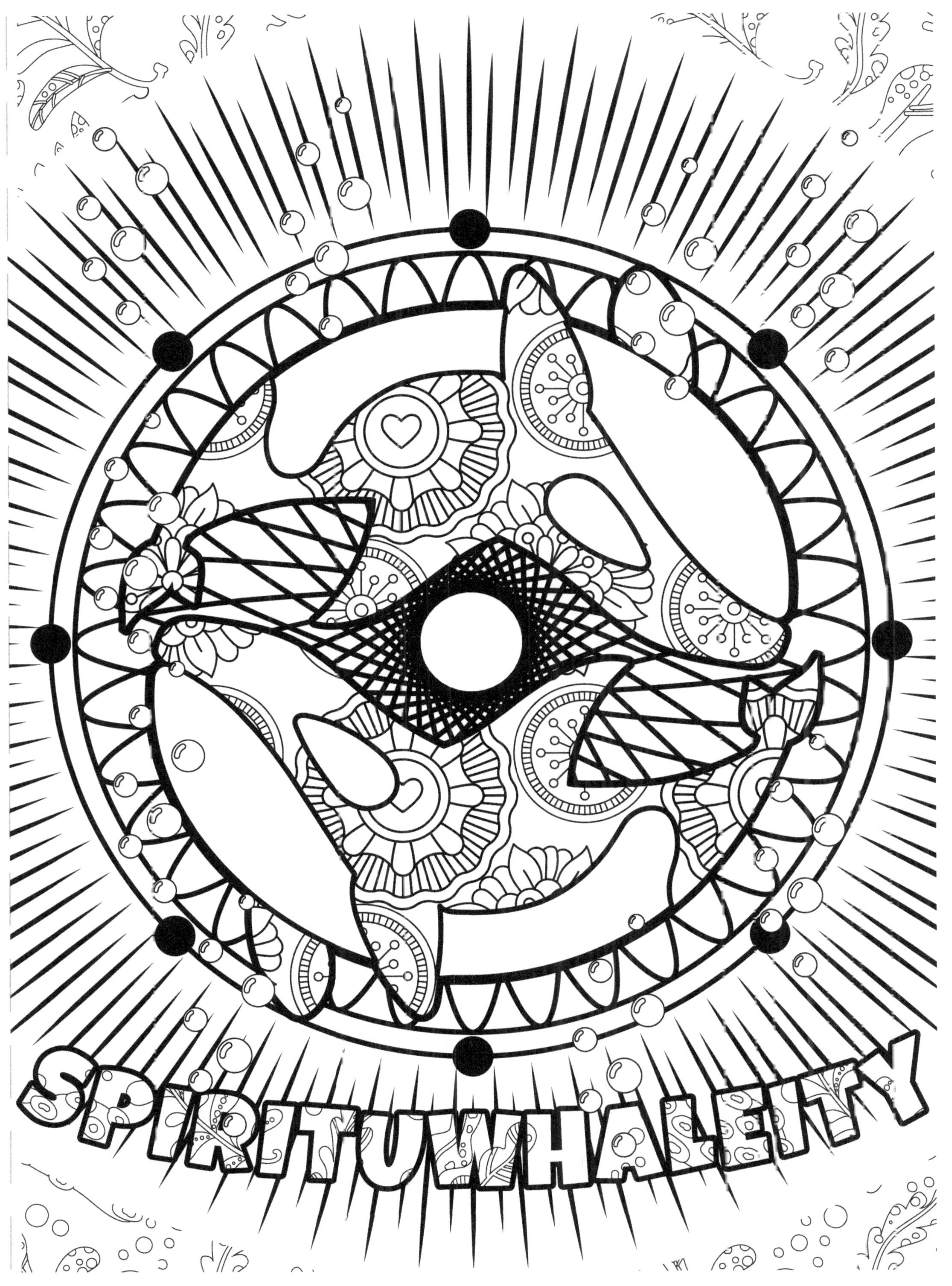
SPIRITUWHALEITY

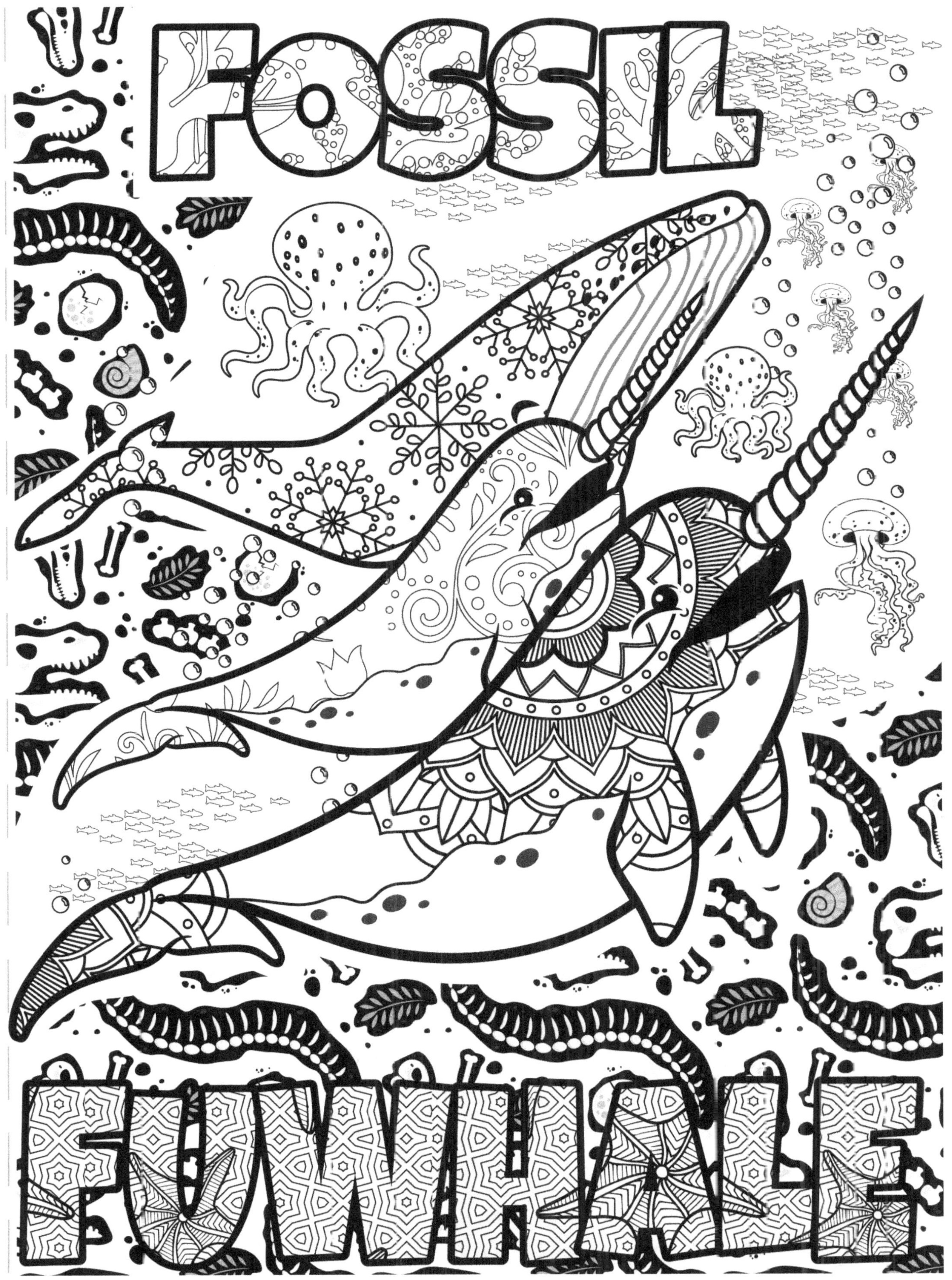

FOSSIL
FUN WHALE

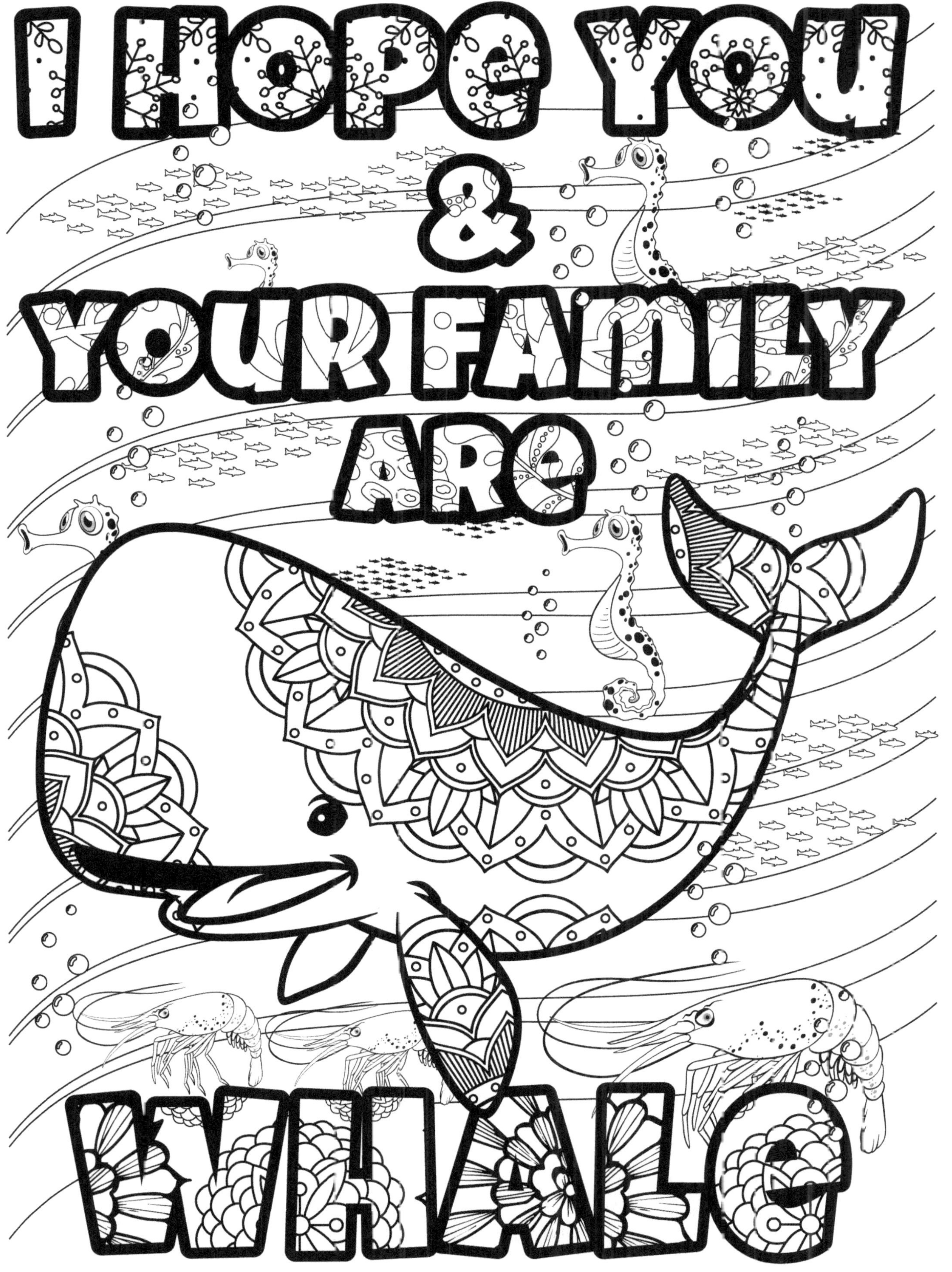

I HOPE YOU
&
YOUR FAMILY
ARE
WHALE

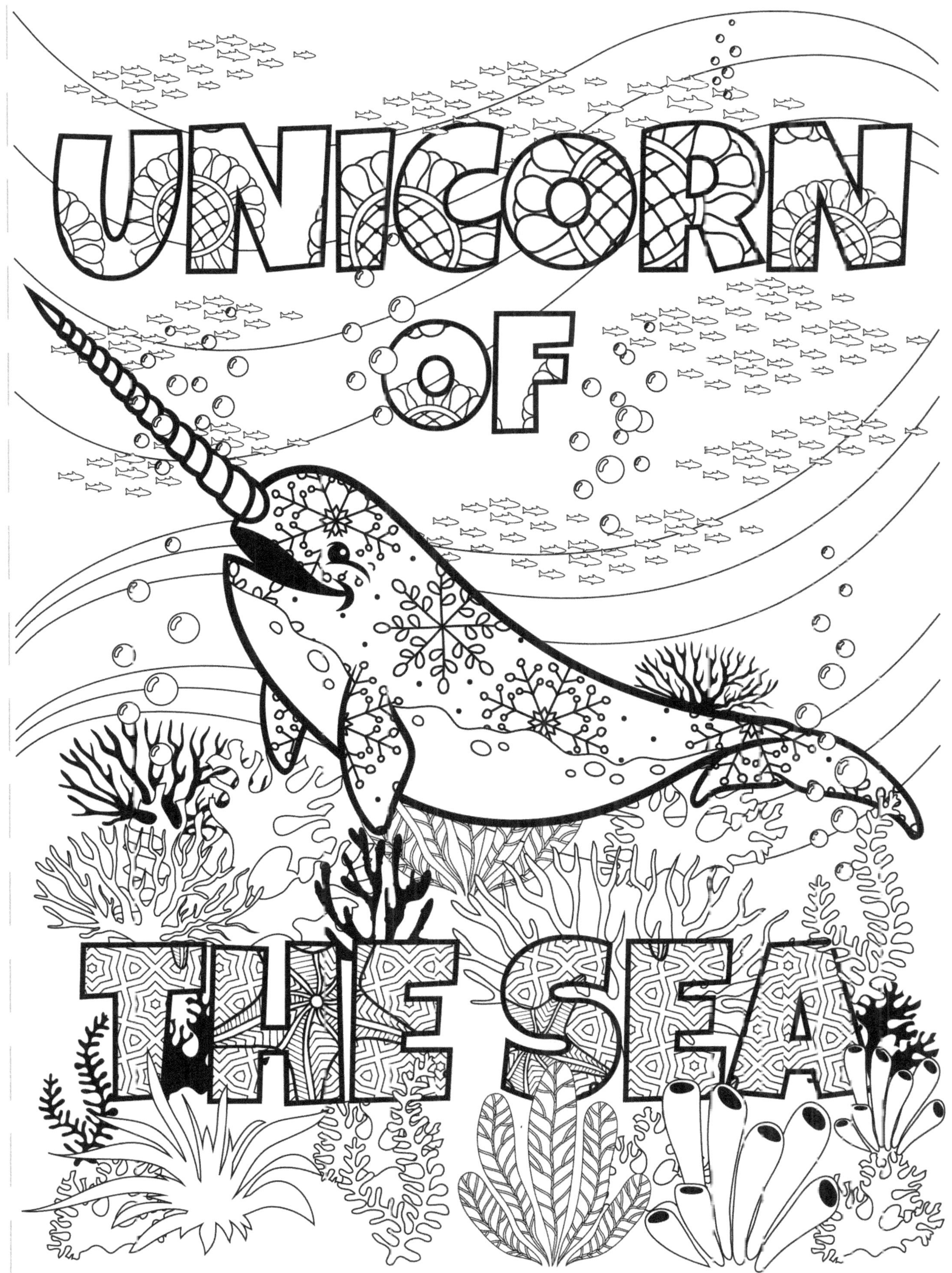

UNICORN
OF
THE SEA

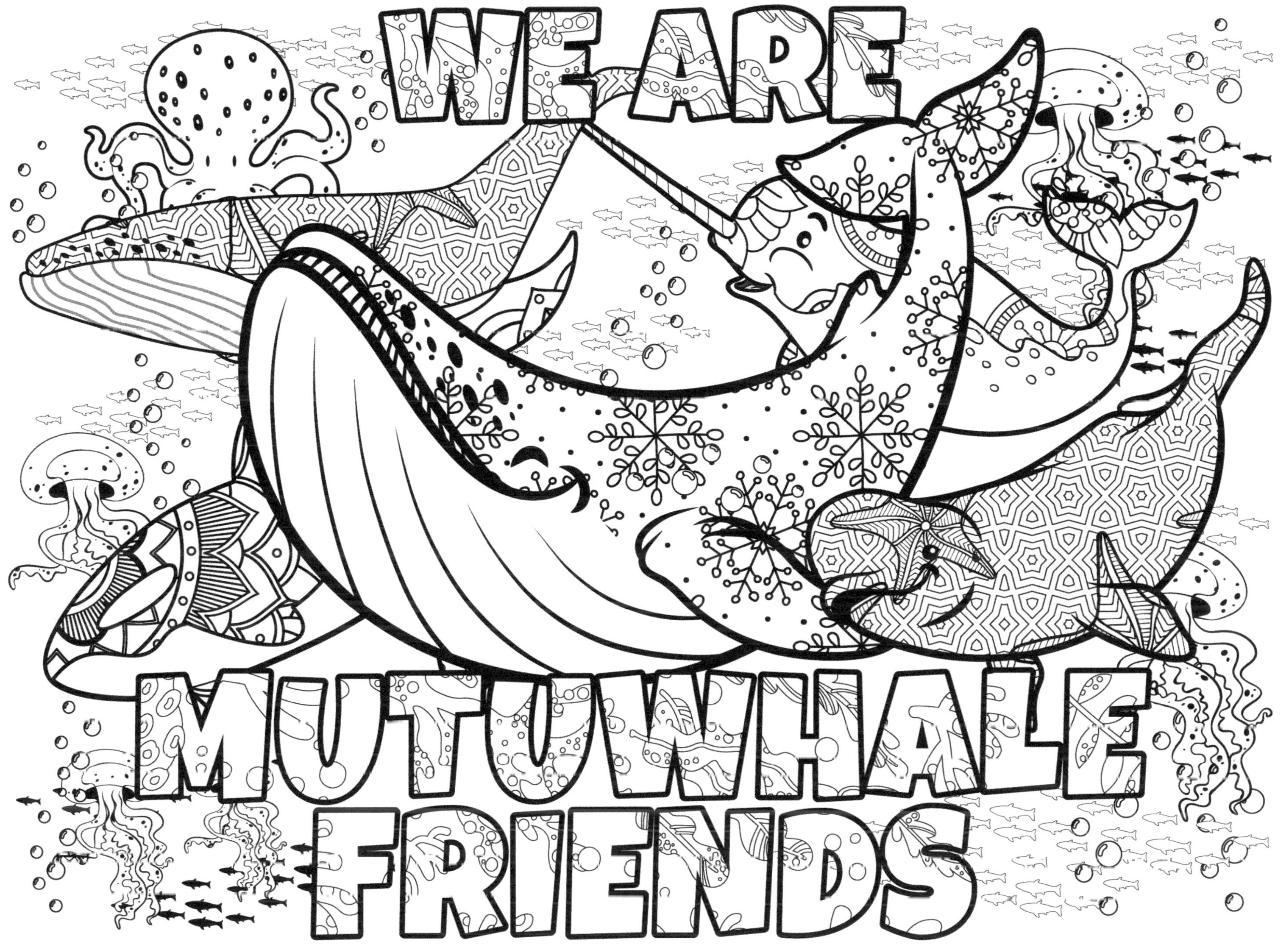

WE ARE
MUTUWHALE
FRIENDS

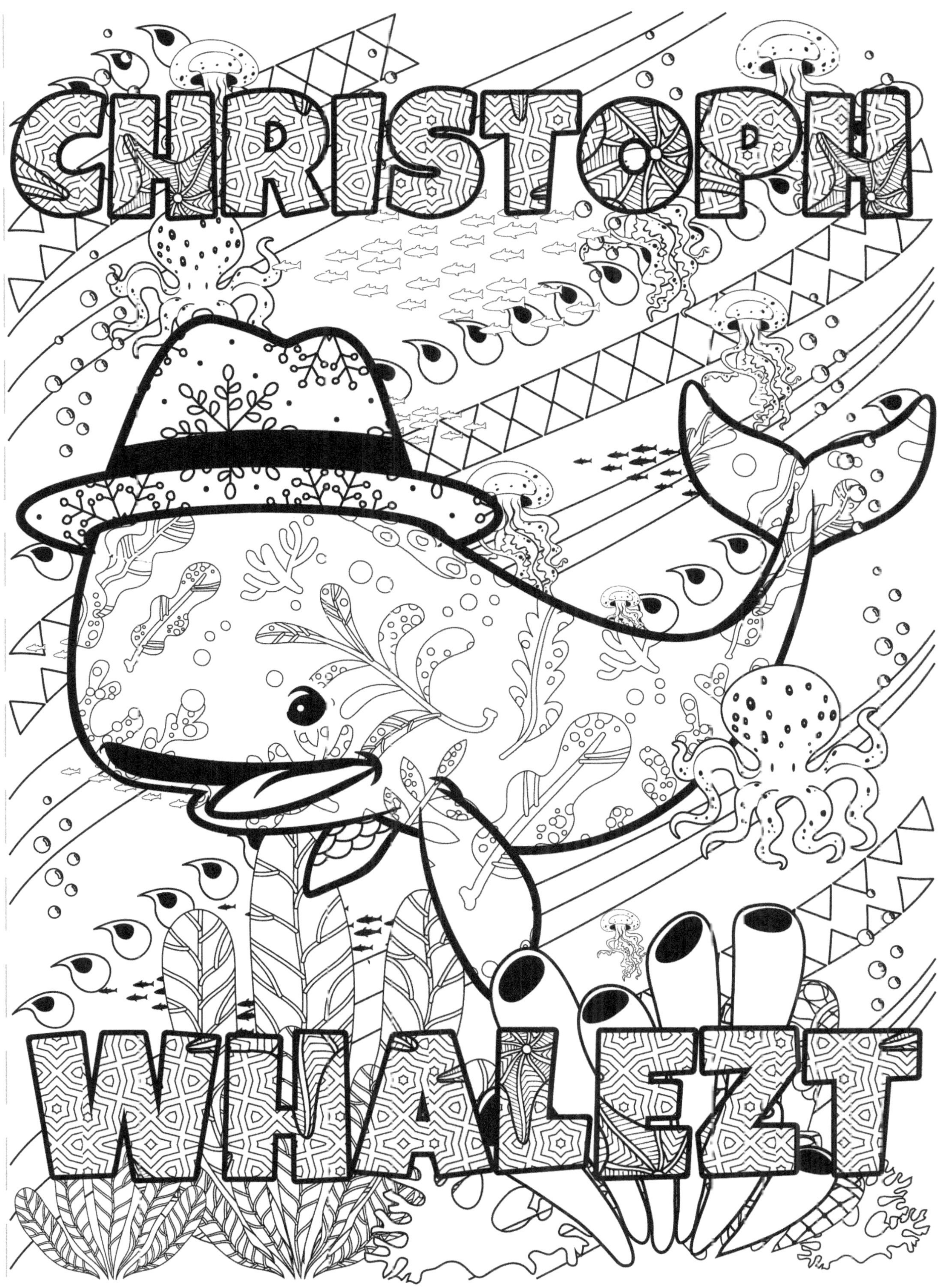

CHRISTOPH
WHALEZT

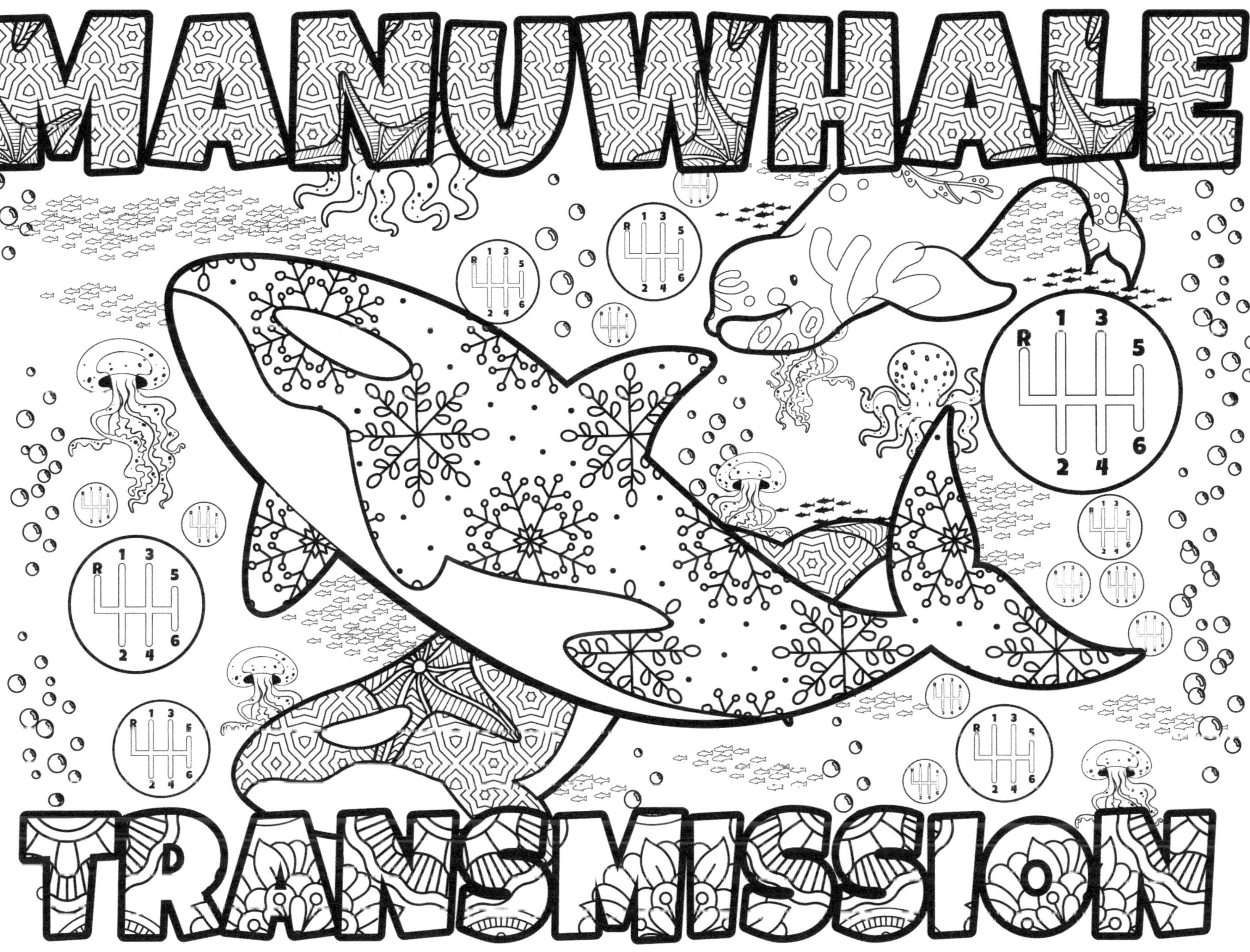
MANUWHALE
TRANSMISSION

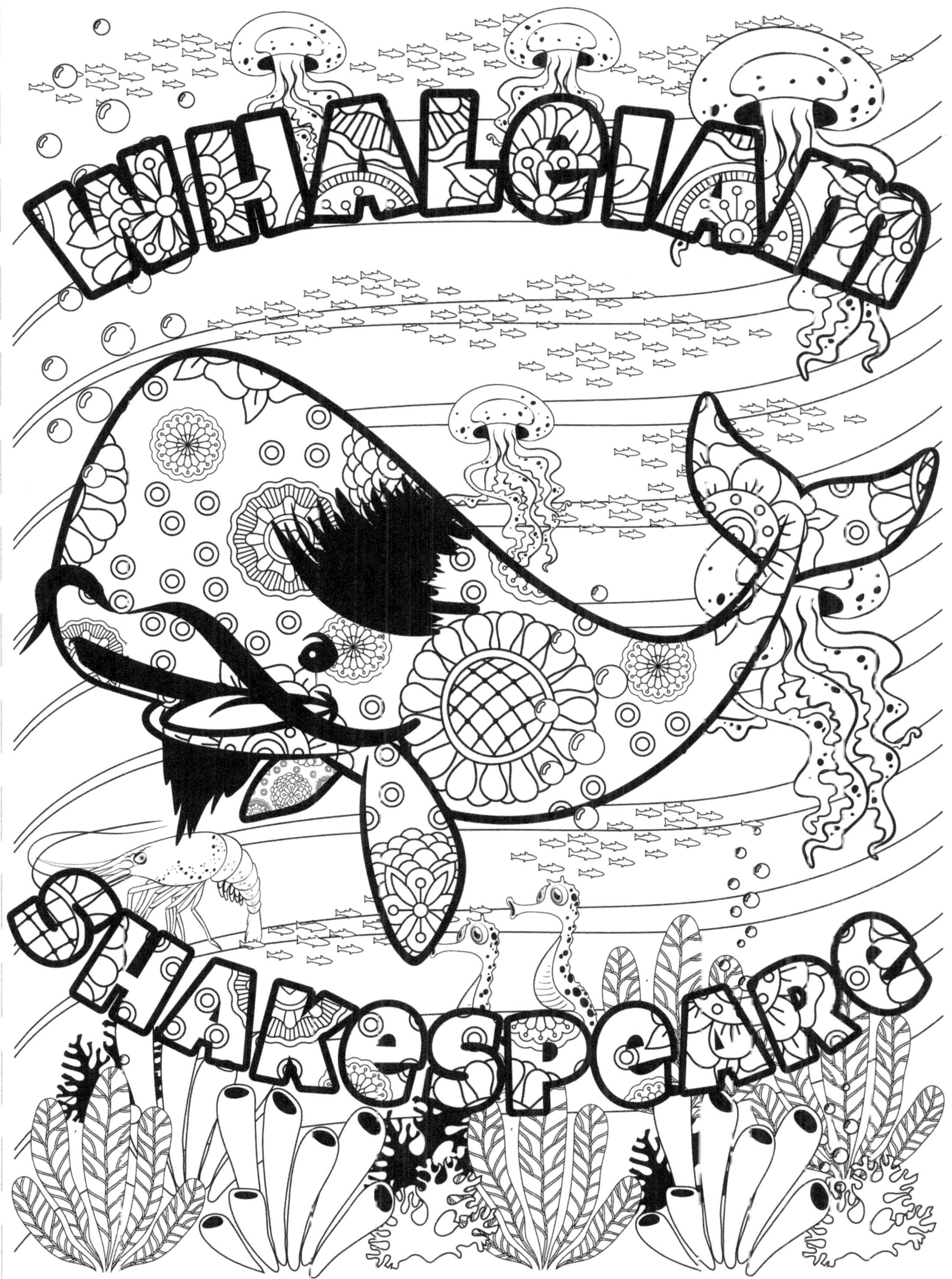

WHALGIAH
SHAKESPEARE

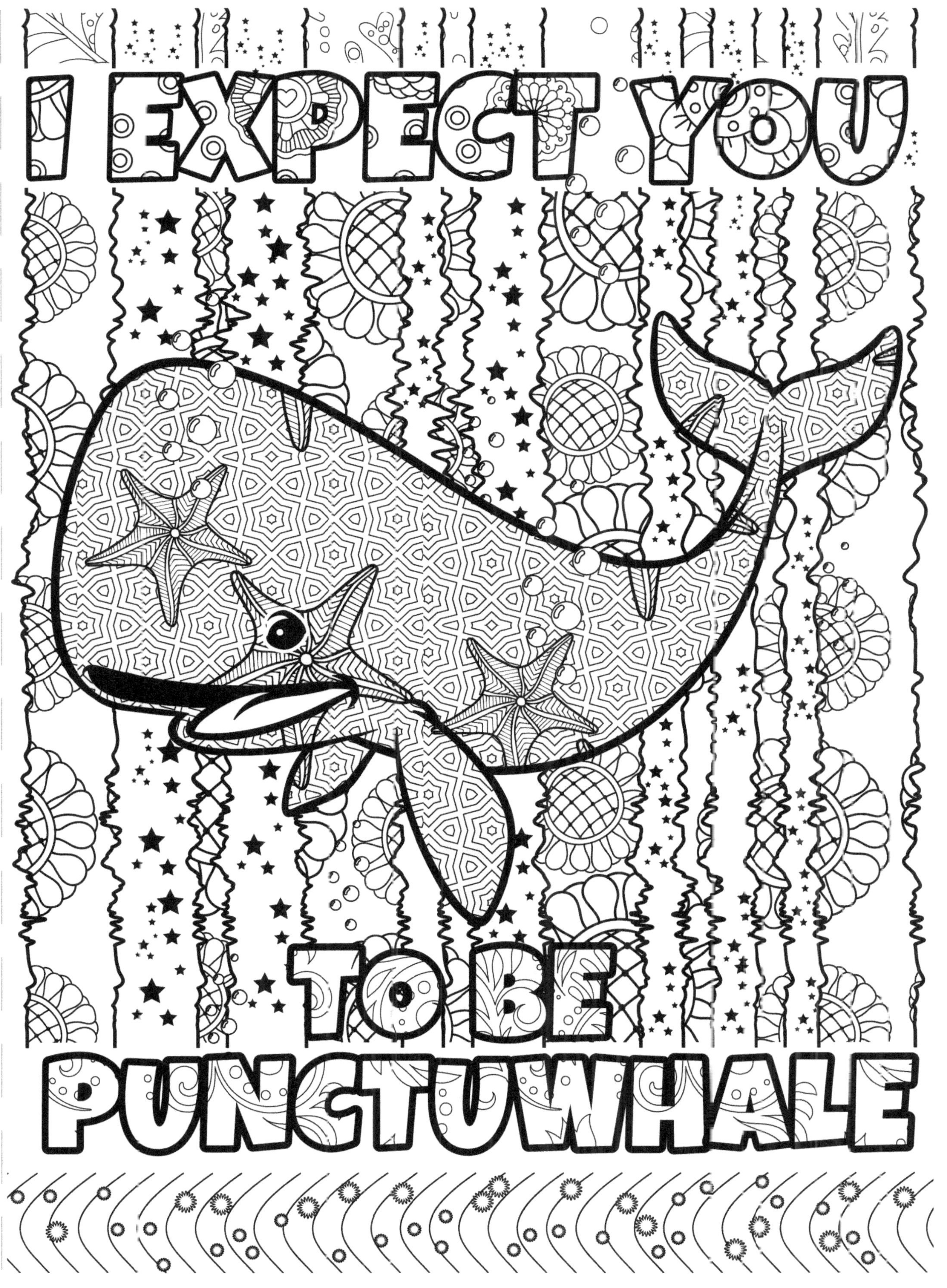

I EXPECT YOU
TO BE
PUNCTUWHALE

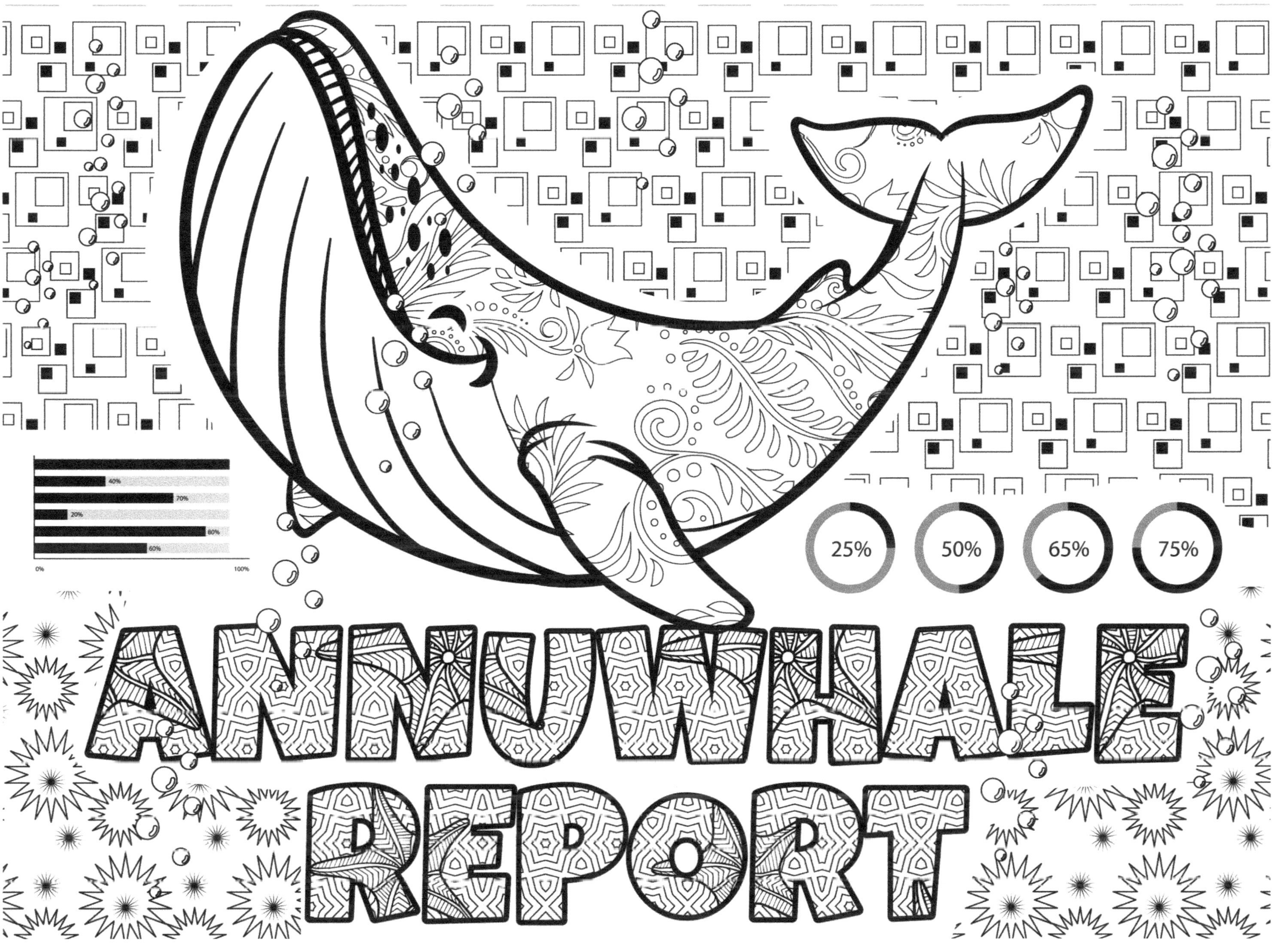

40%
70%
20%
80%
60%
0%
100%
25%
50%
65%
75%
ANNUWHALE
REPORT

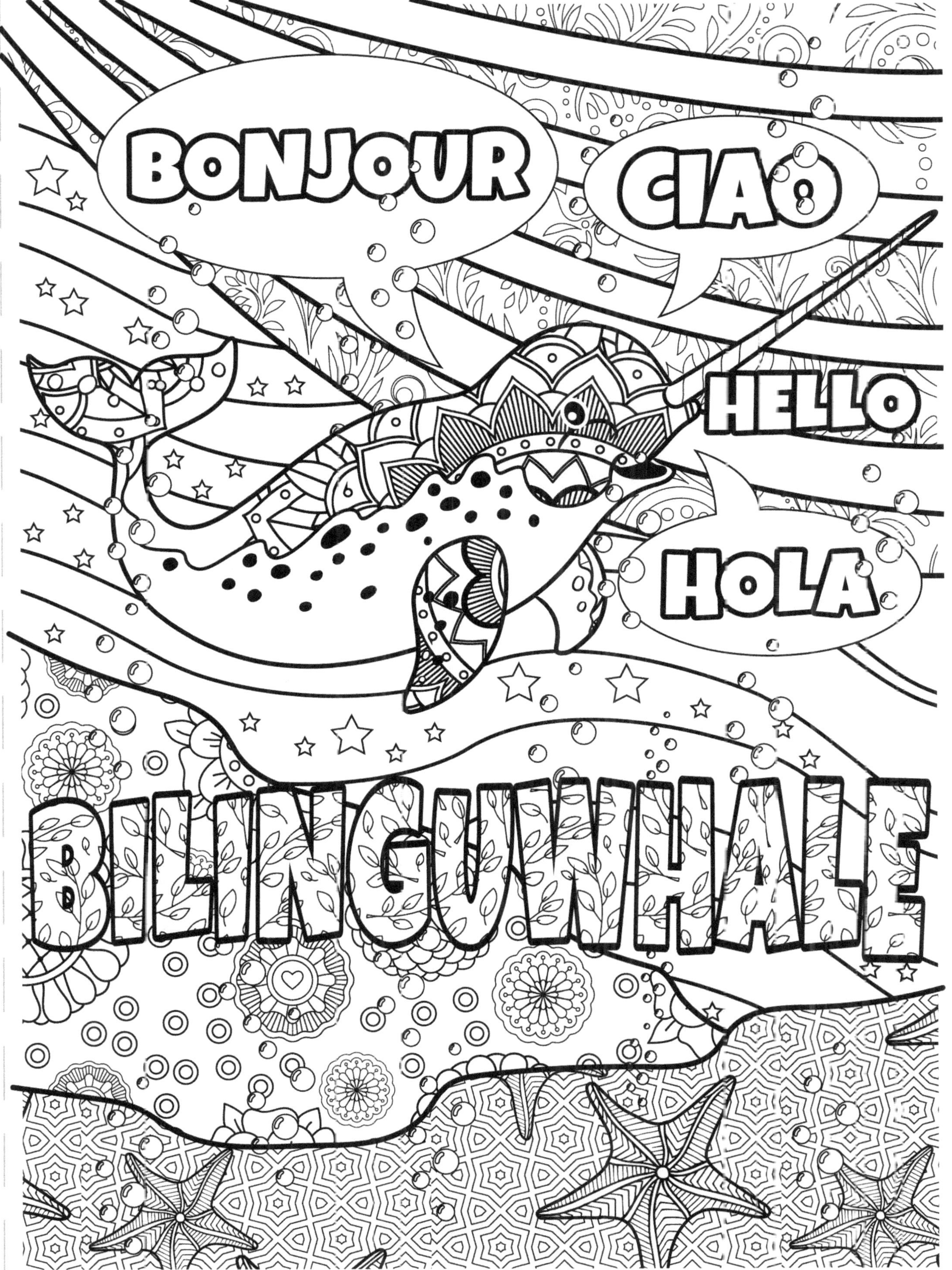

BONJOUR
CIAO
HELLO
HOLA
BILINGUWHALE

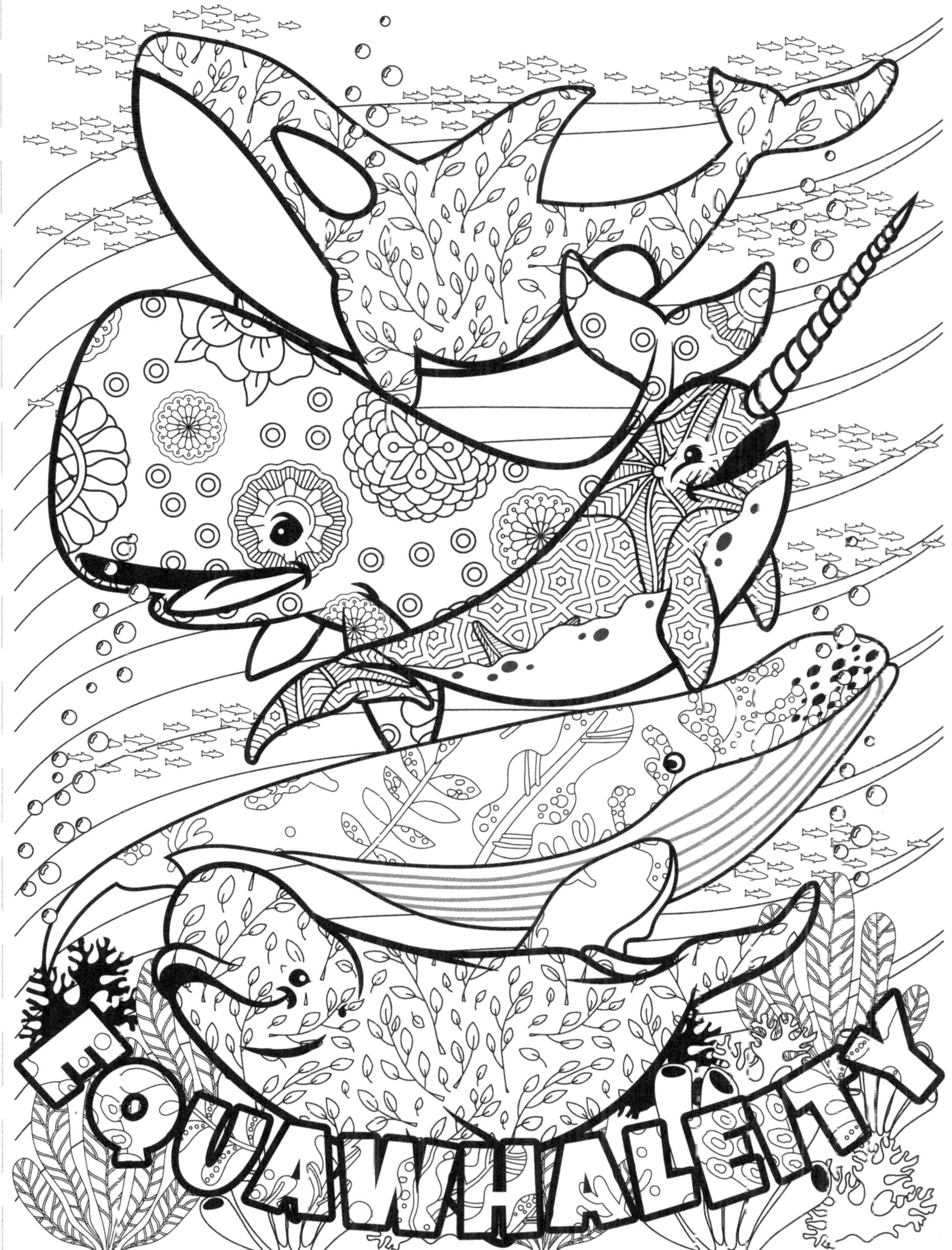
EQUAWHALEITY

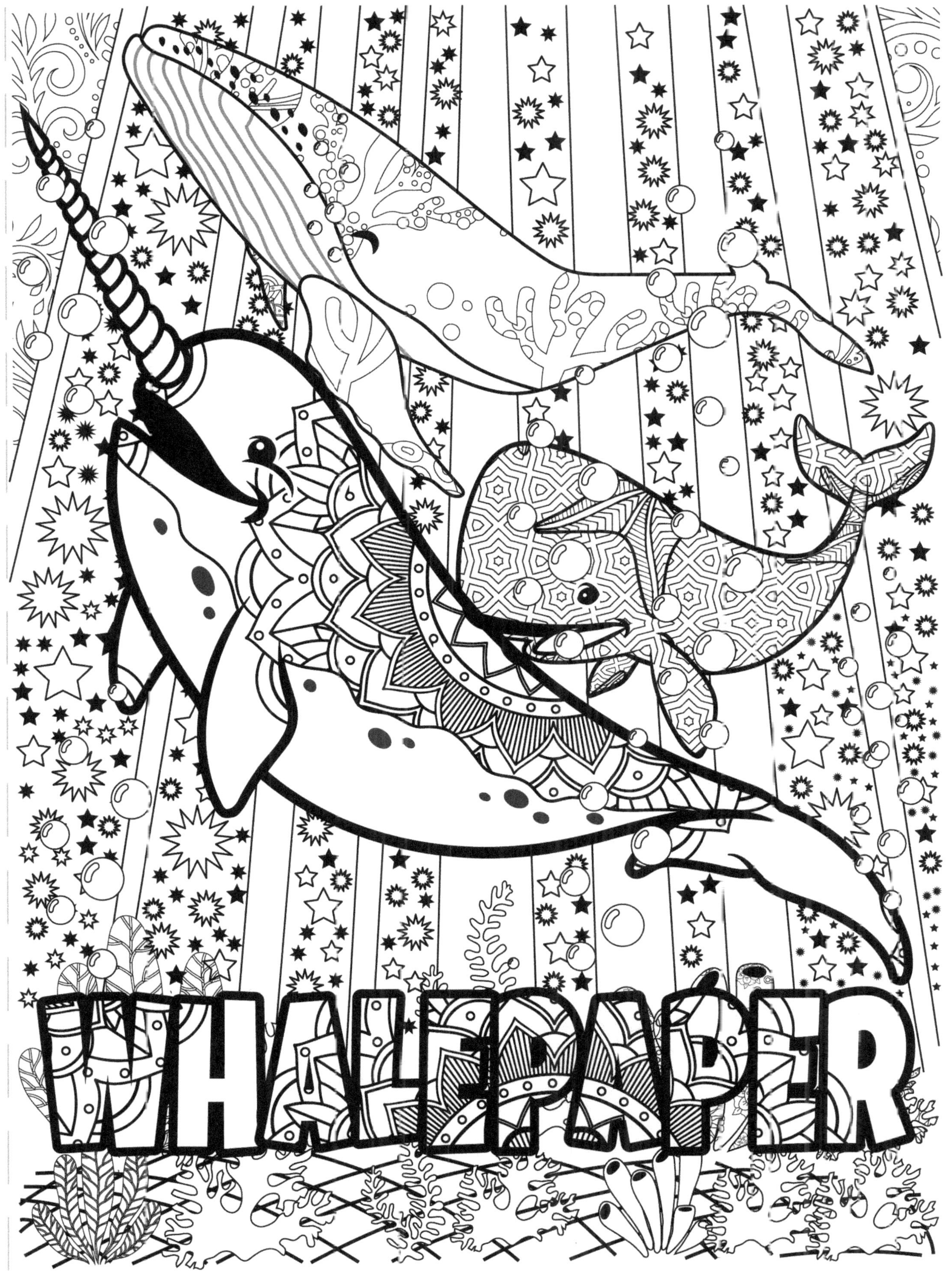
WHALEPAPER

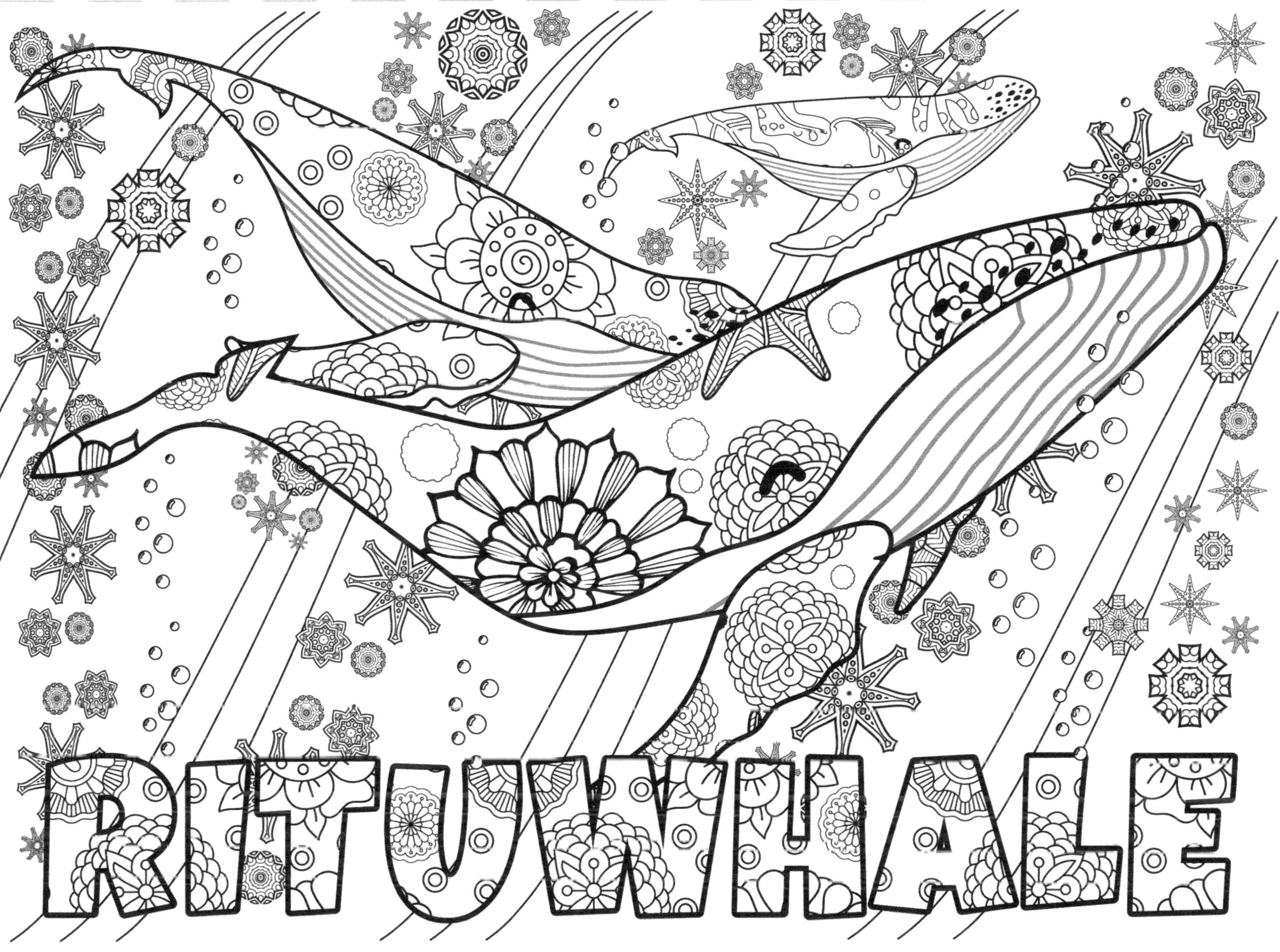
RITUWHALE

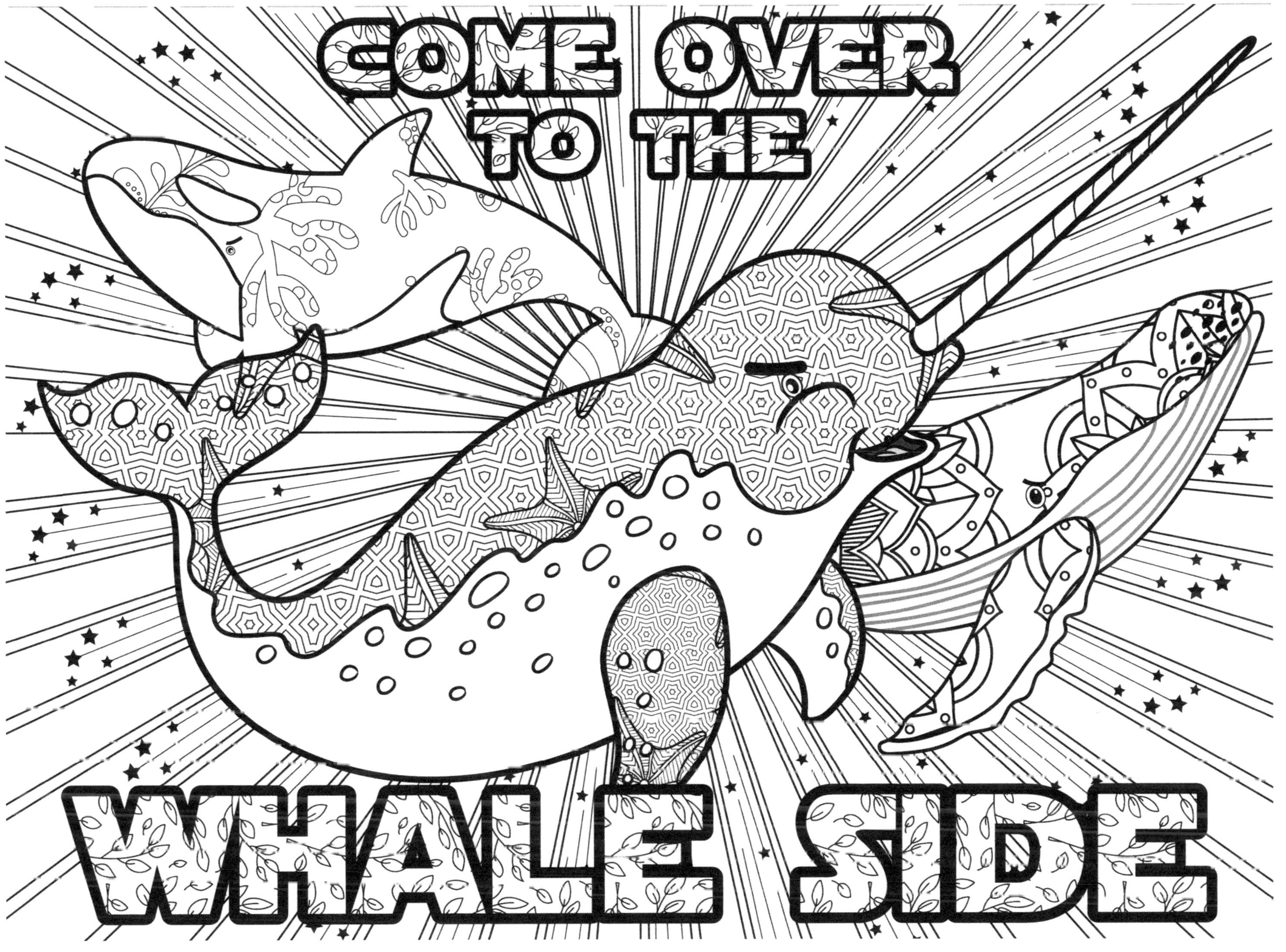

COME OVER
TO THE
WHALE SIDE

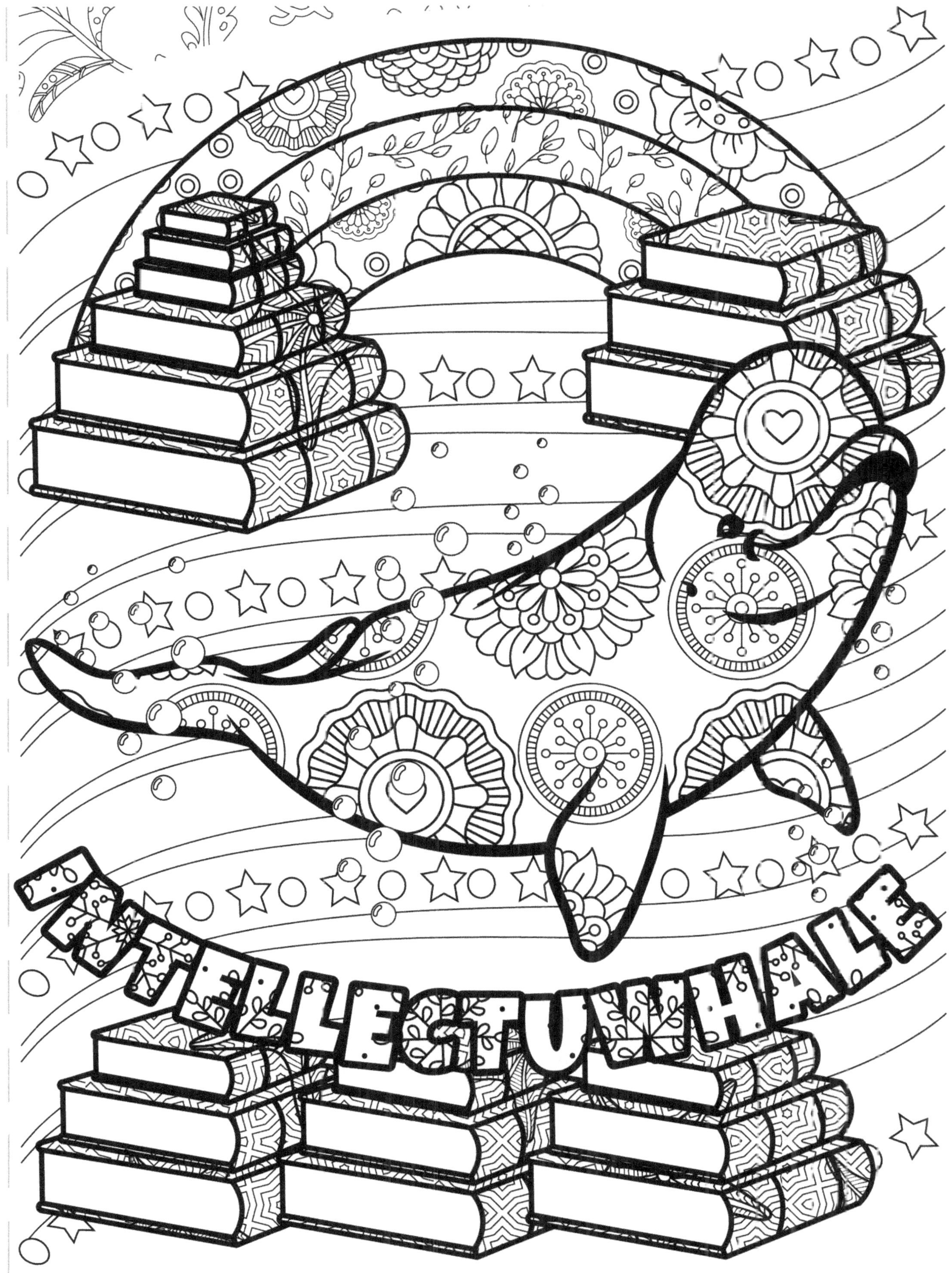
I'D TELL YOU A WHALE

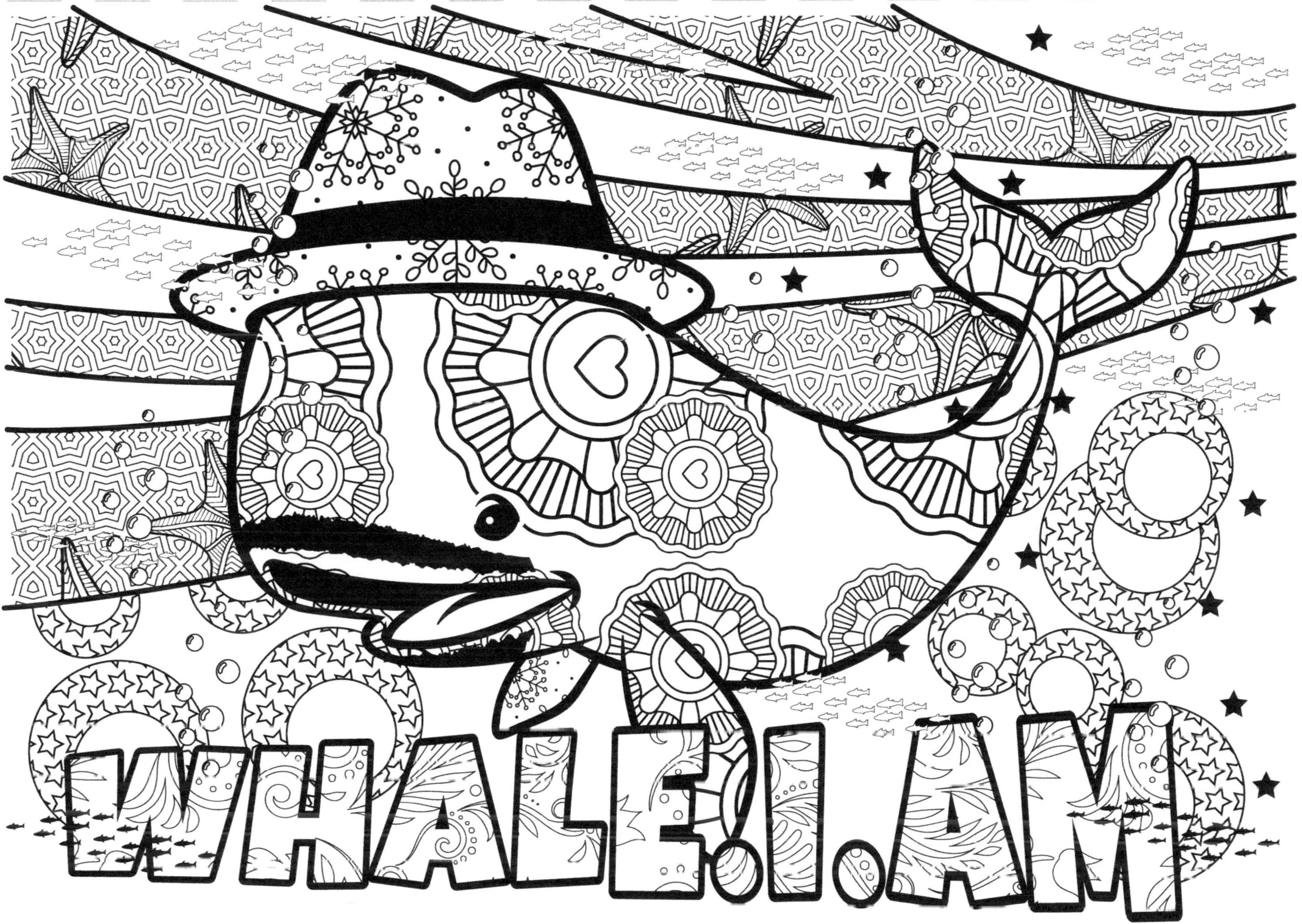

WHALE.I.AM

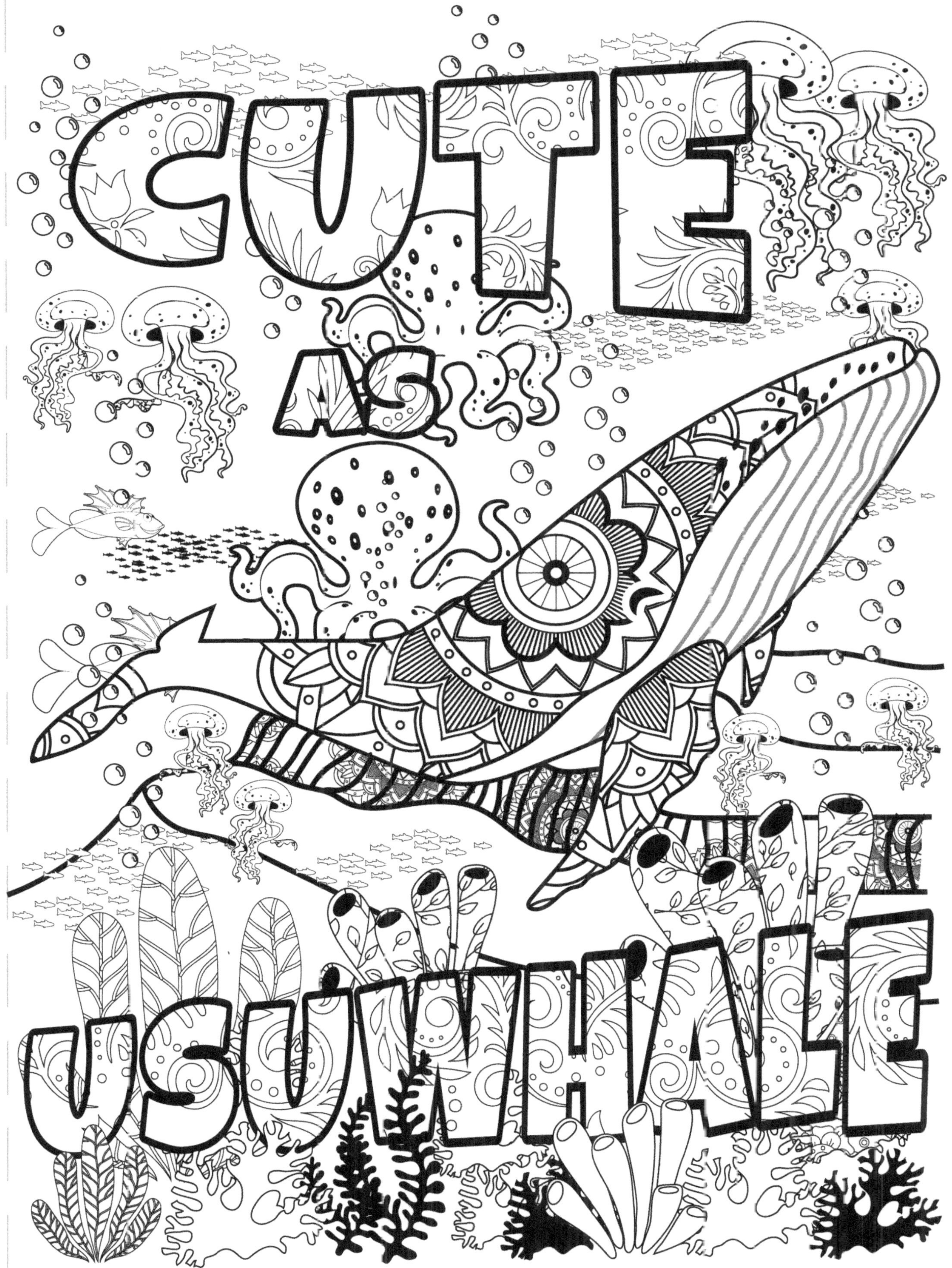

CUTE
AS
US UWHALE

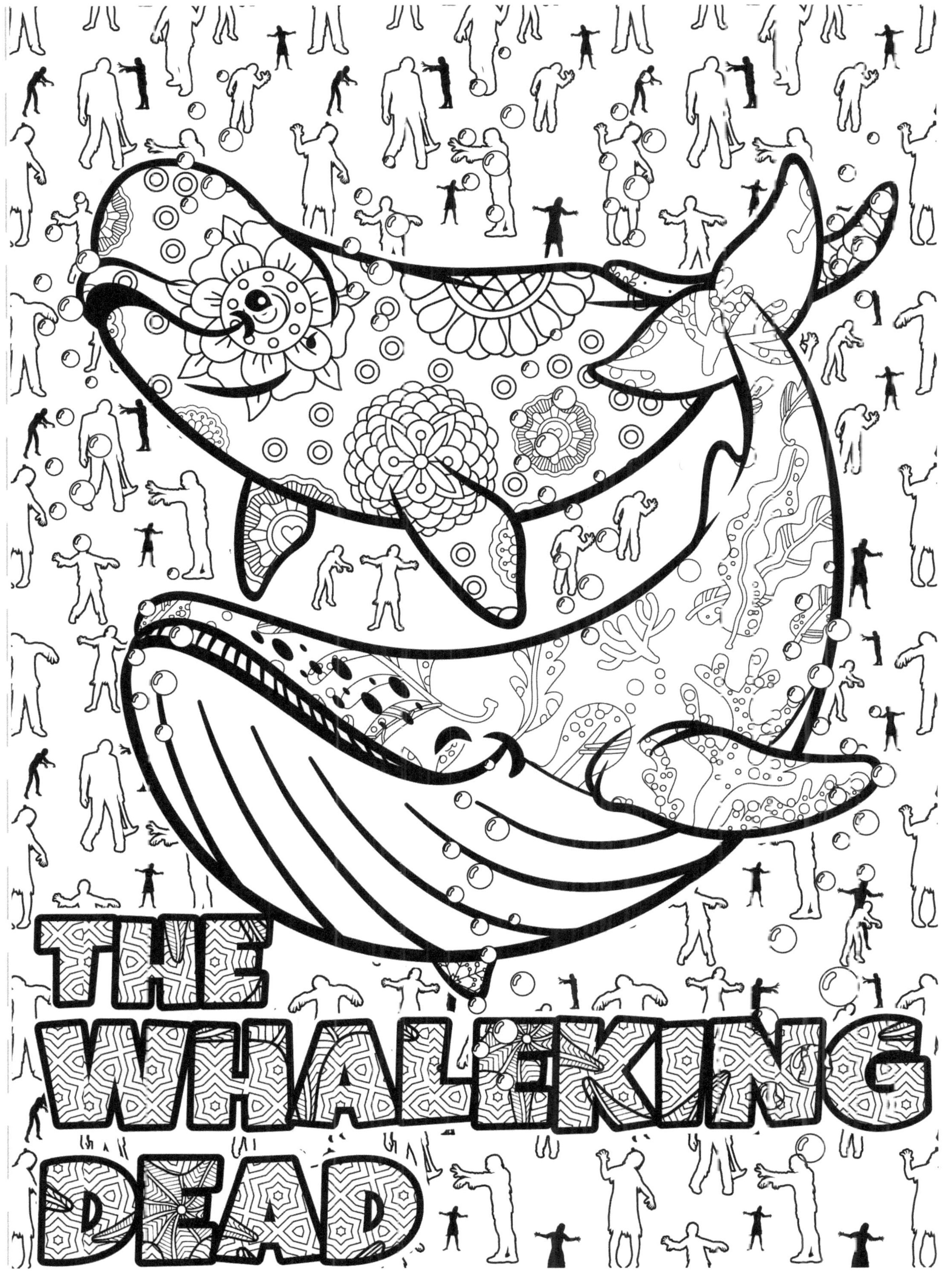

THE
WHALE-KING
DEAD

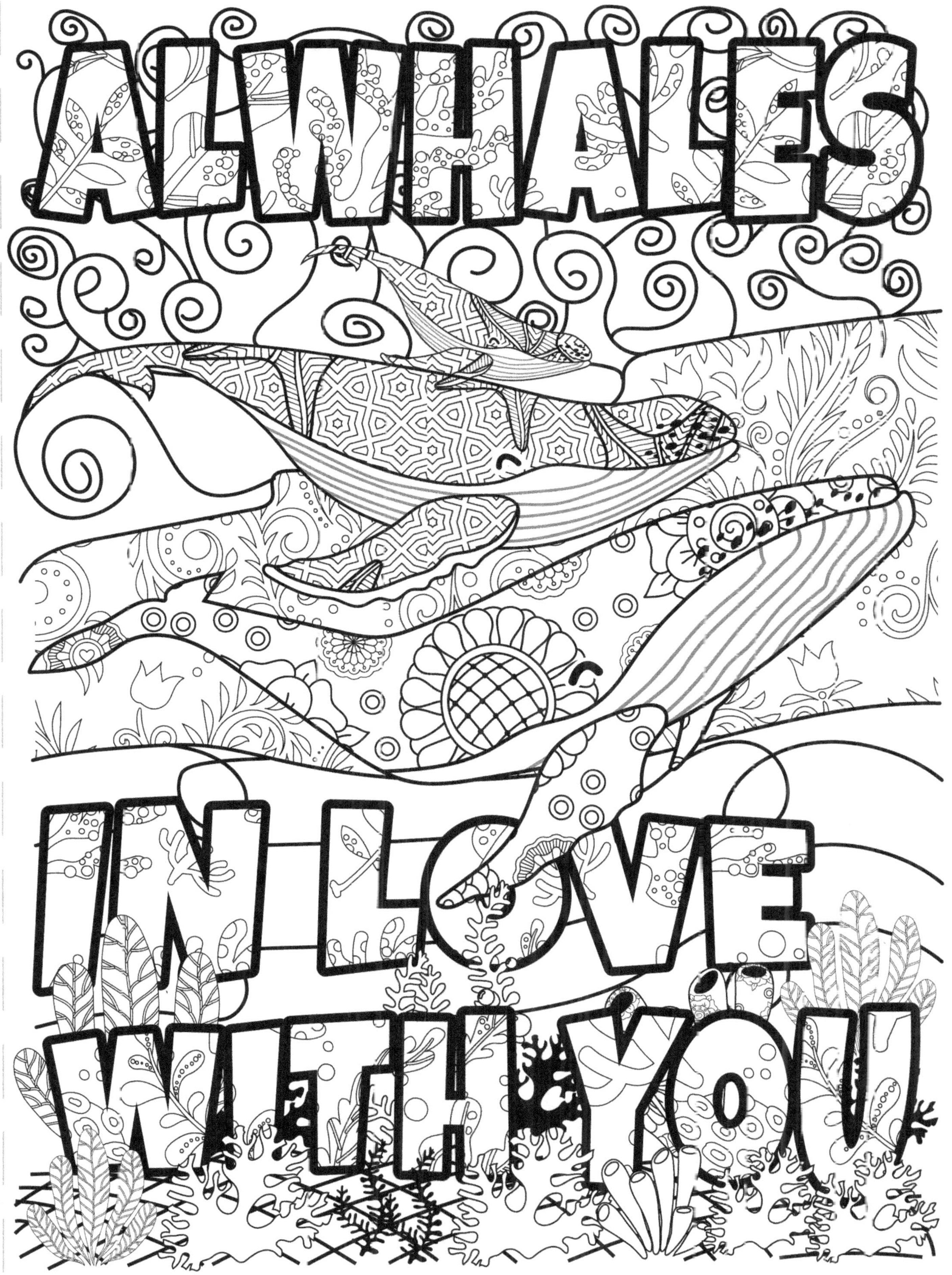
A WHALES
IN LOVE
WITH YOU

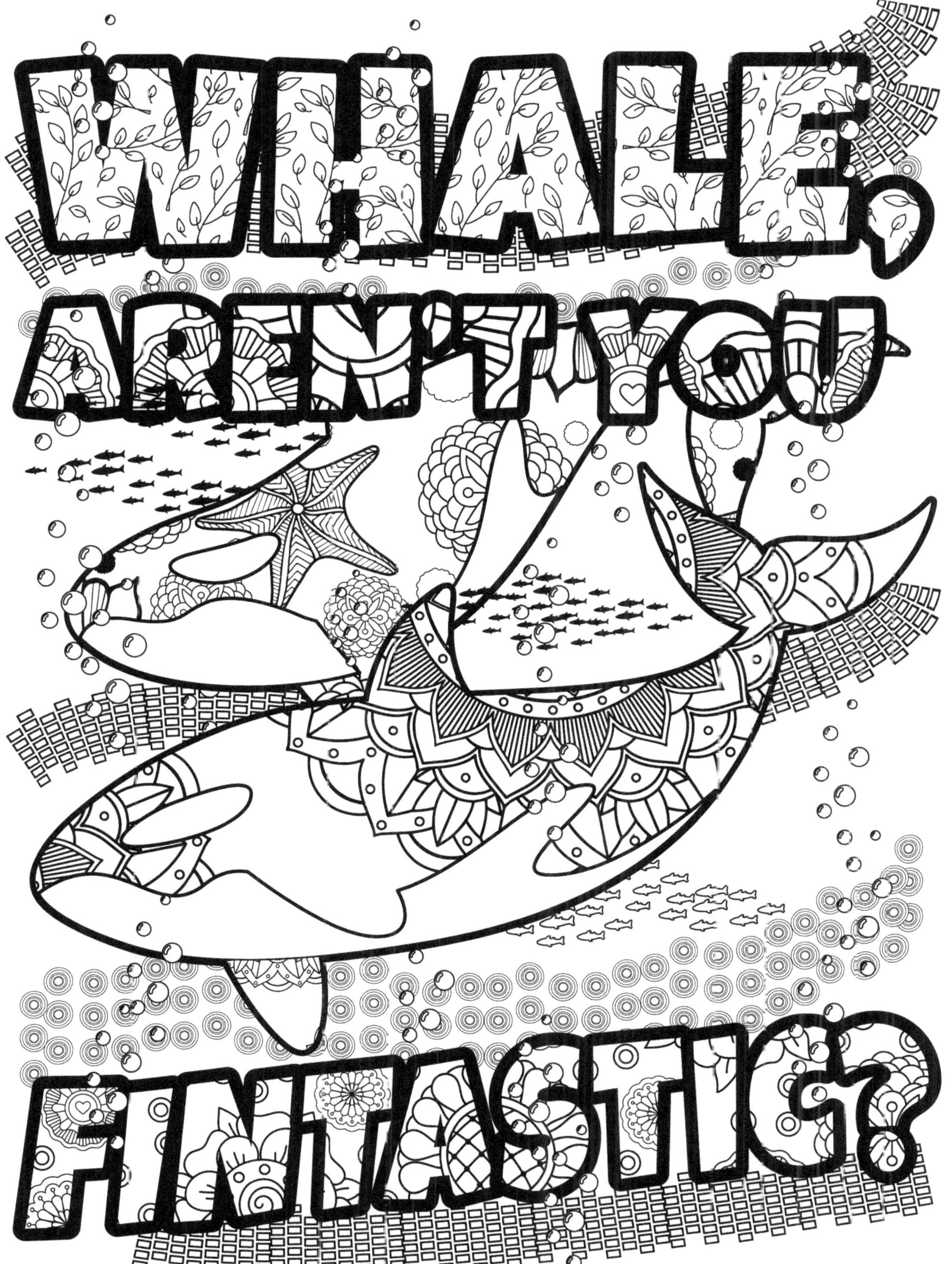
WHALE,
AREN'T YOU
FINTASTIC?

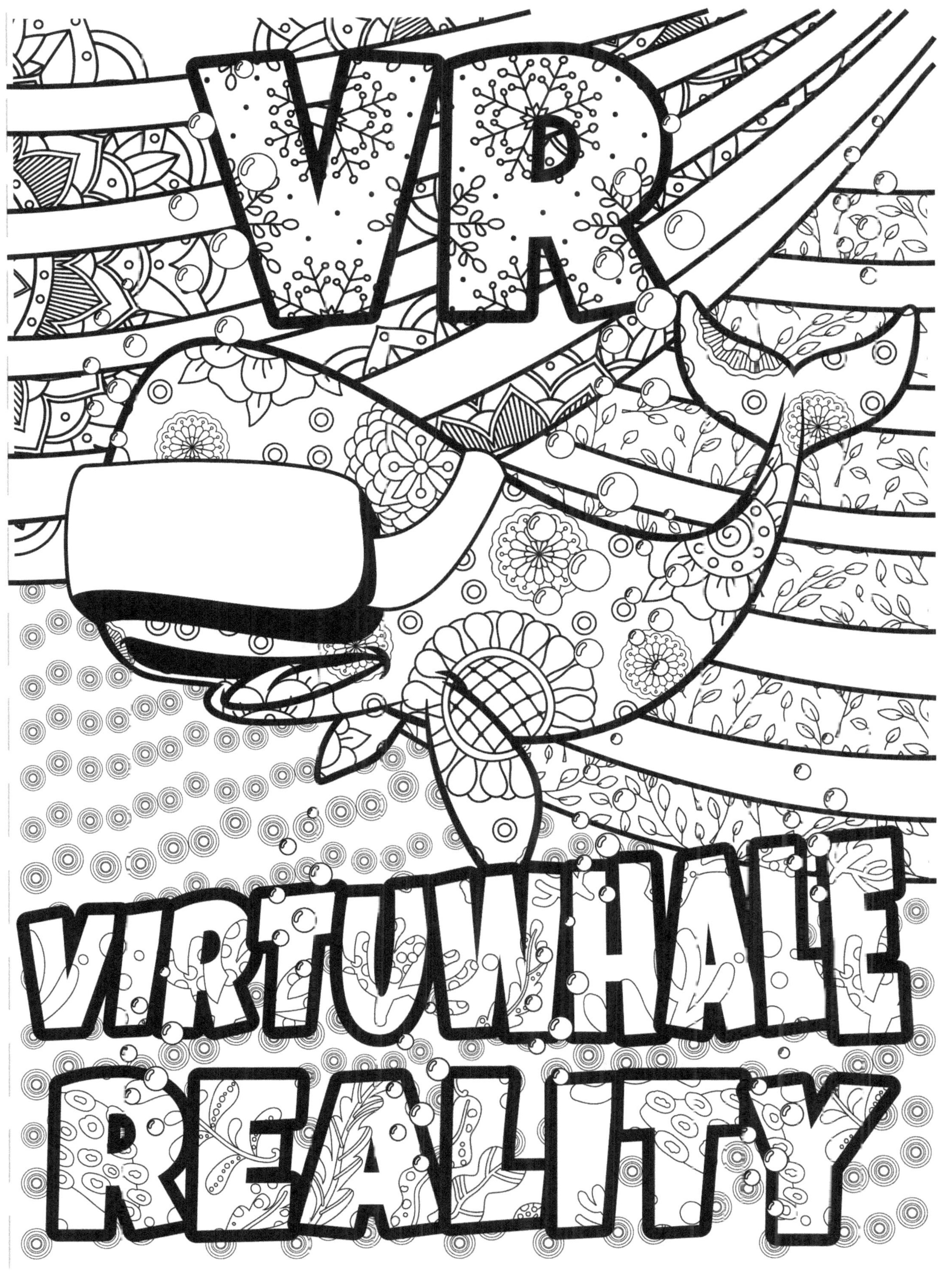

VR
VIRTUWHALE
REALITY

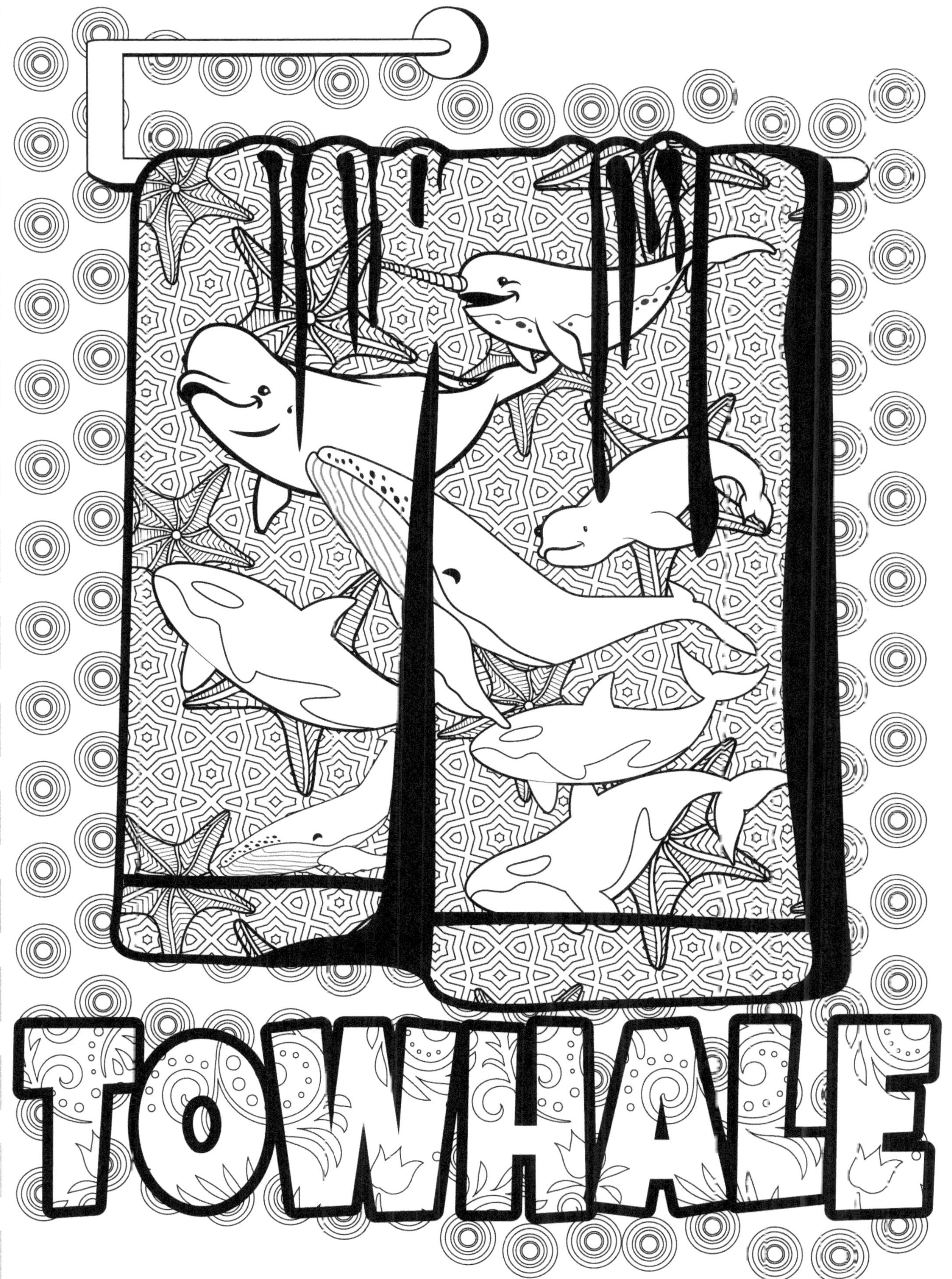
TOWHALE

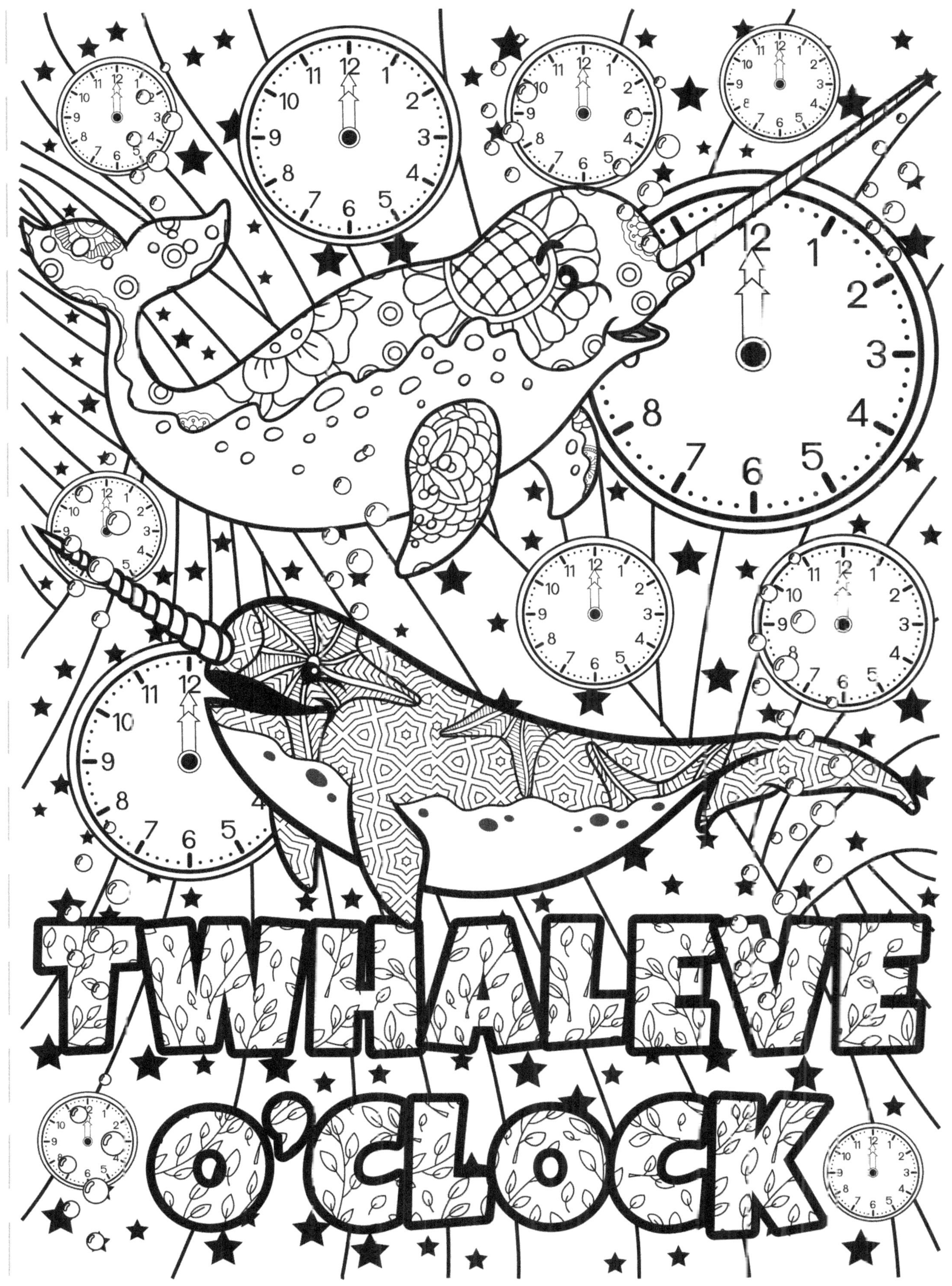

TWHALEVE
O'CLOCK

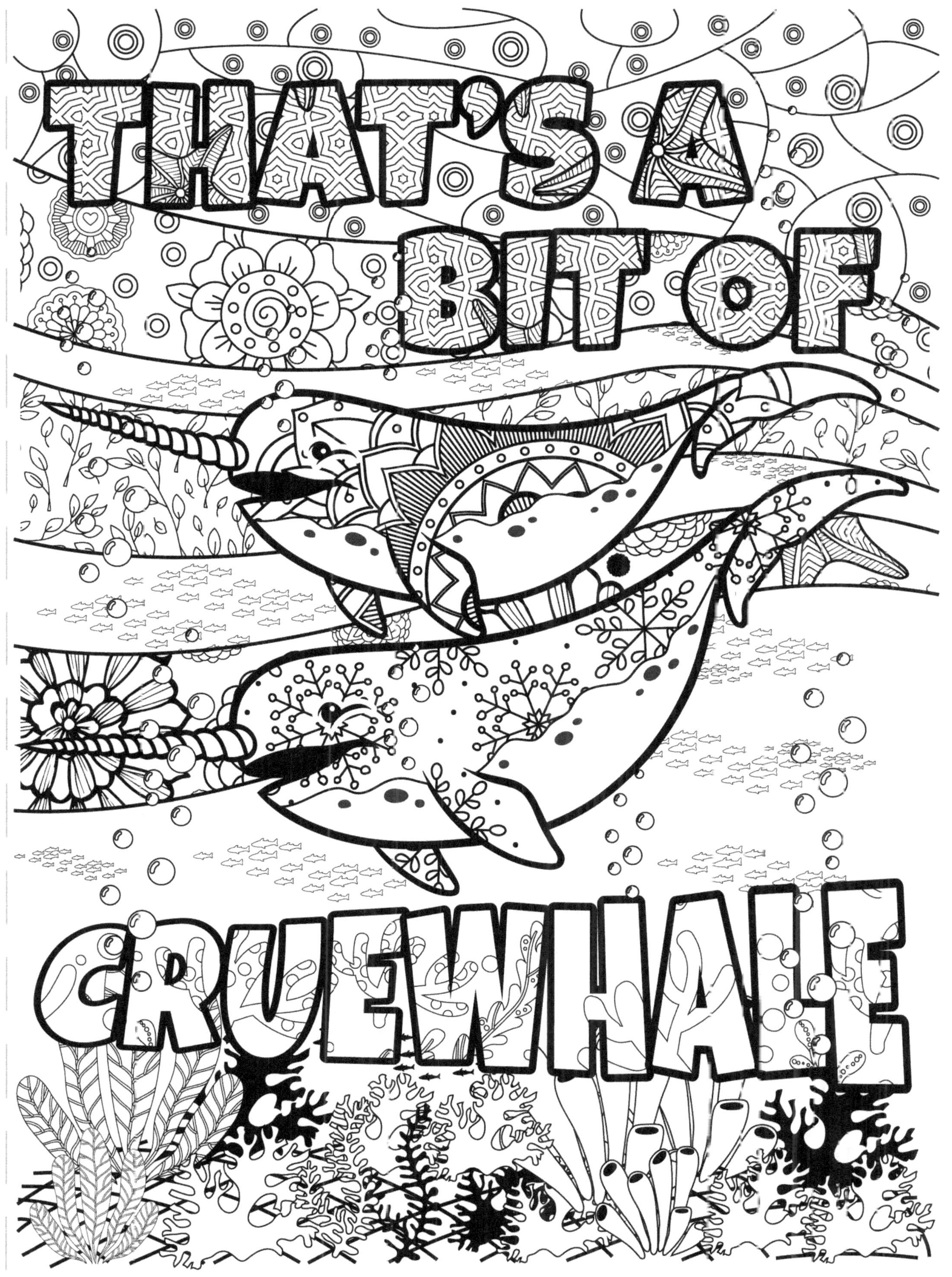

THAT'S A BIT OF
CRUEWHALE

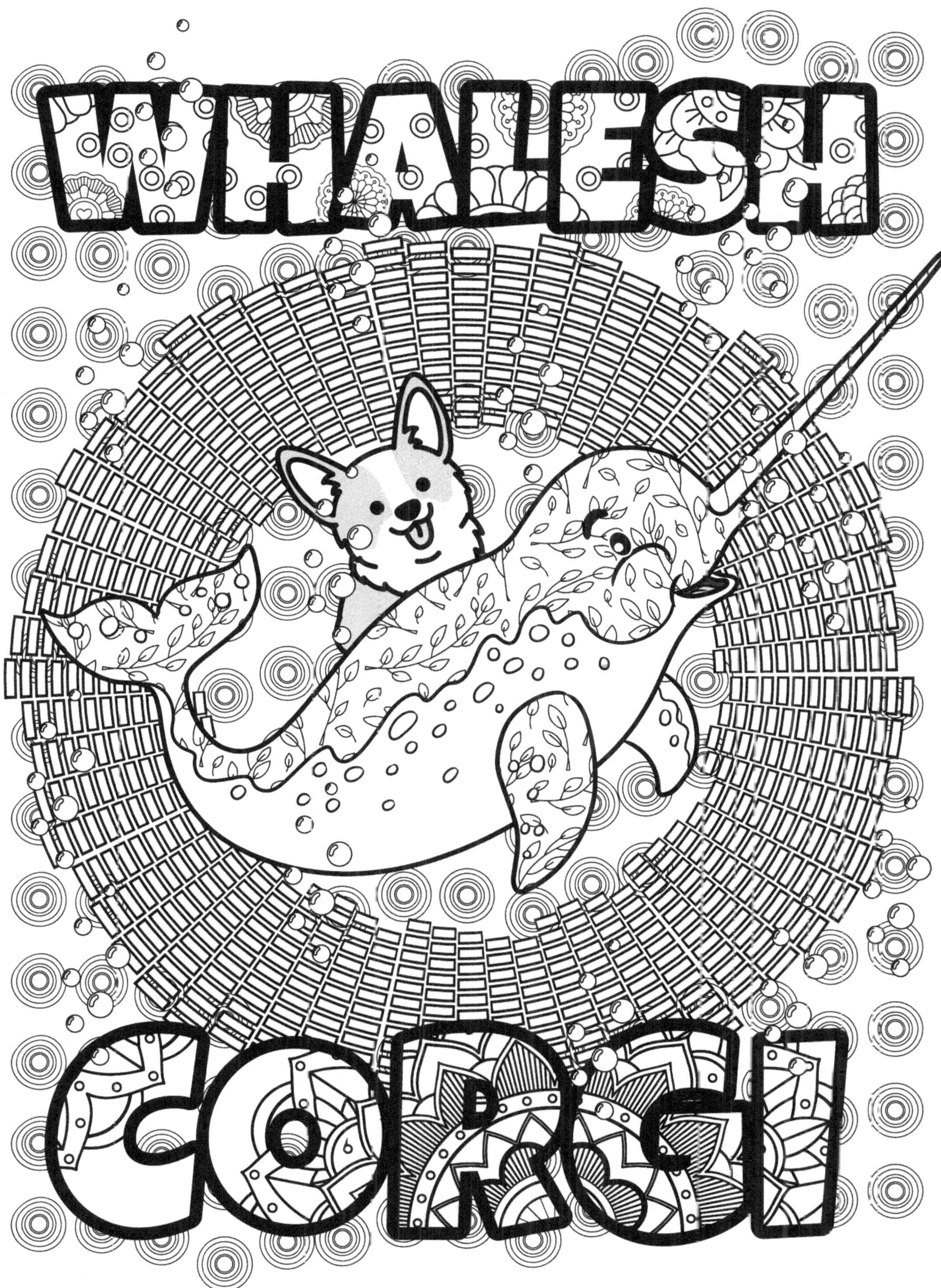

WHALESH
CORGI

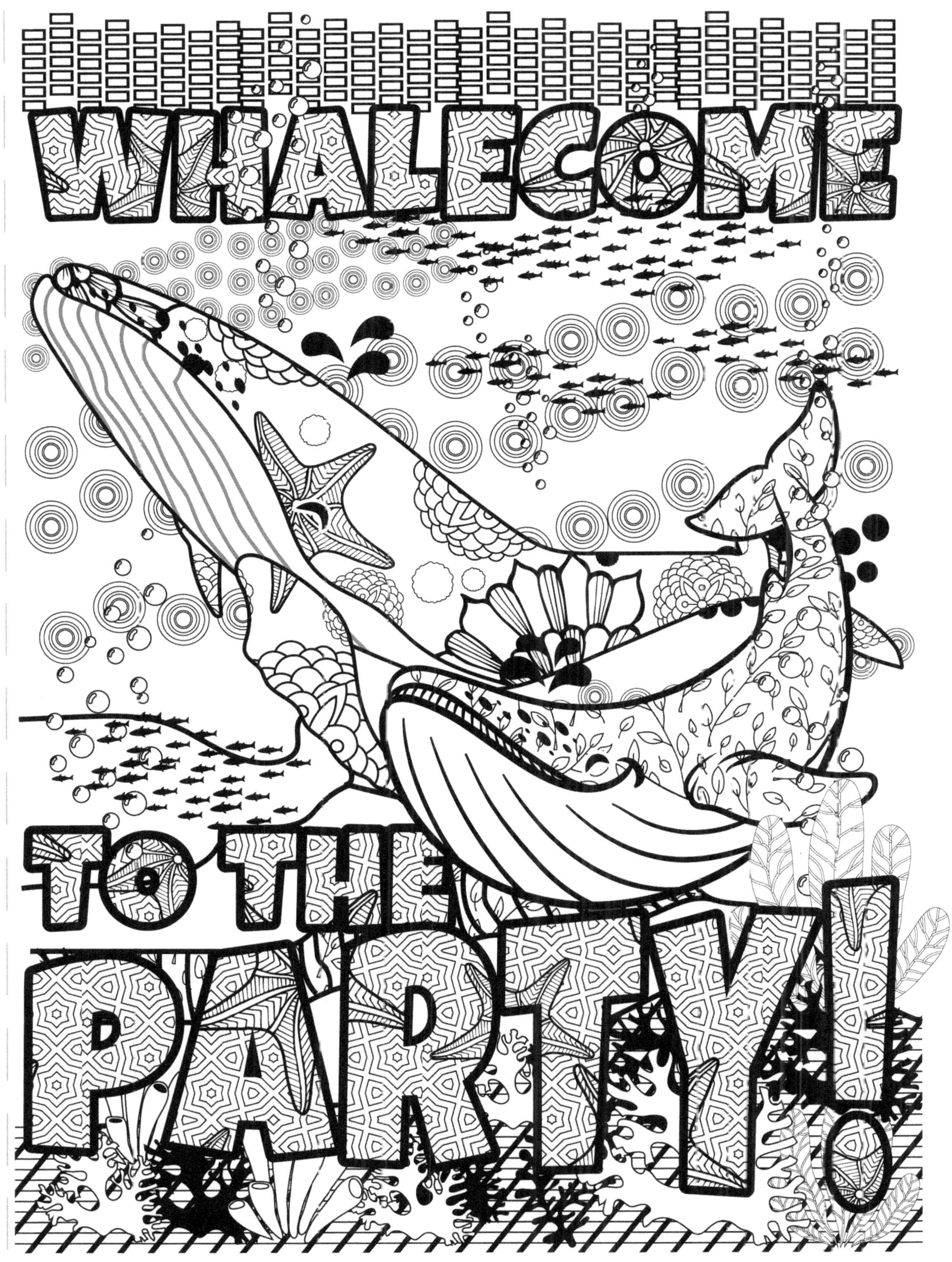
WHALECOME
TO THE
PARTY!

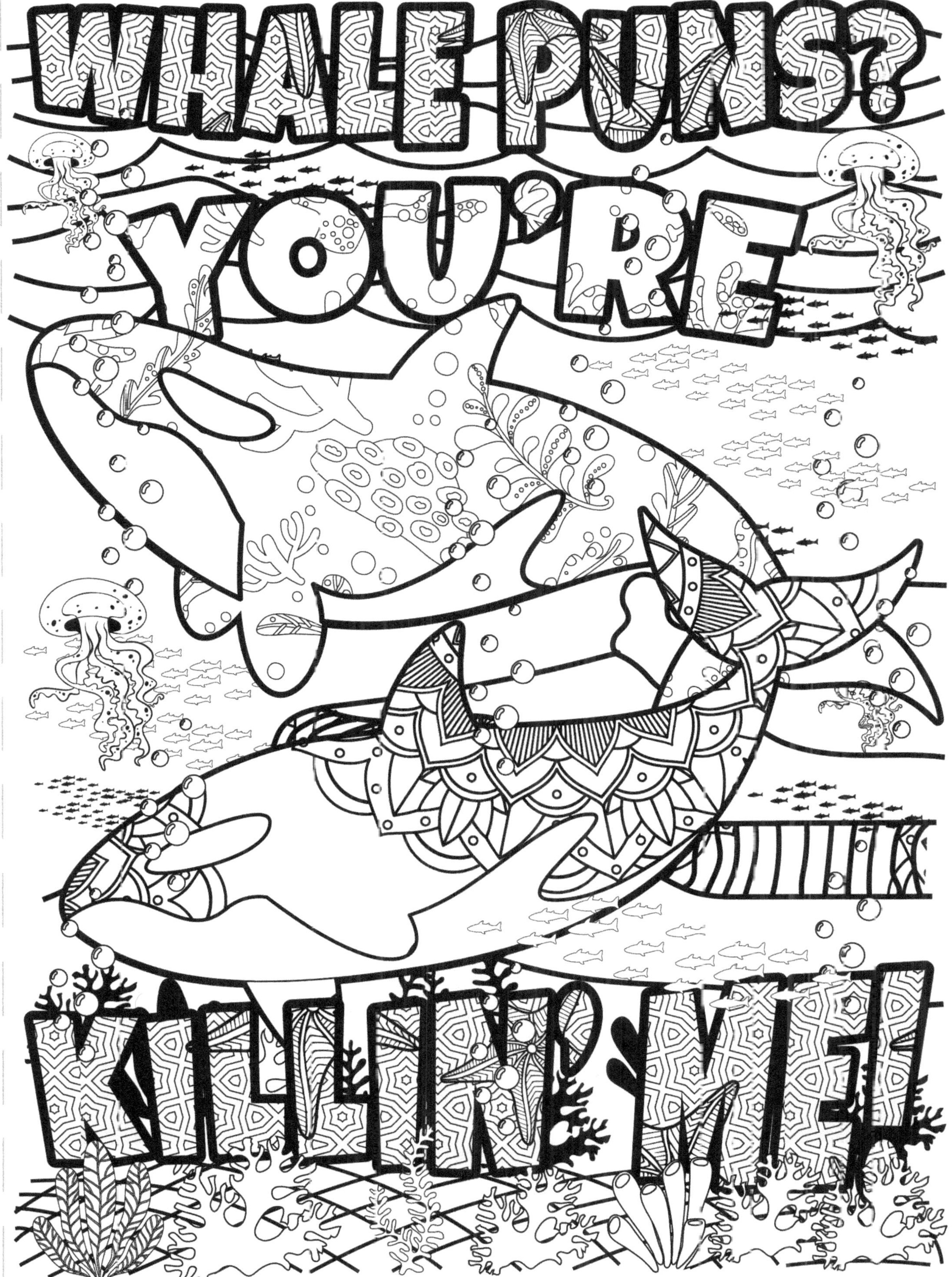

WHALE PUNS? YOU'RE KILLIN' ME!

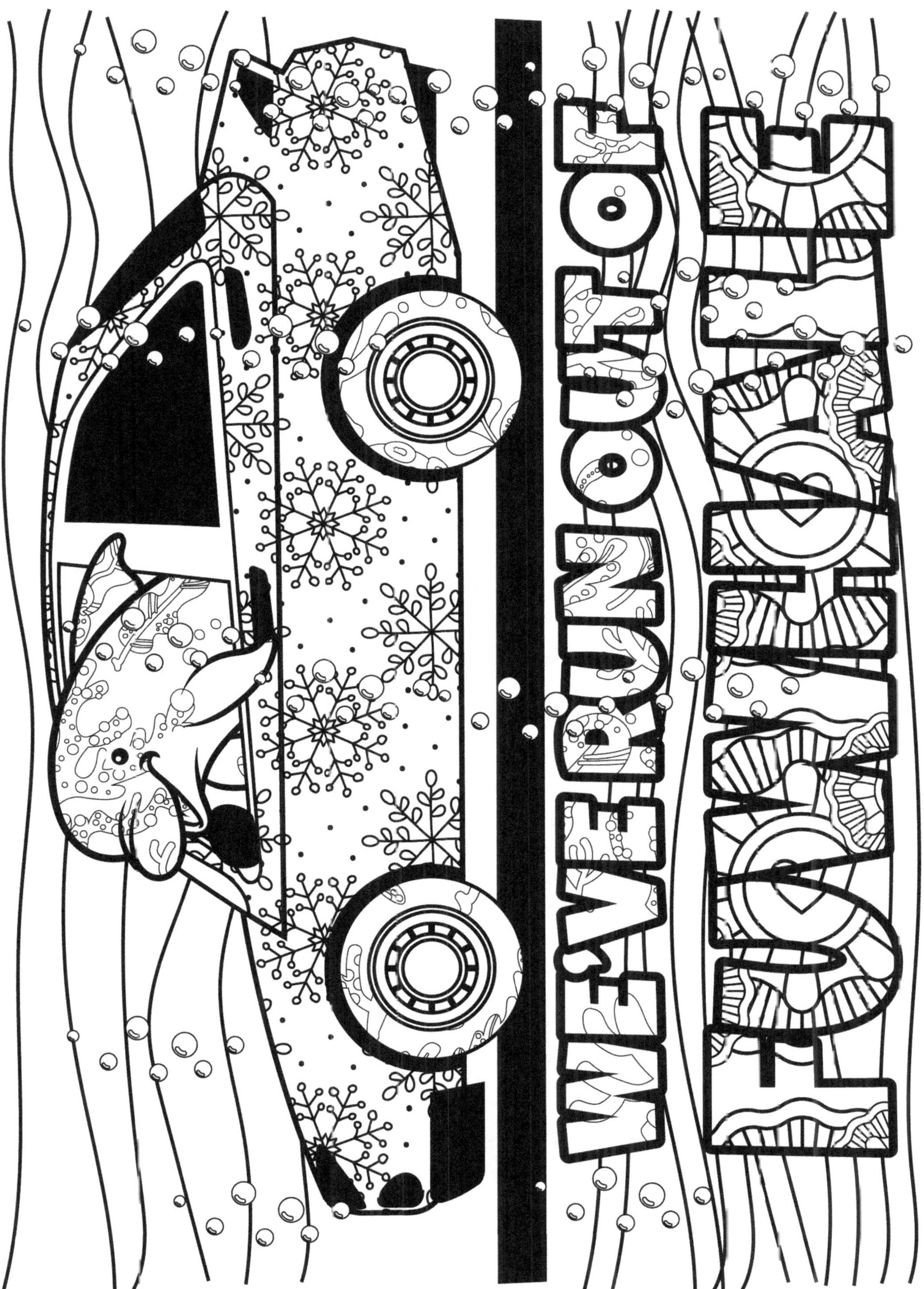

WE'VE RUN OUT OF FUCKS TO GIVE

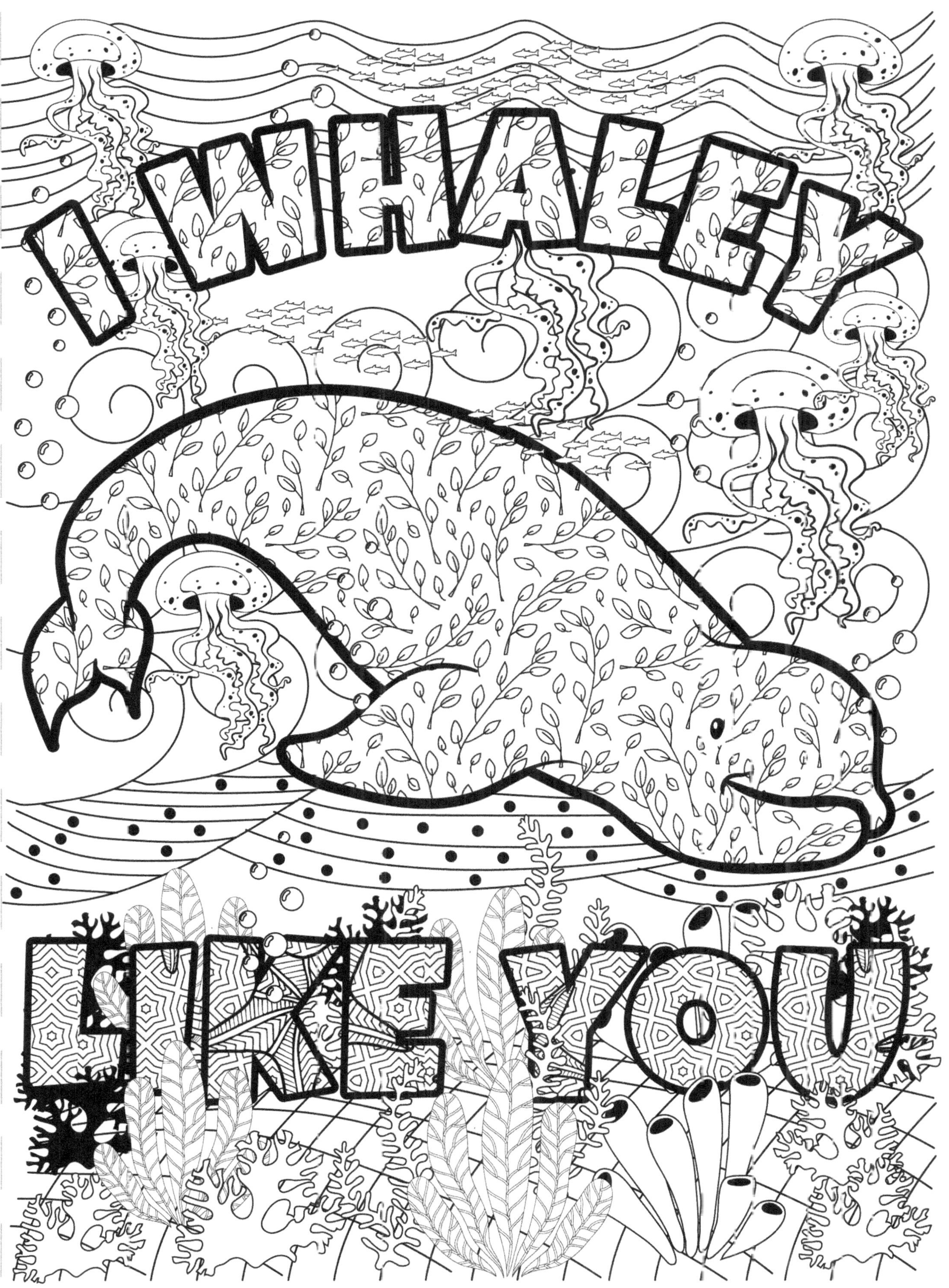

I WHALEY
LIKE YOU

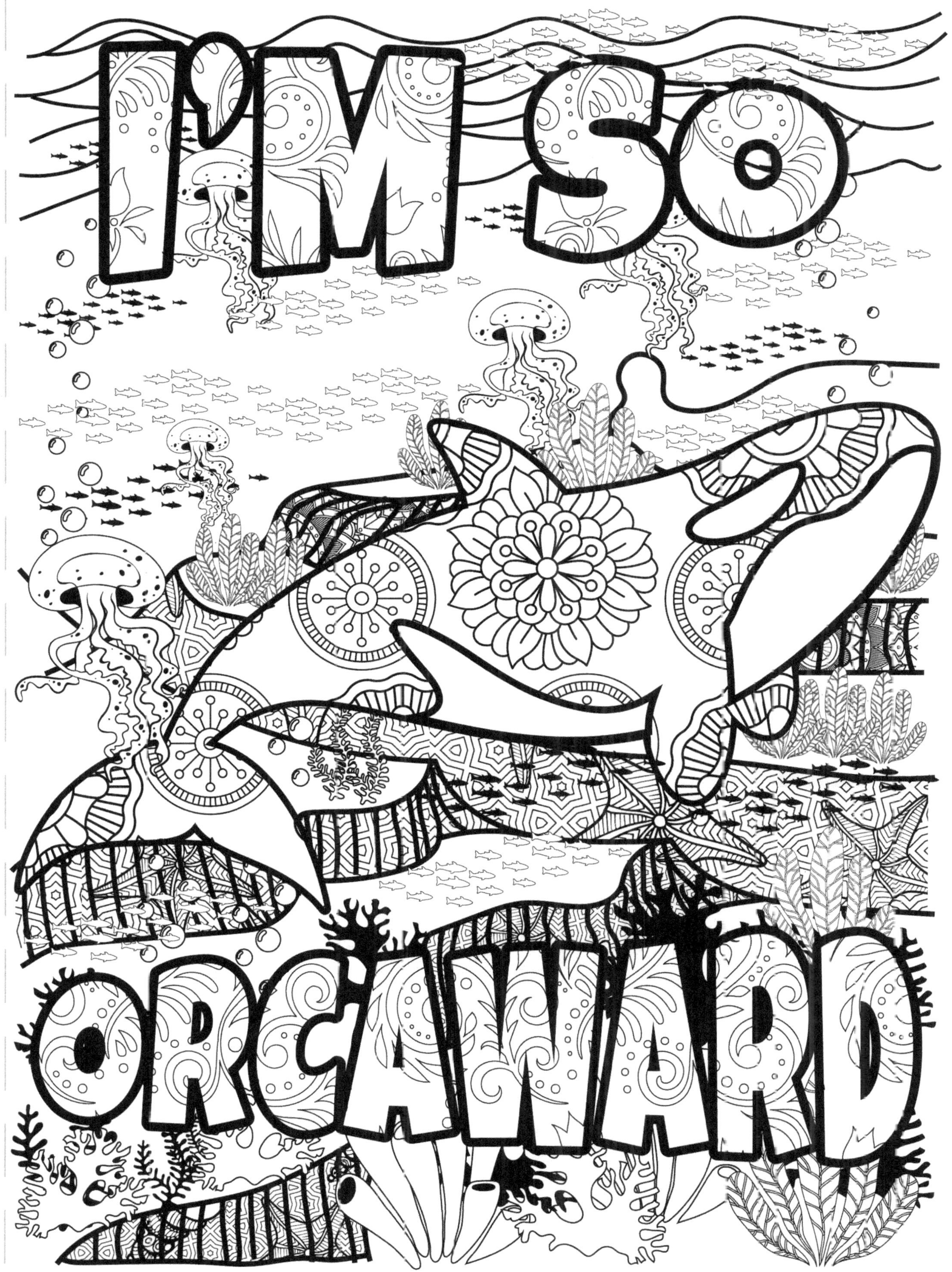

I'M SO
ORCAWARD

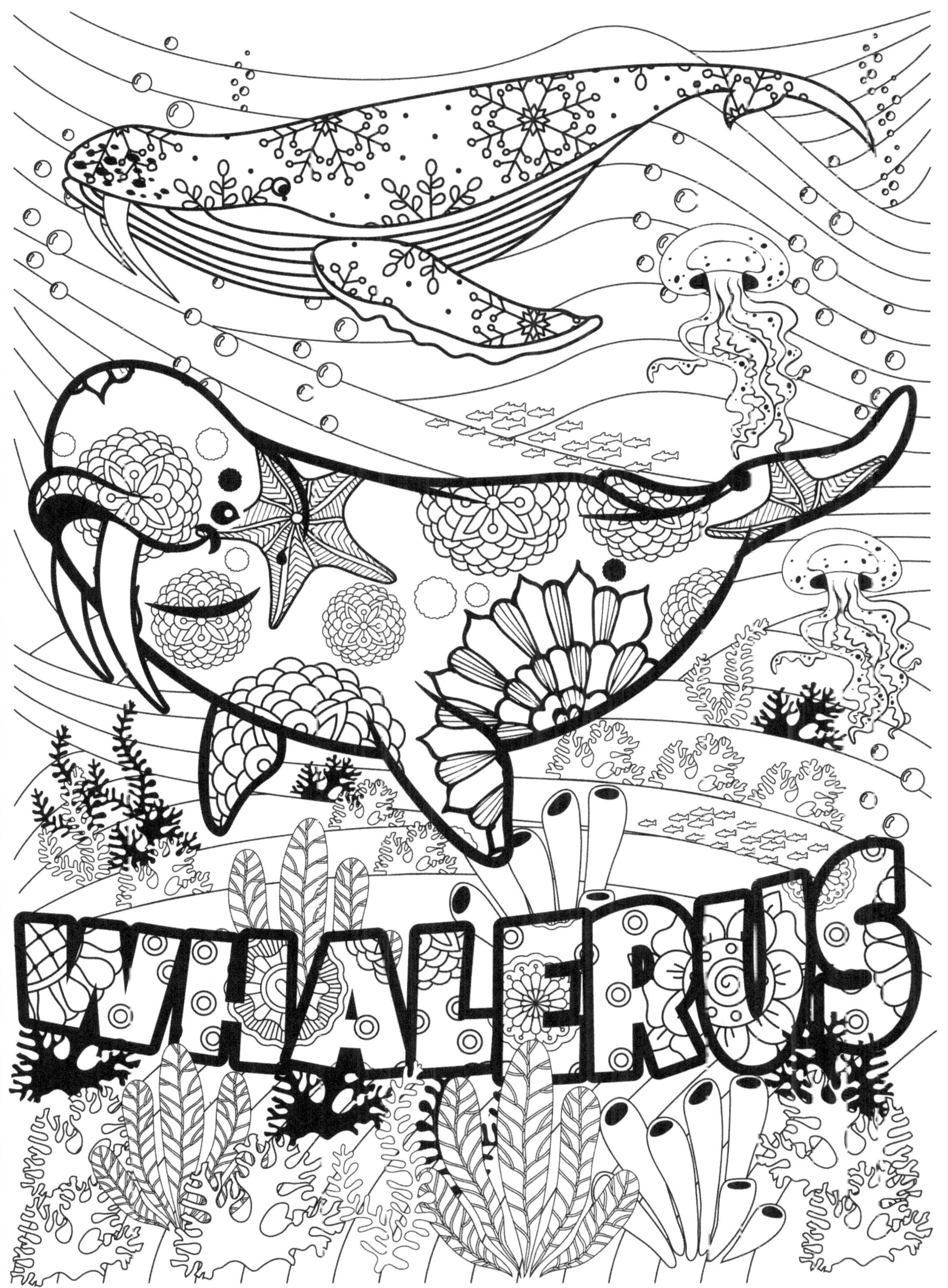
WHALERUS

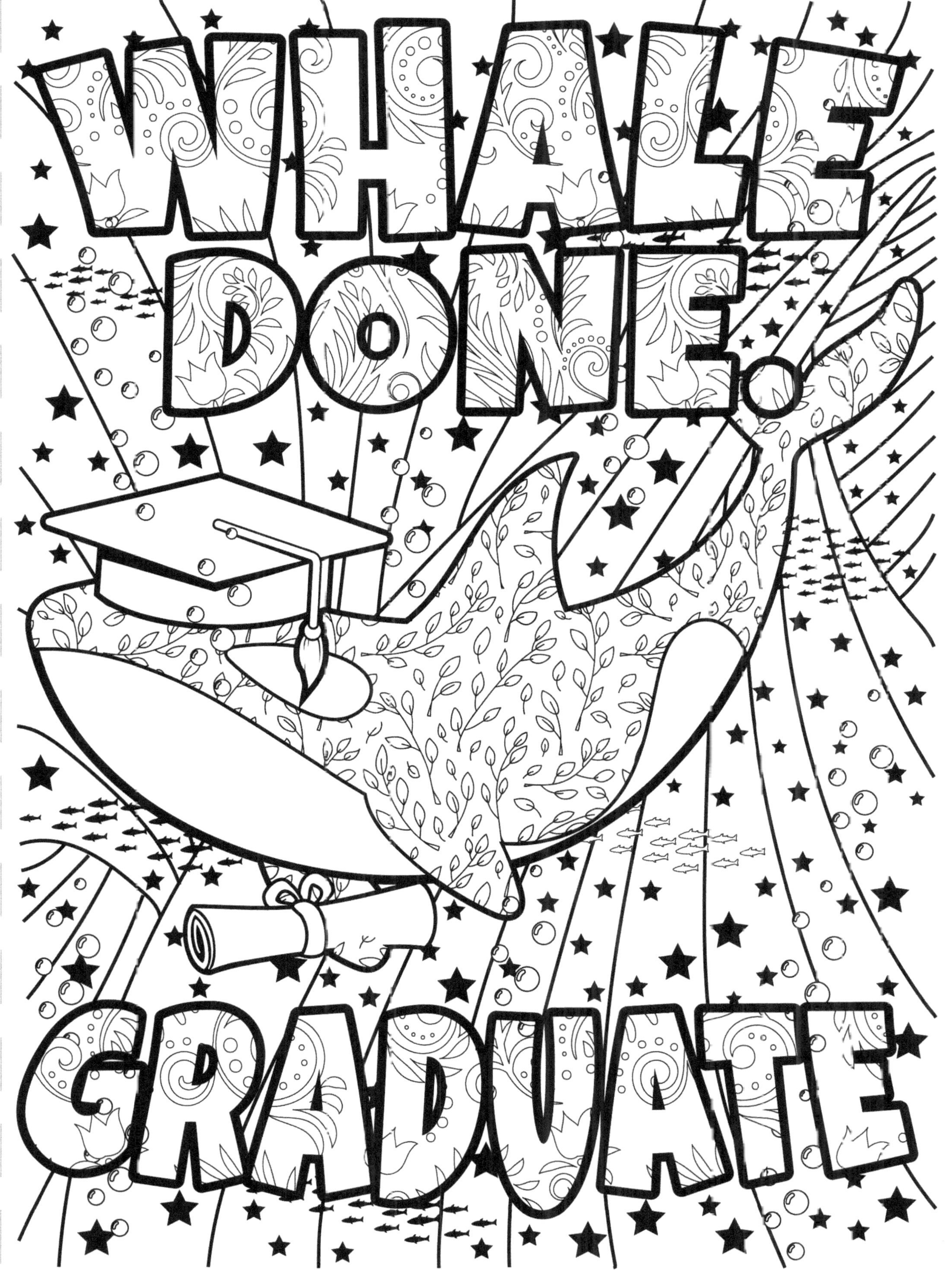

WHALE DONE.
GRADUATE

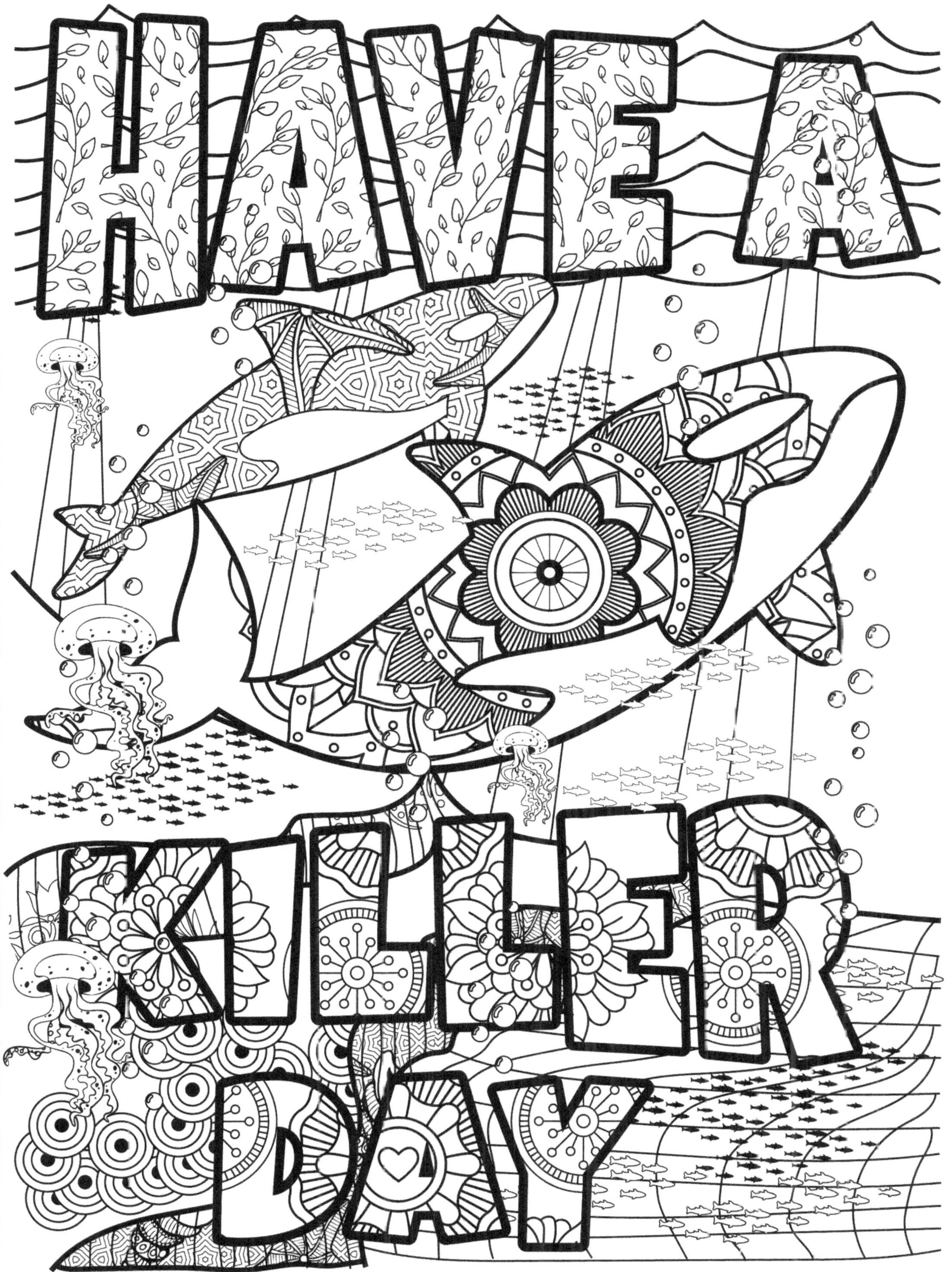

HAVE A
KILLER
DAY

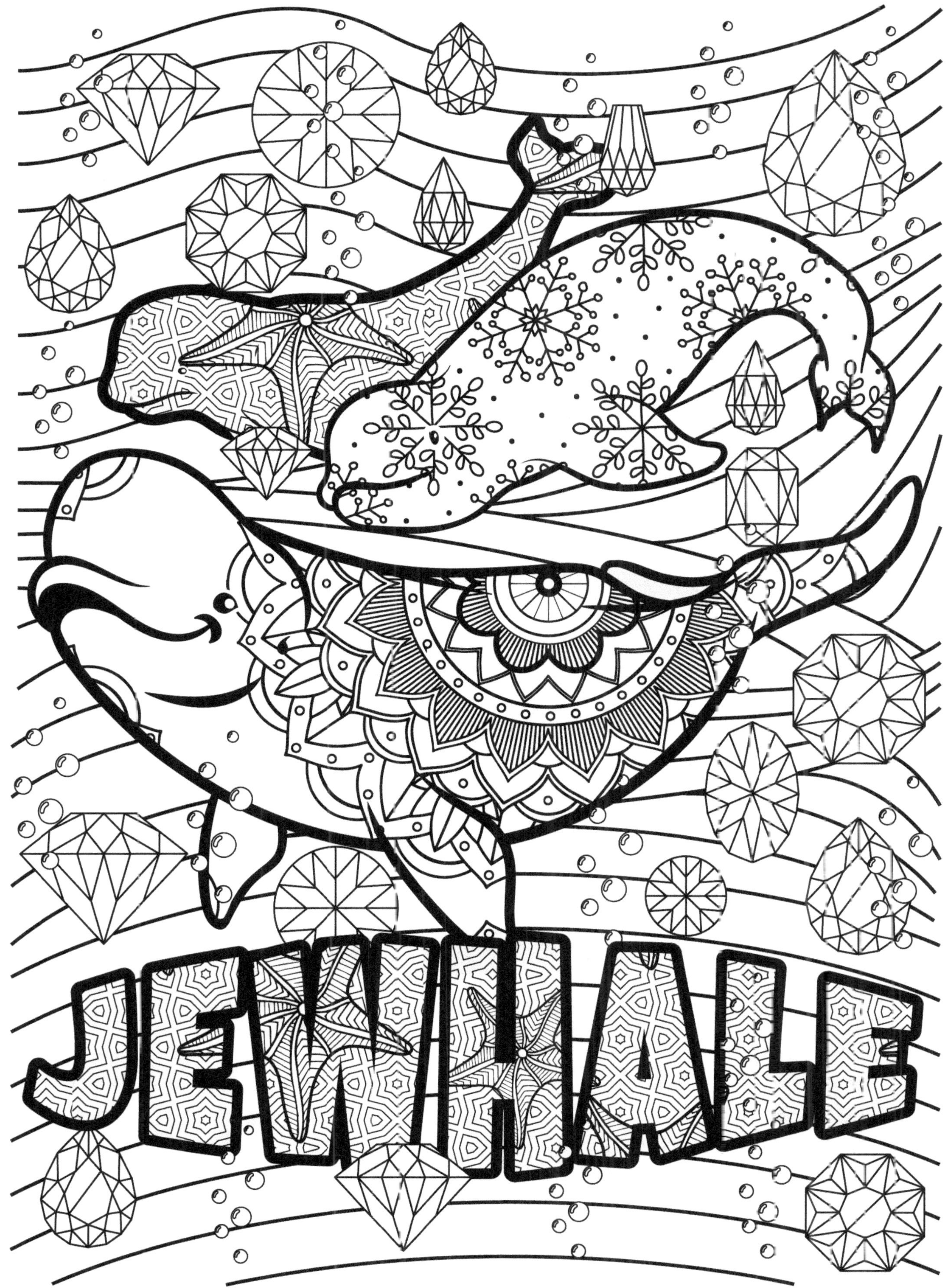

JEWHALE

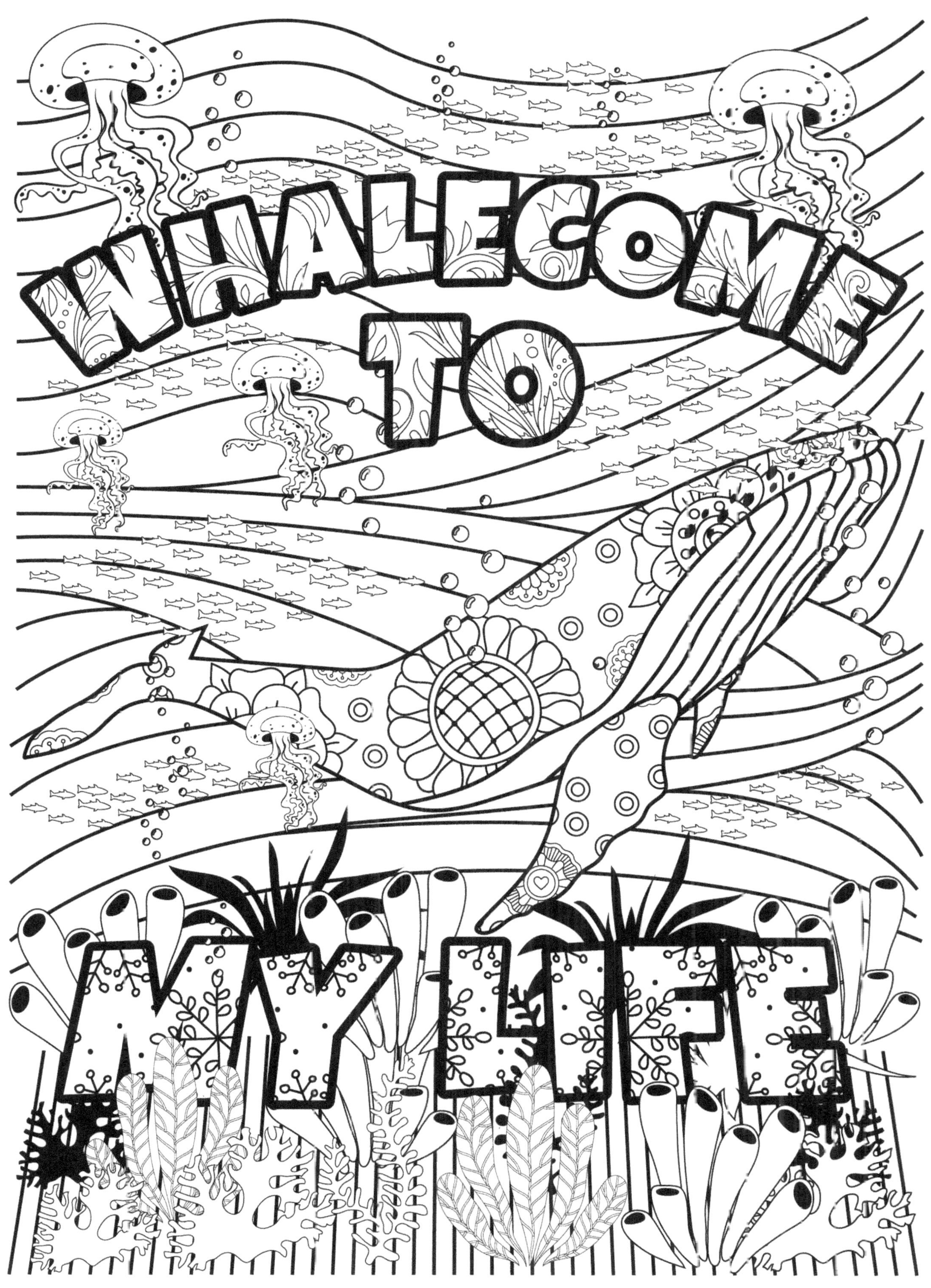

WHALECOME TO
MY LIFE

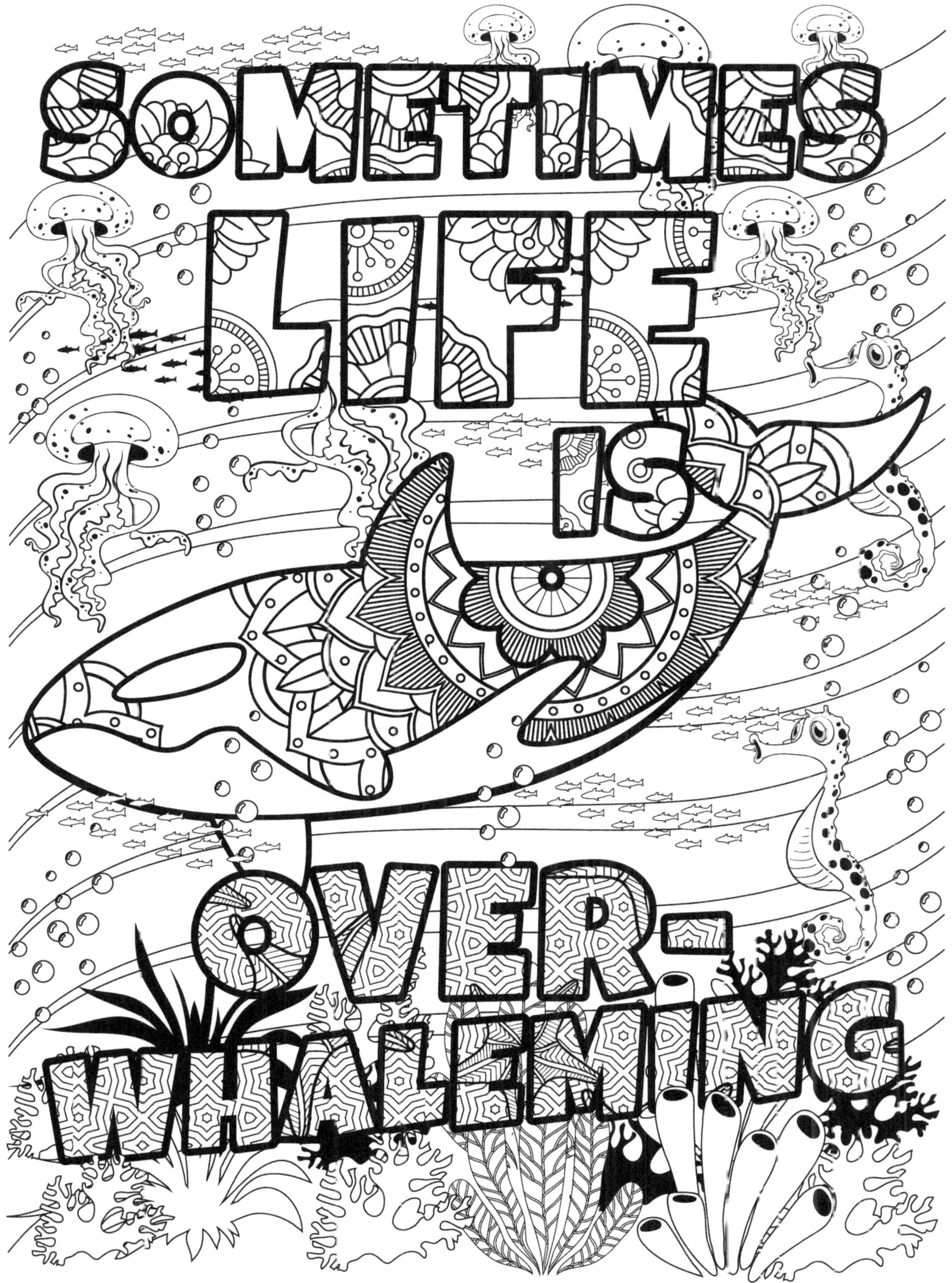

SOMETIMES
LIFE
IS
OVER-
WHALEMING

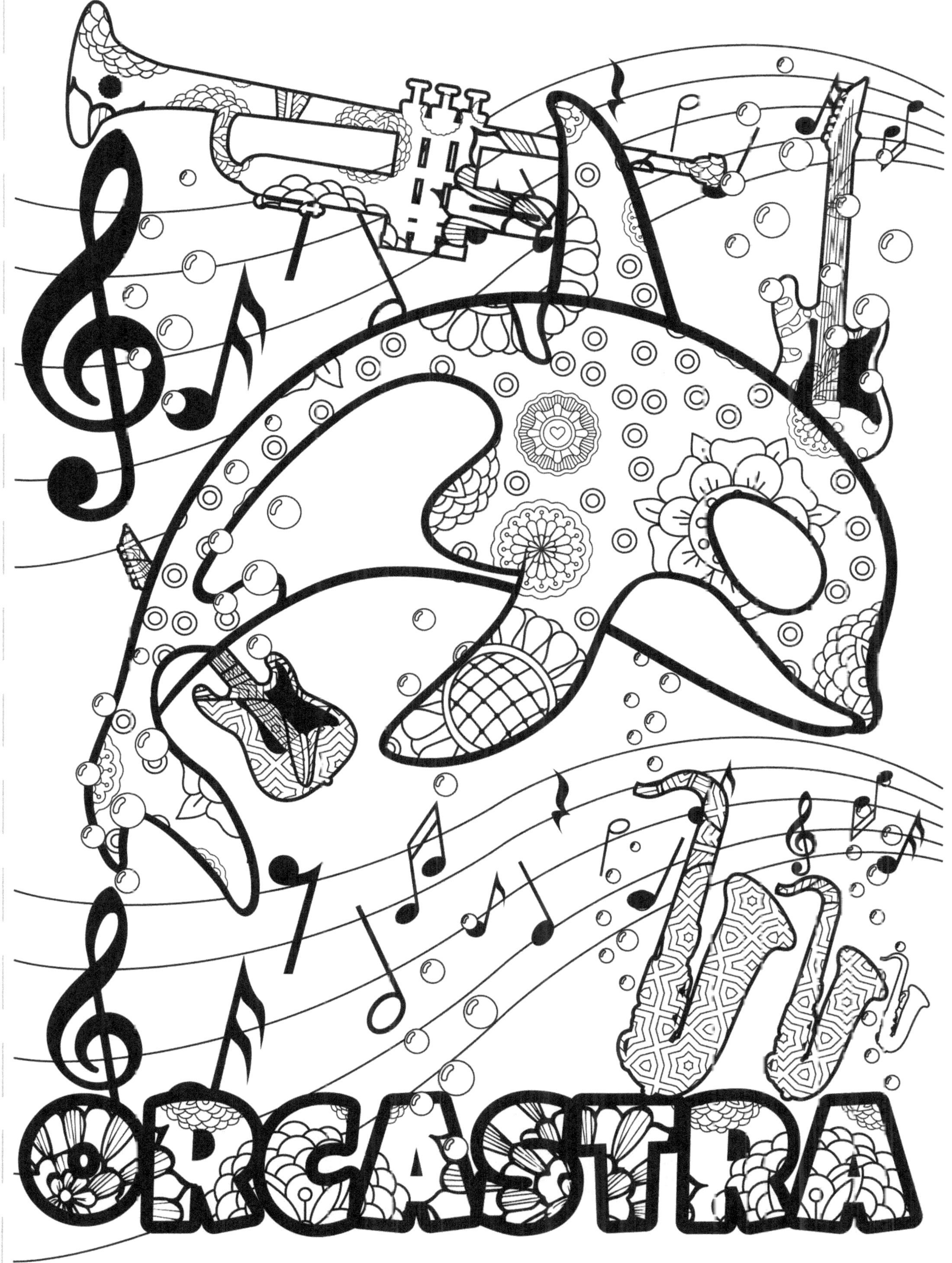
ORCASTRA

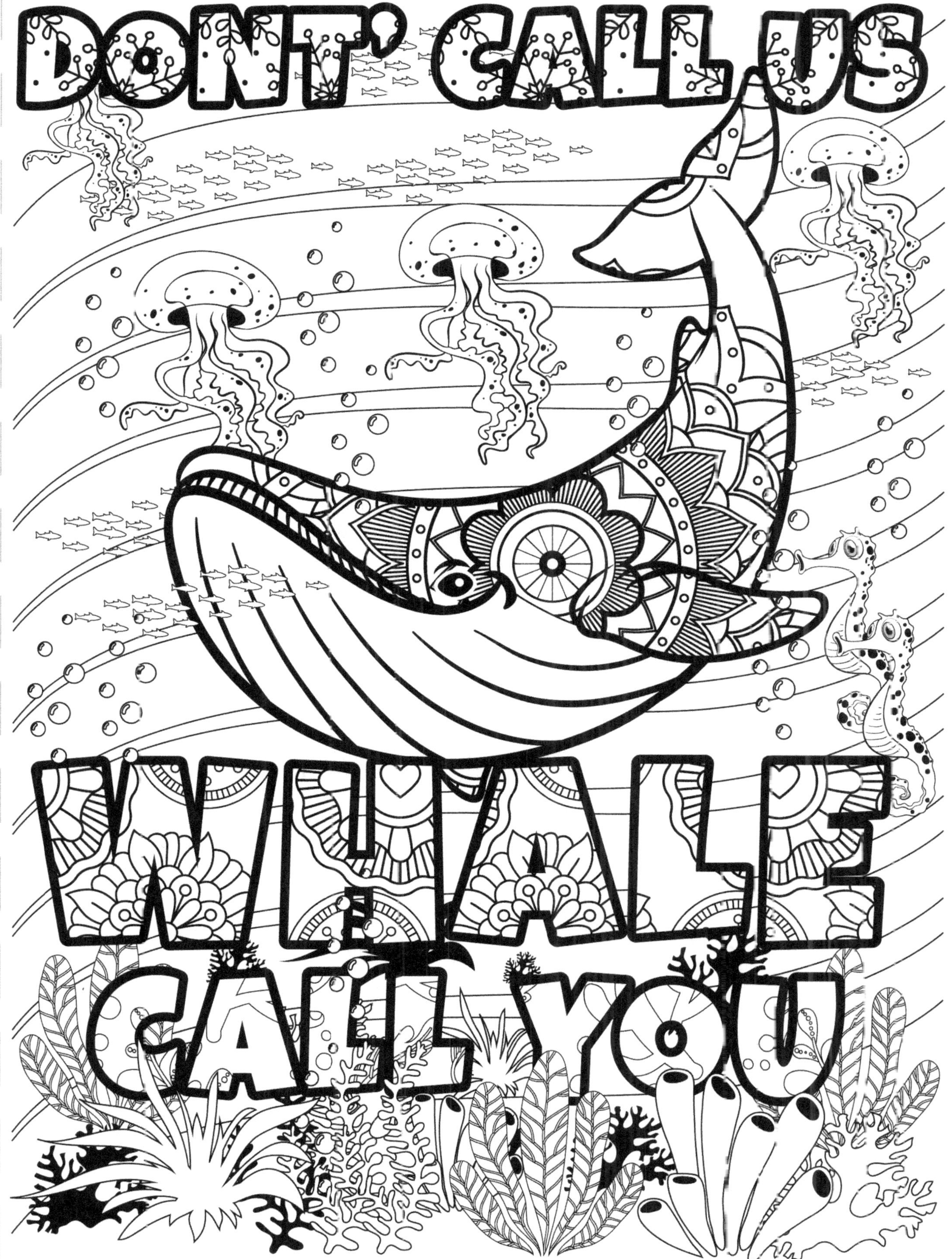

DONT' CALL US
WHALE
CALL YOU

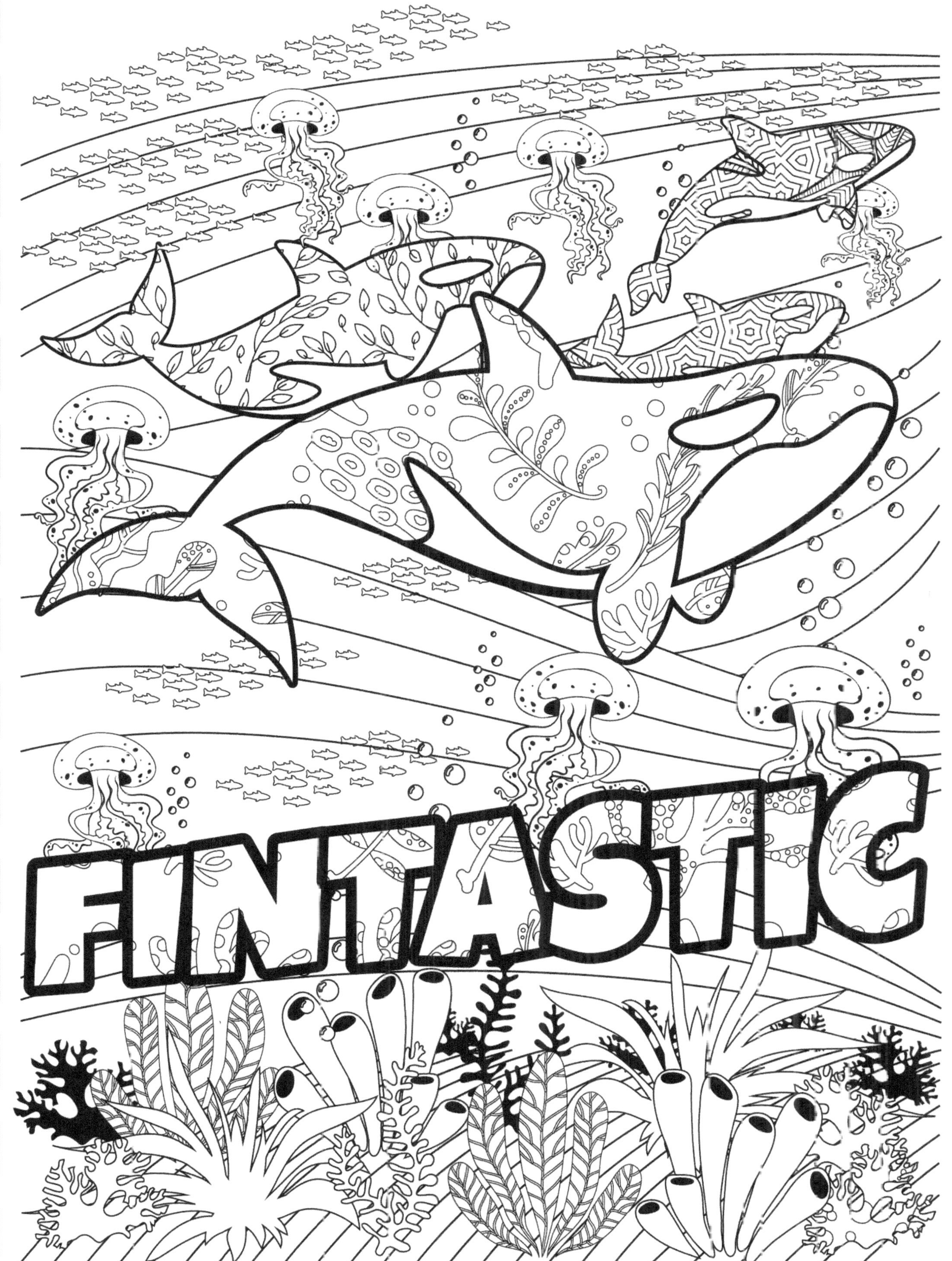
FINTASTIC

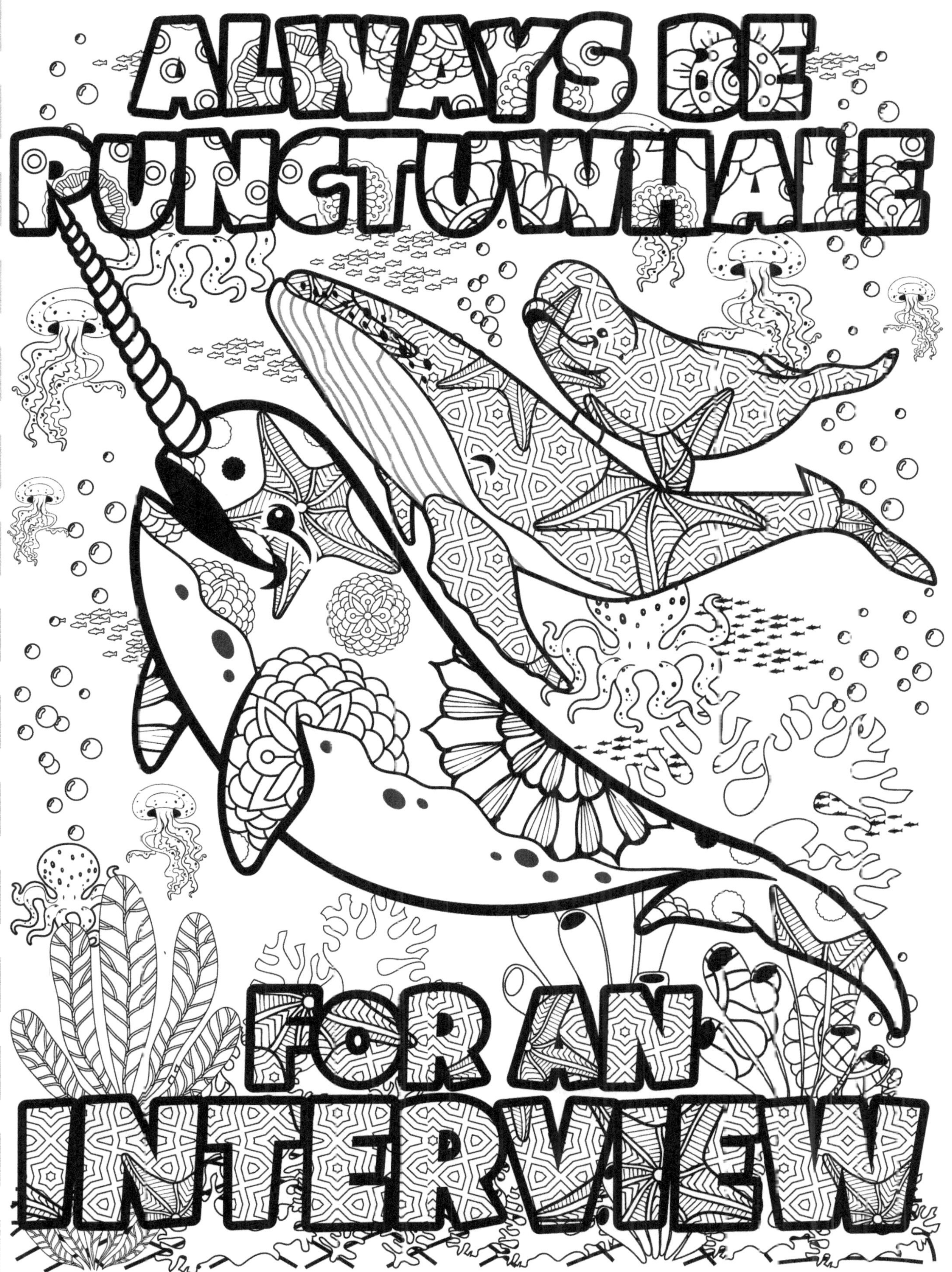

ALWAYS BE PUNCTUWHALE
FOR AN INTERVIEW

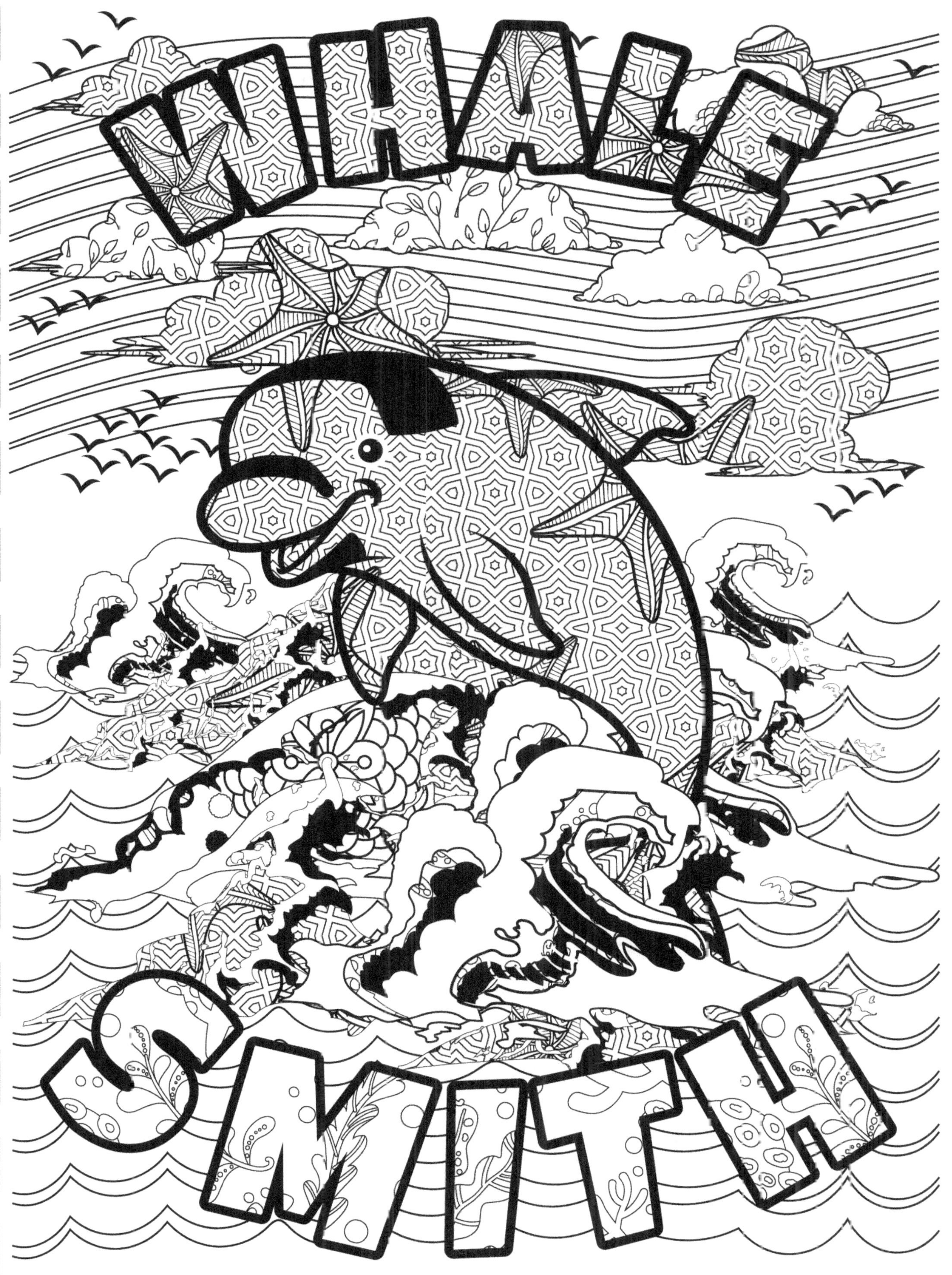

WHALE
SMITH

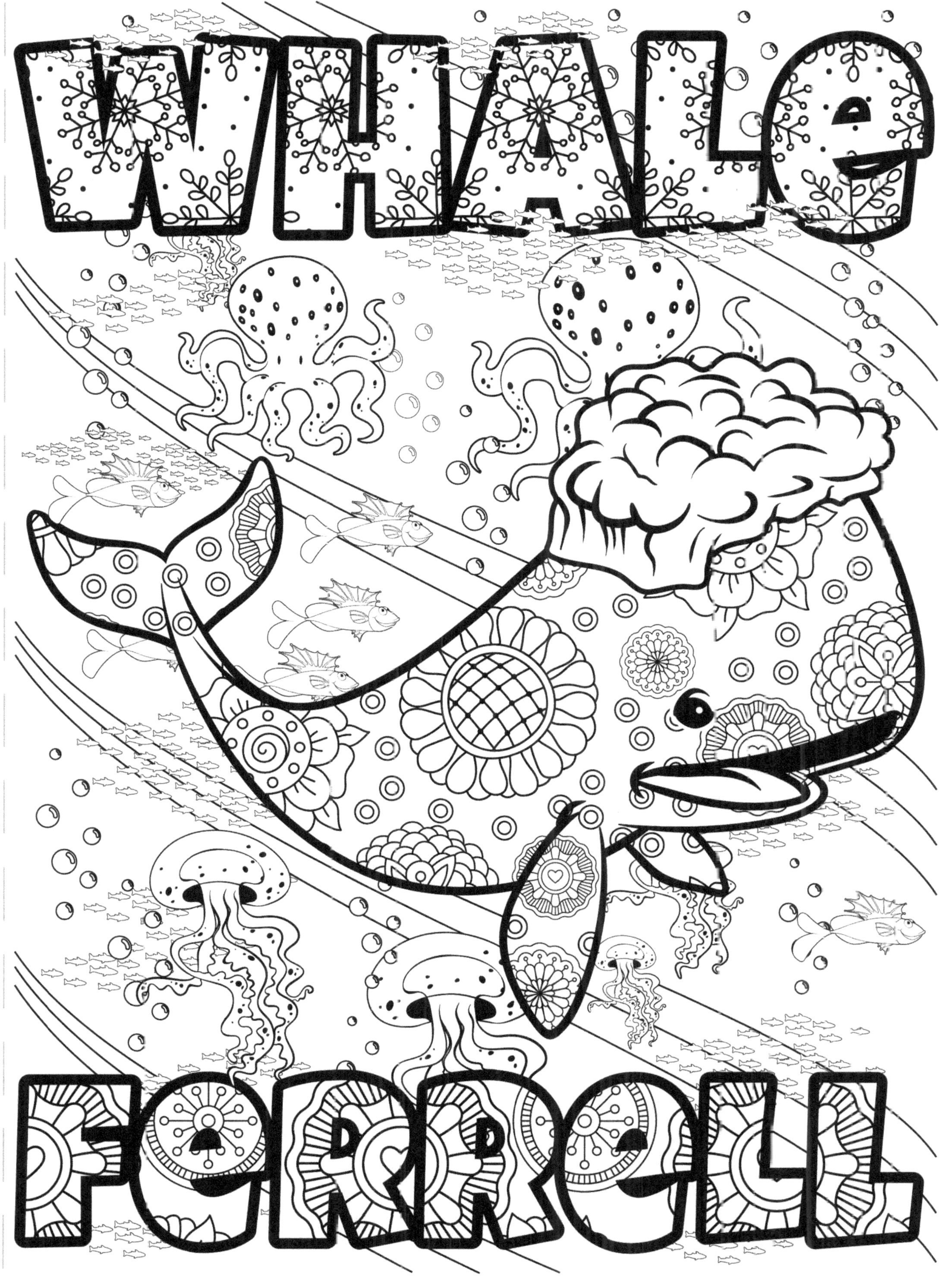
WHALE
FARRELL

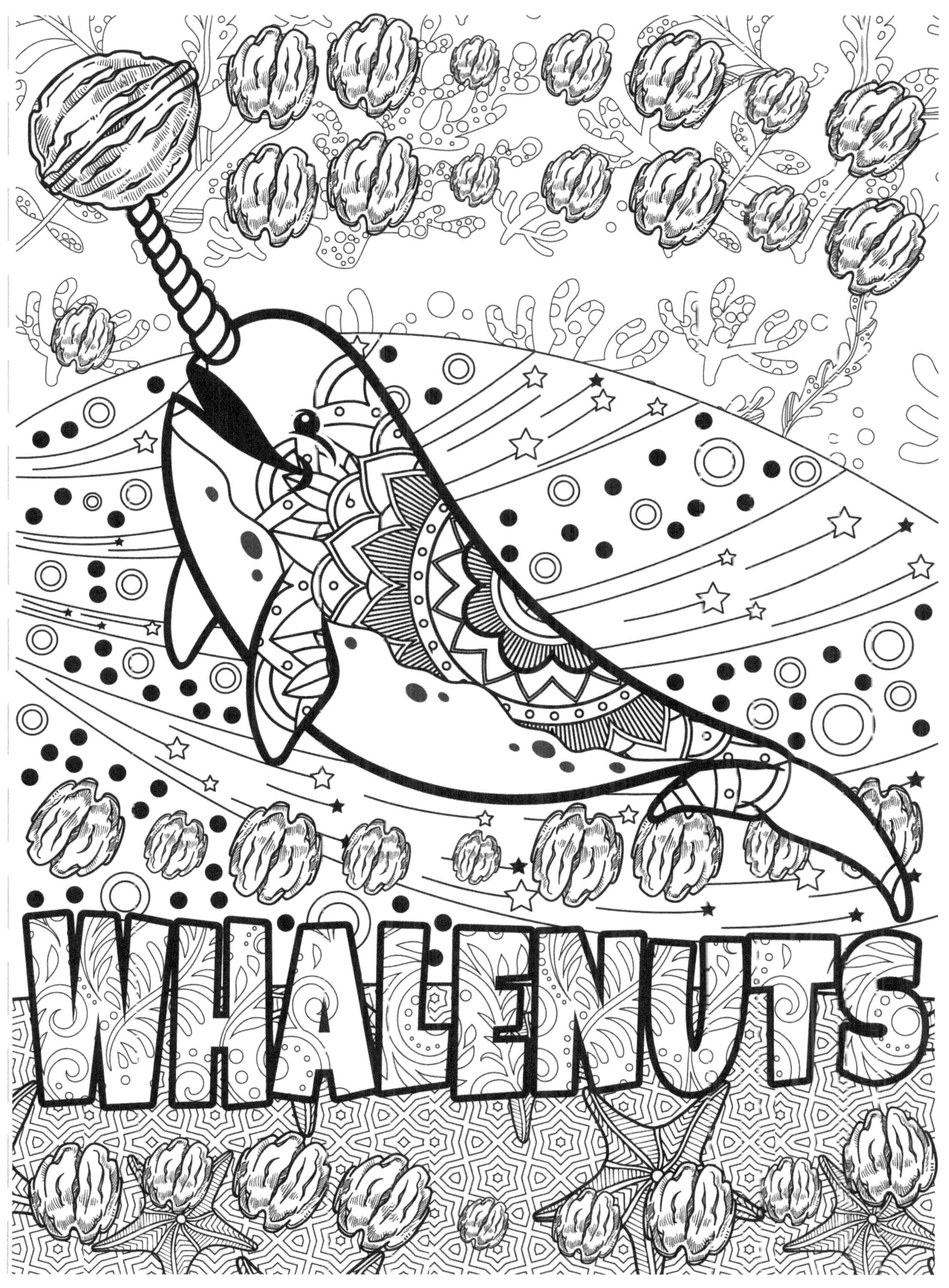

WHALENUTS

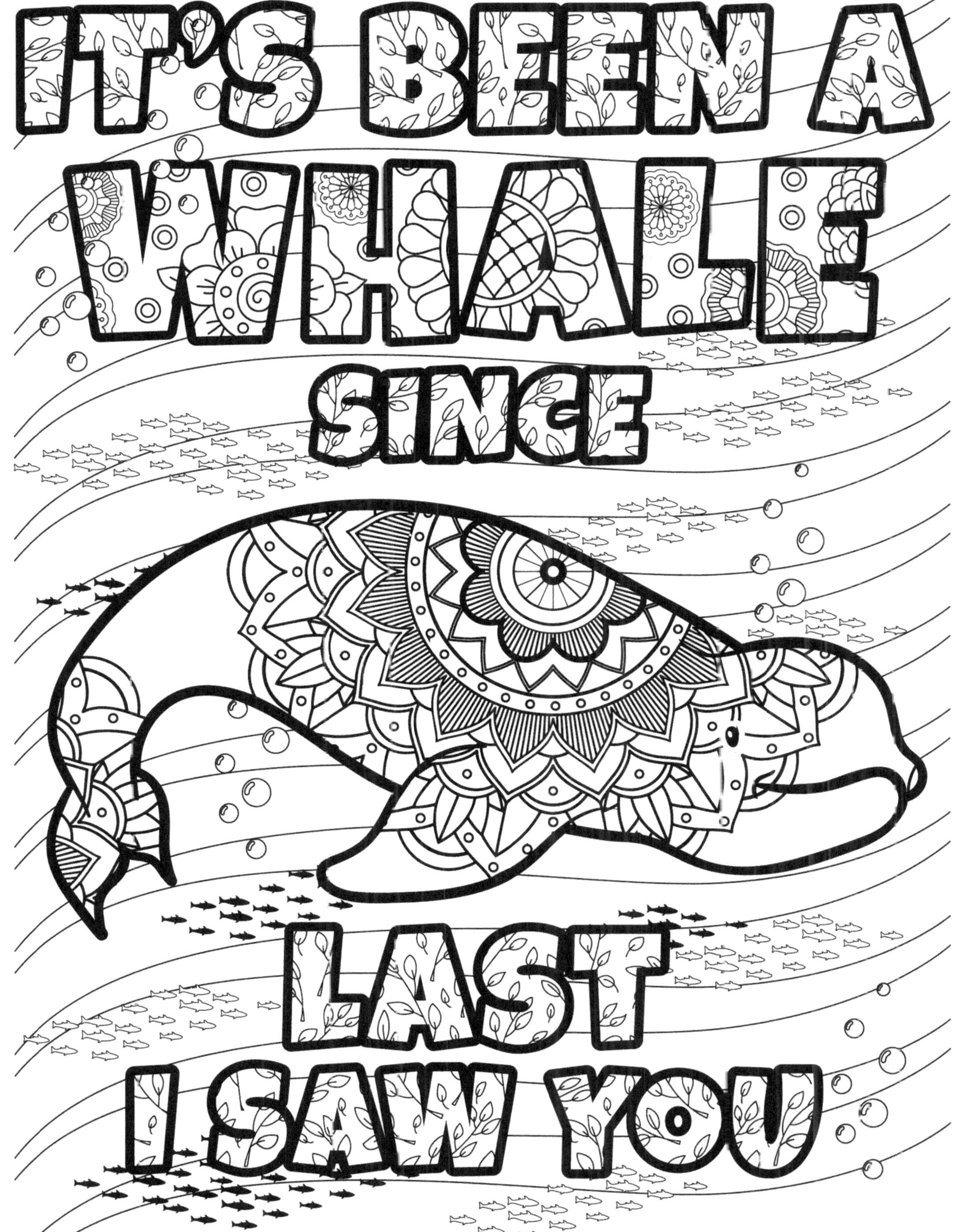

IT'S BEEN A
WHALE
SINCE
LAST
I SAW YOU

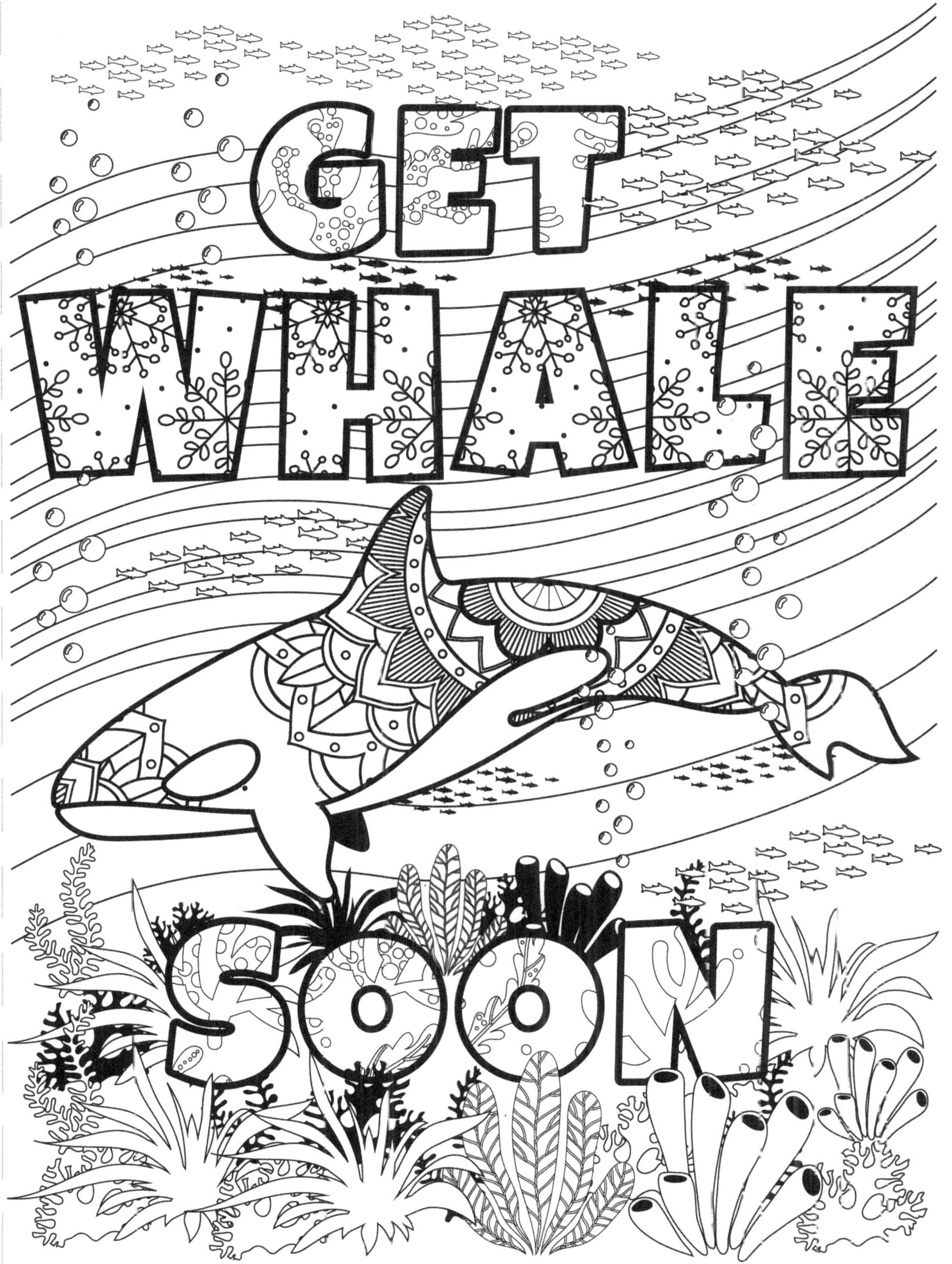

GET
WHALE
SOON

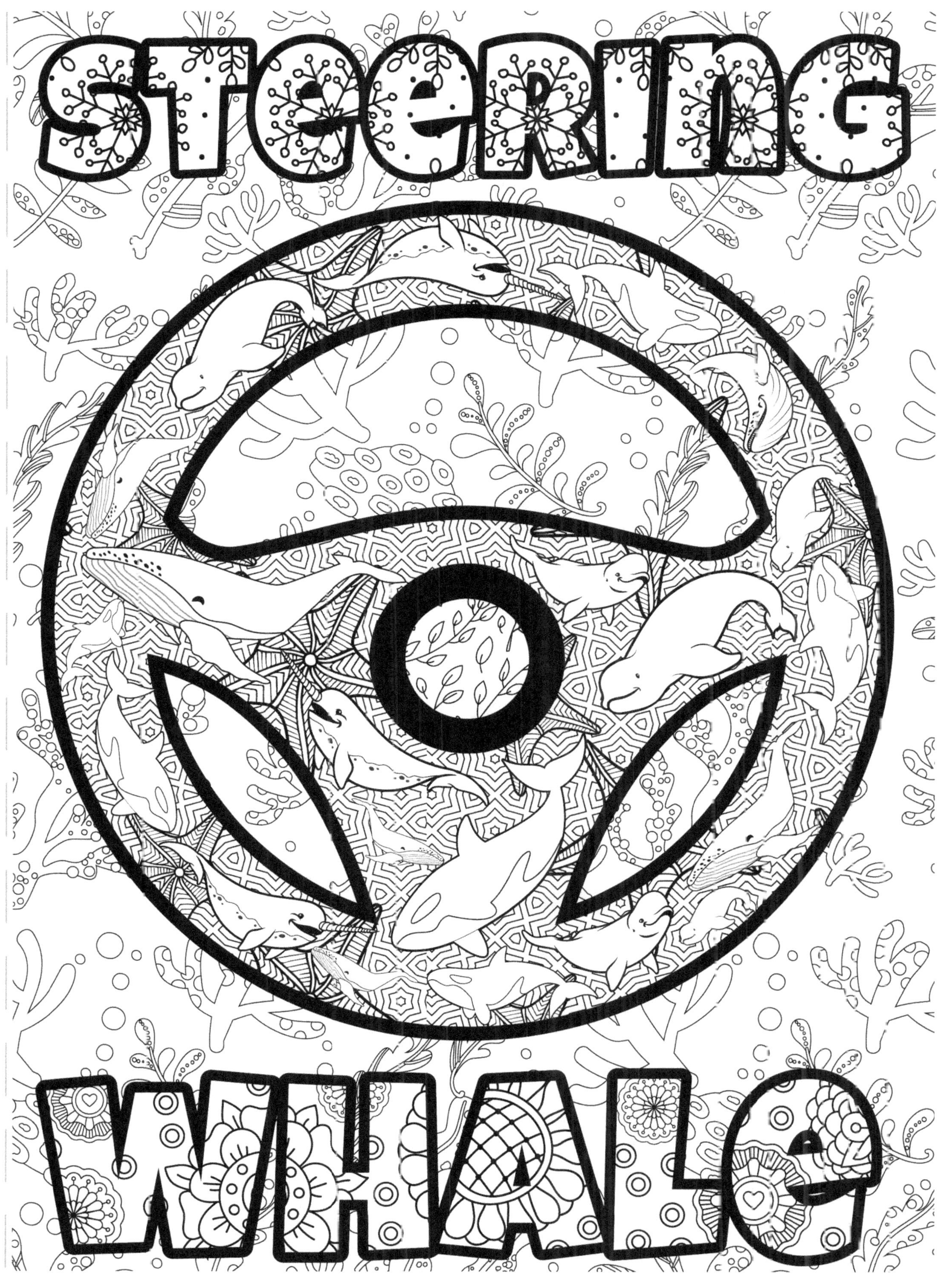

STEERING
WHALE

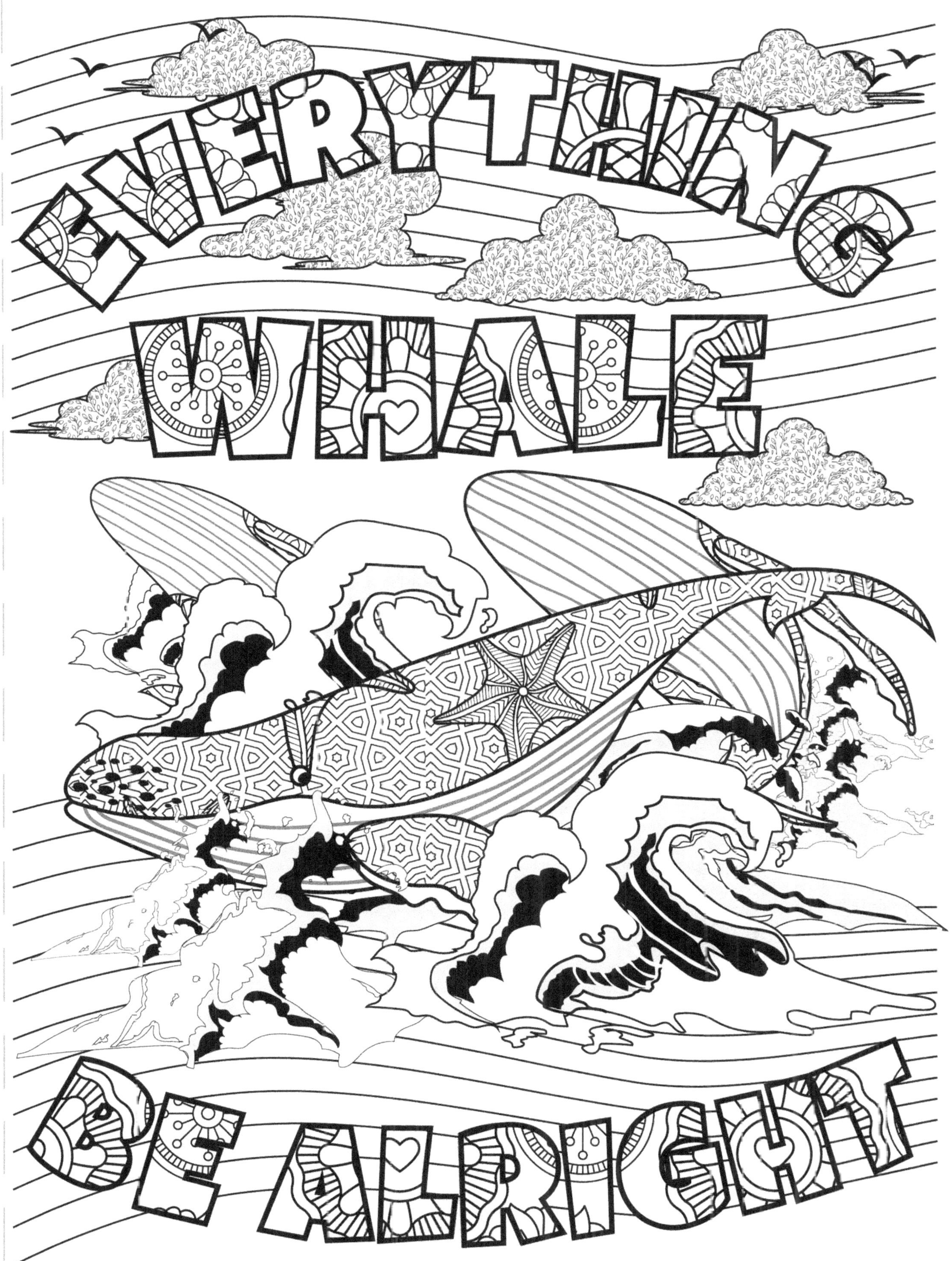

EVERYTHING
WHALE
BE ALRIGHT

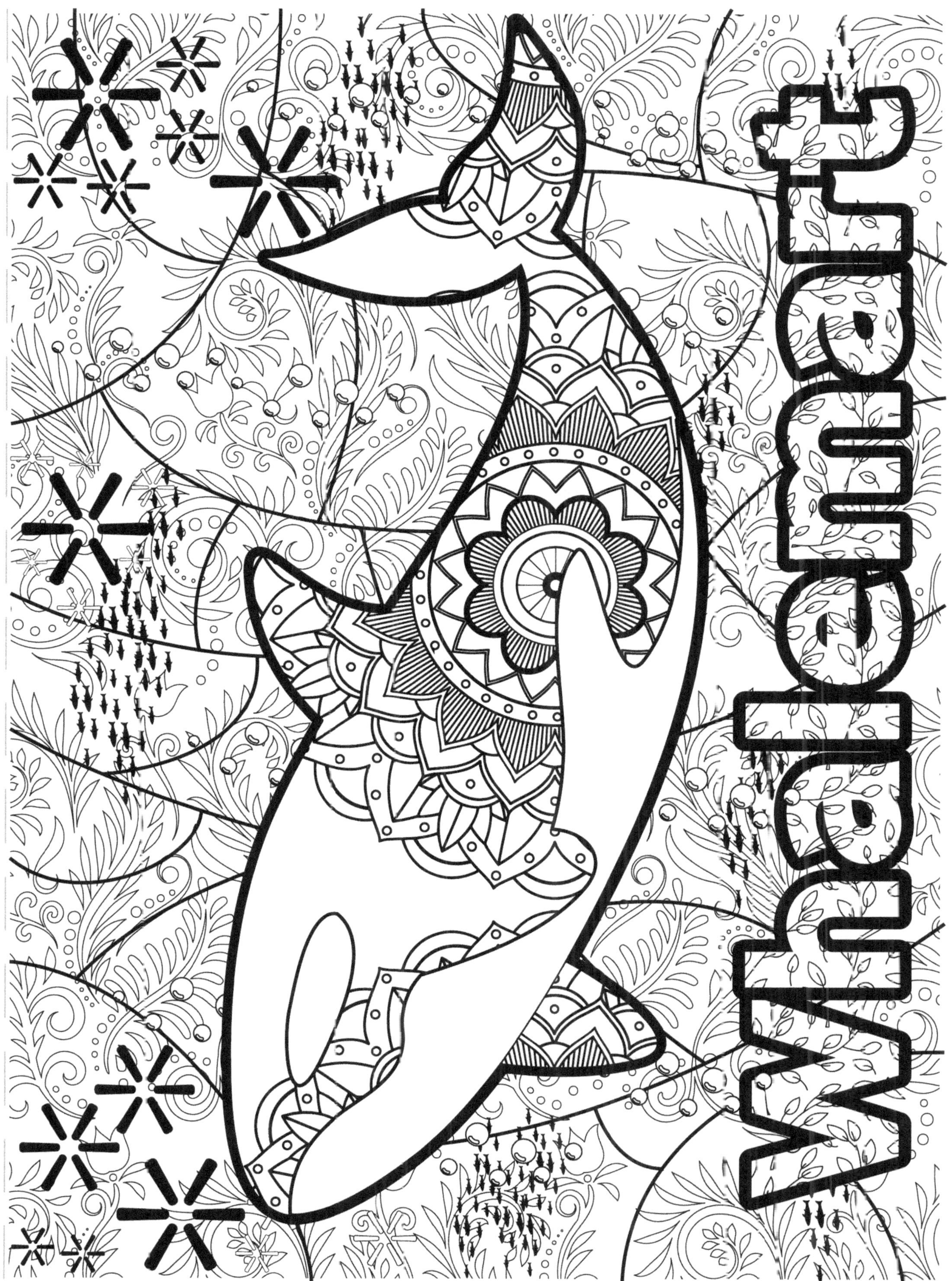

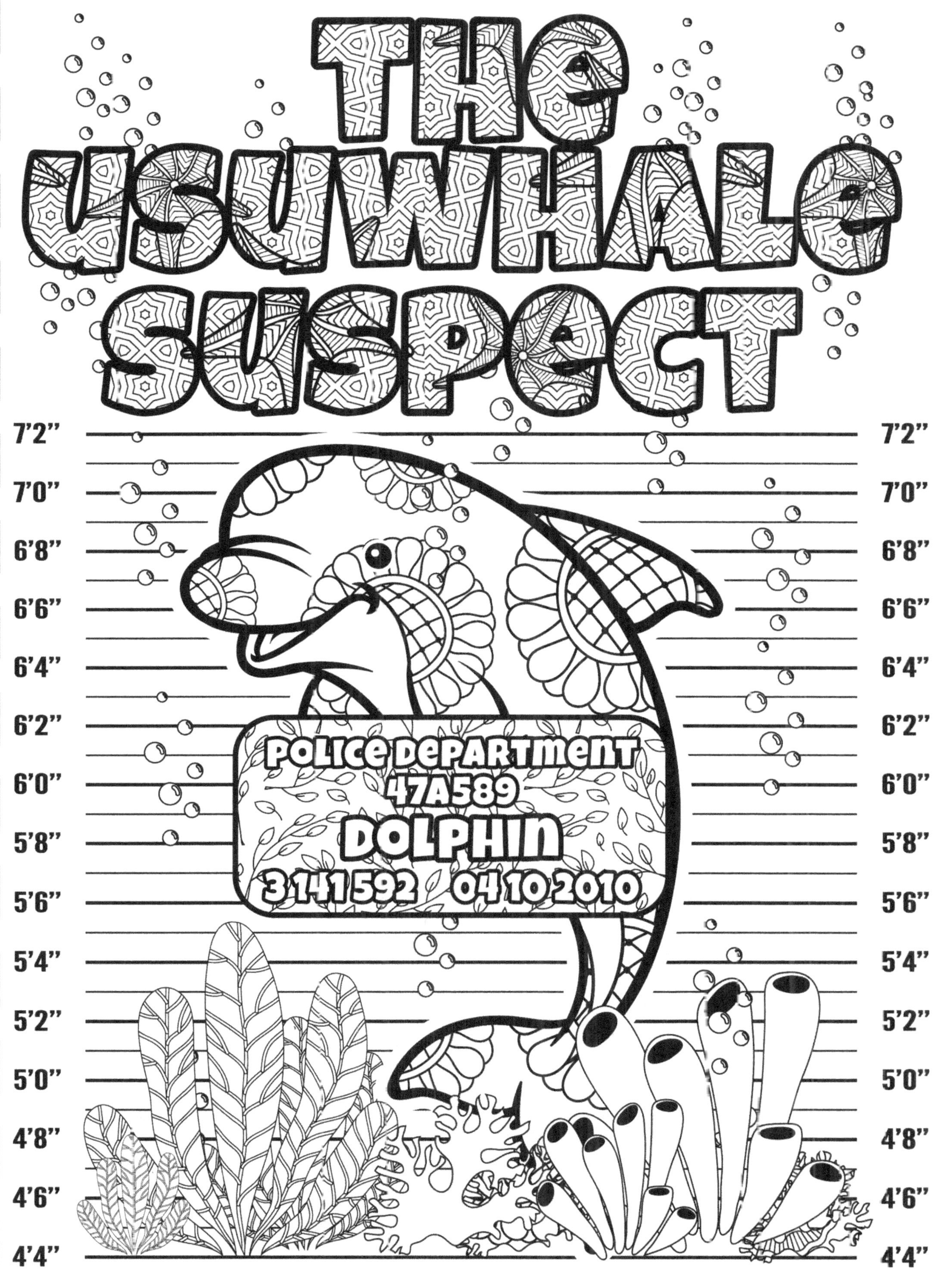

THE USUWHALE SUSPECT
7'2"
7'0"
6'8"
6'6"
6'4"
6'2"
6'0"
5'8"
5'6"
5'4"
5'2"
5'0"
4'8"
4'6"
4'4"
POLICE DEPARTMENT
47A589
DOLPHIN
3 141 592   04 10 2010

www.ingramcontent.com/pod-product-compliance
Lightning Source LLC
Chambersburg PA
CBHW081312250726
48662CB00008B/2525

ZOMBIE COLORING BOOK

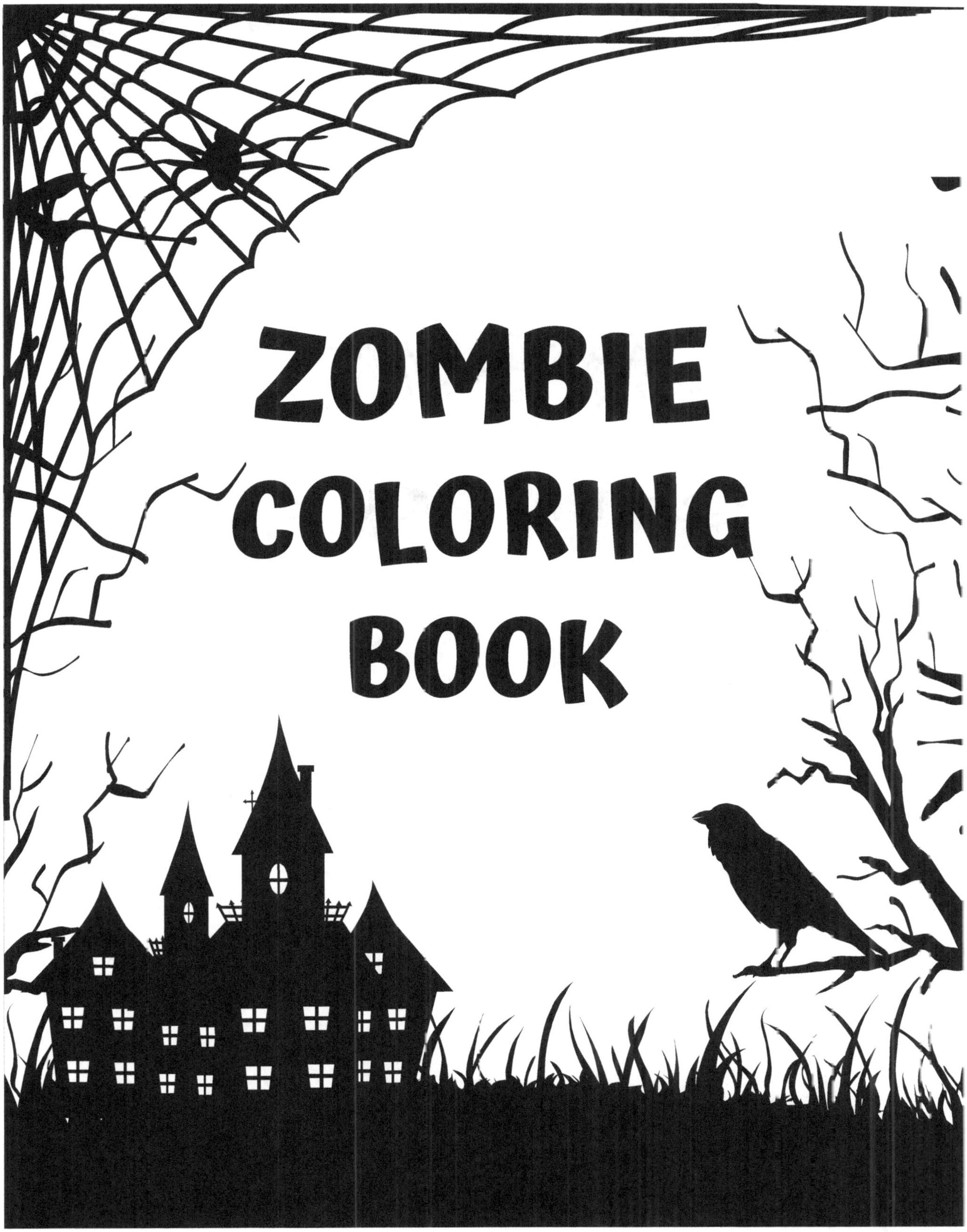

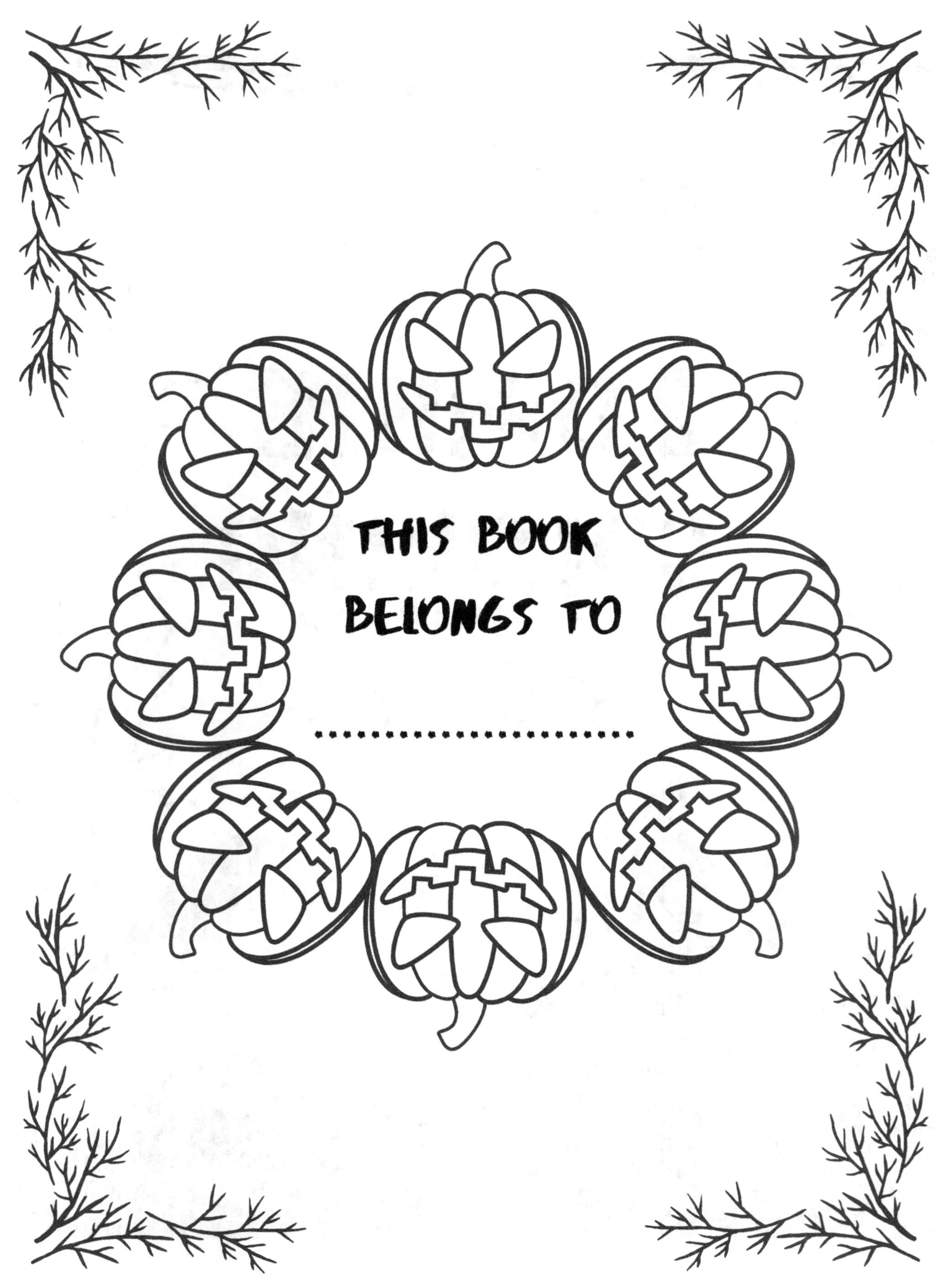
THIS BOOK
BELONGS TO
....

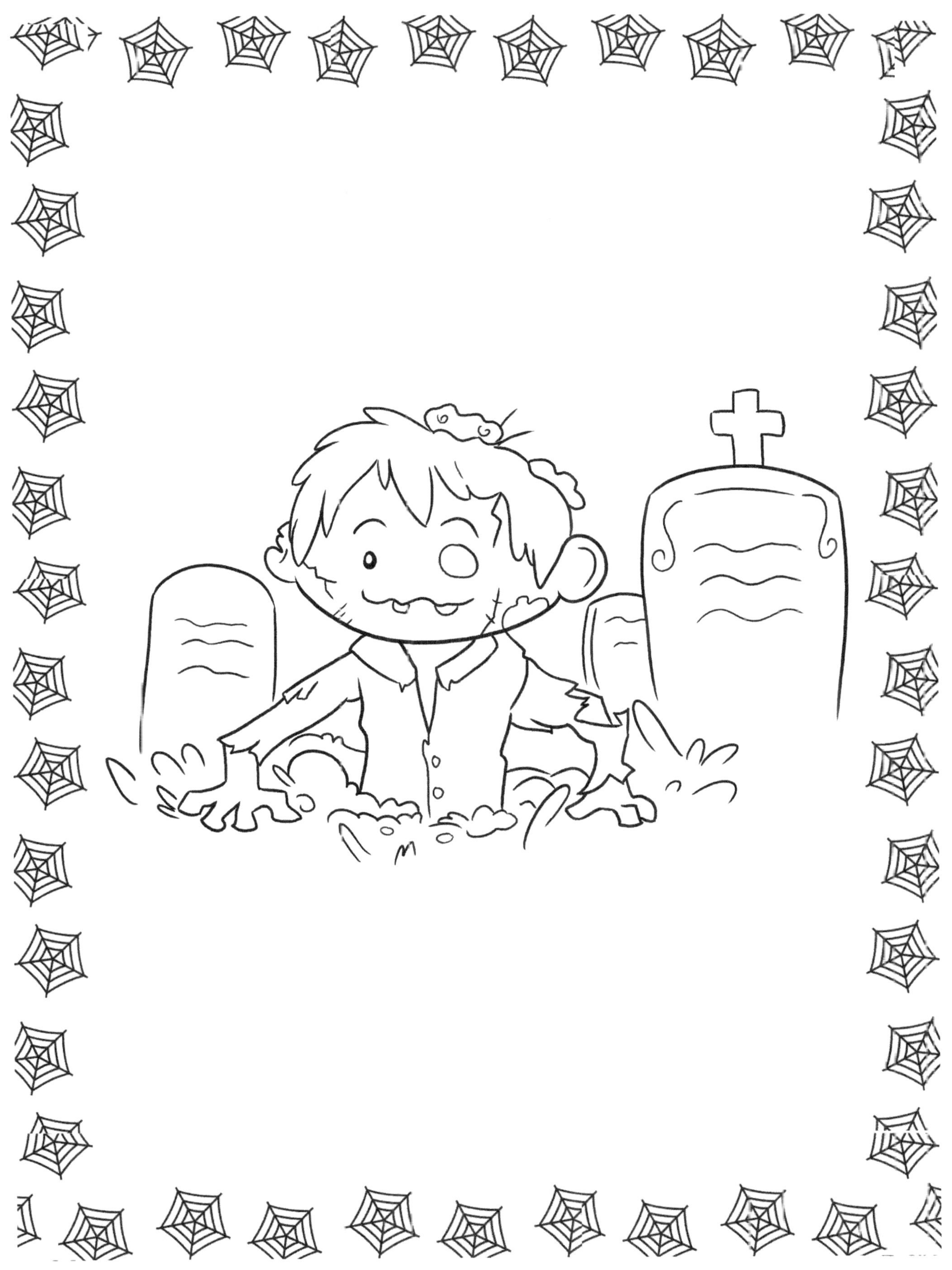

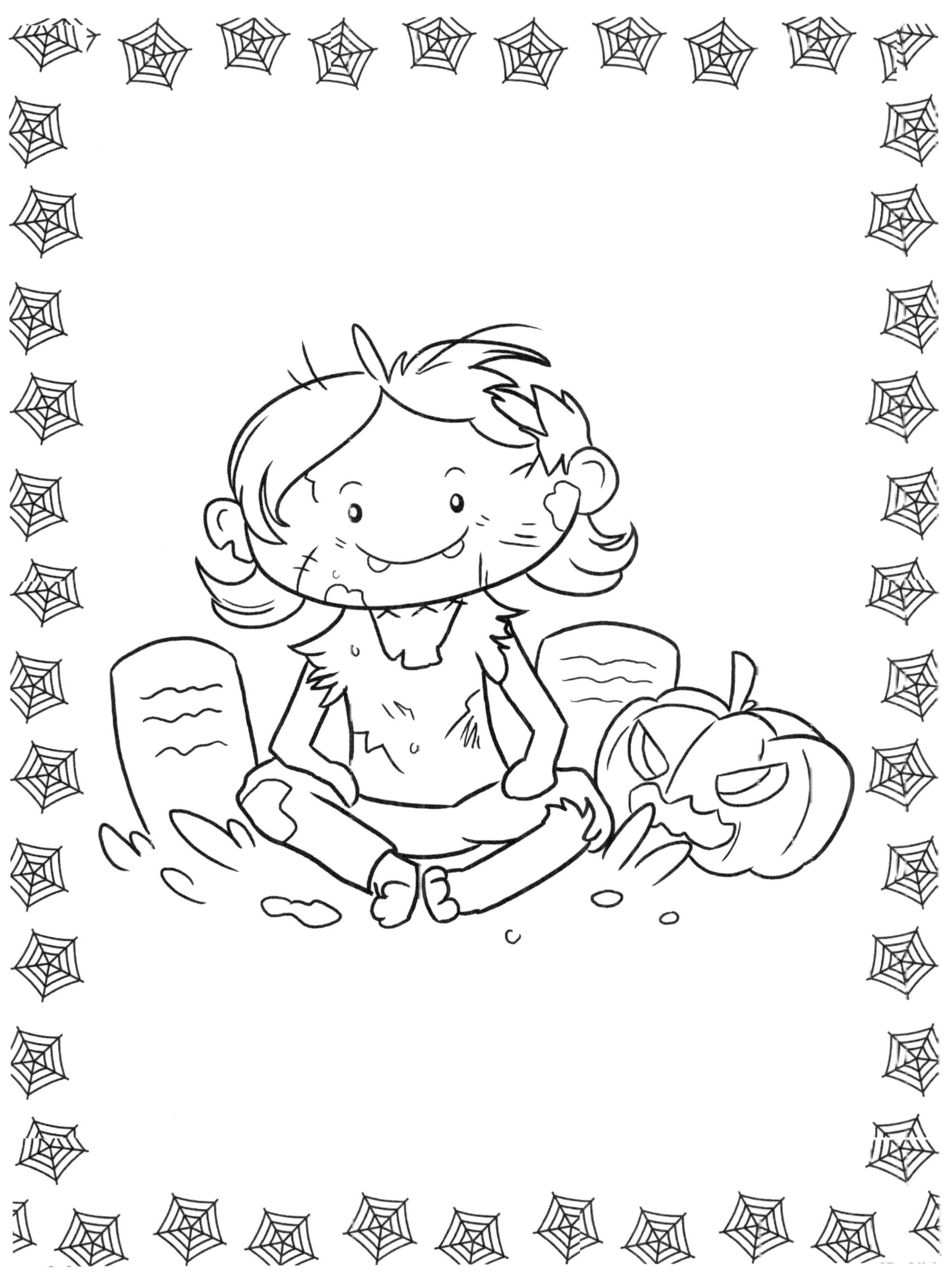

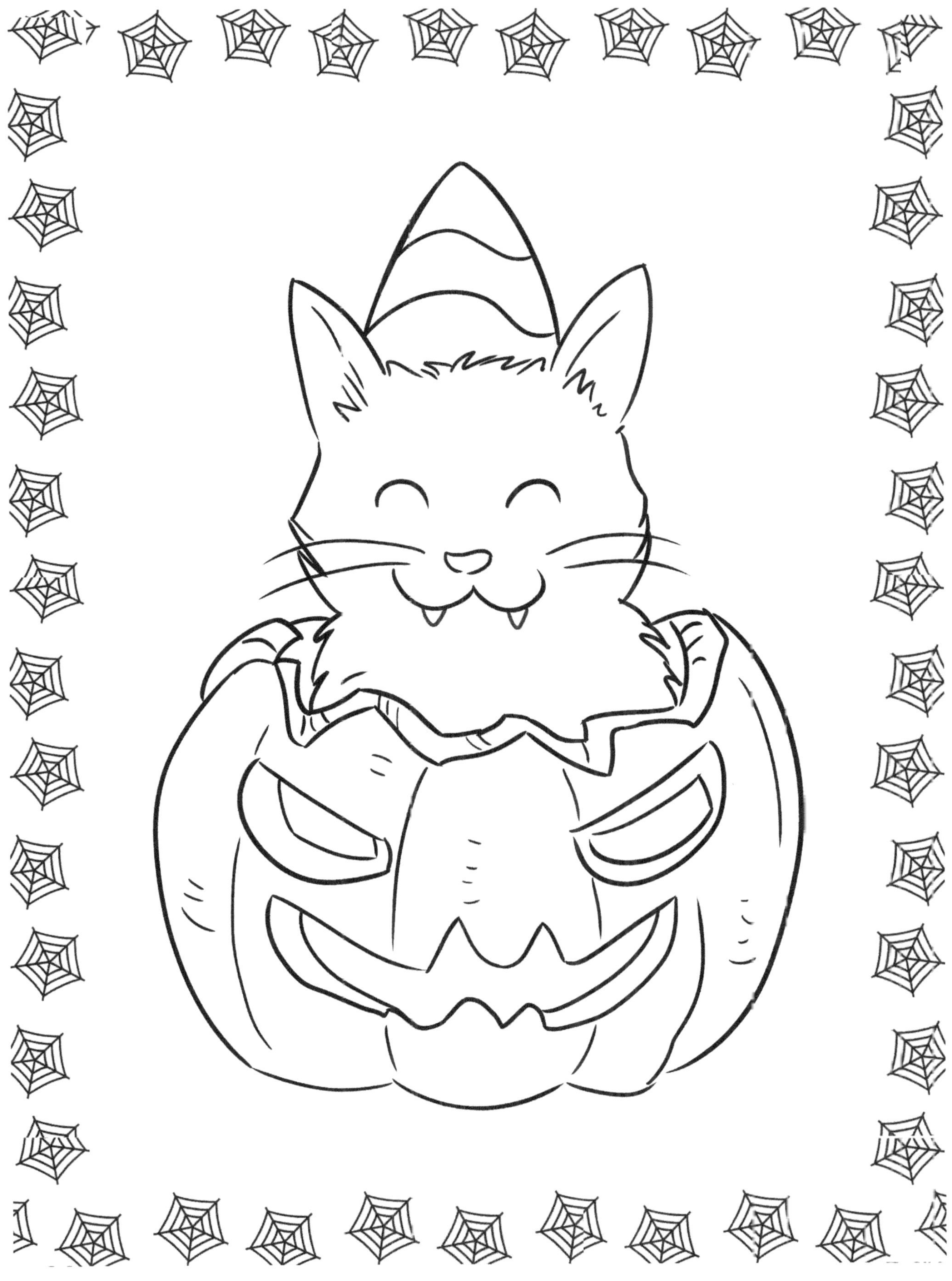

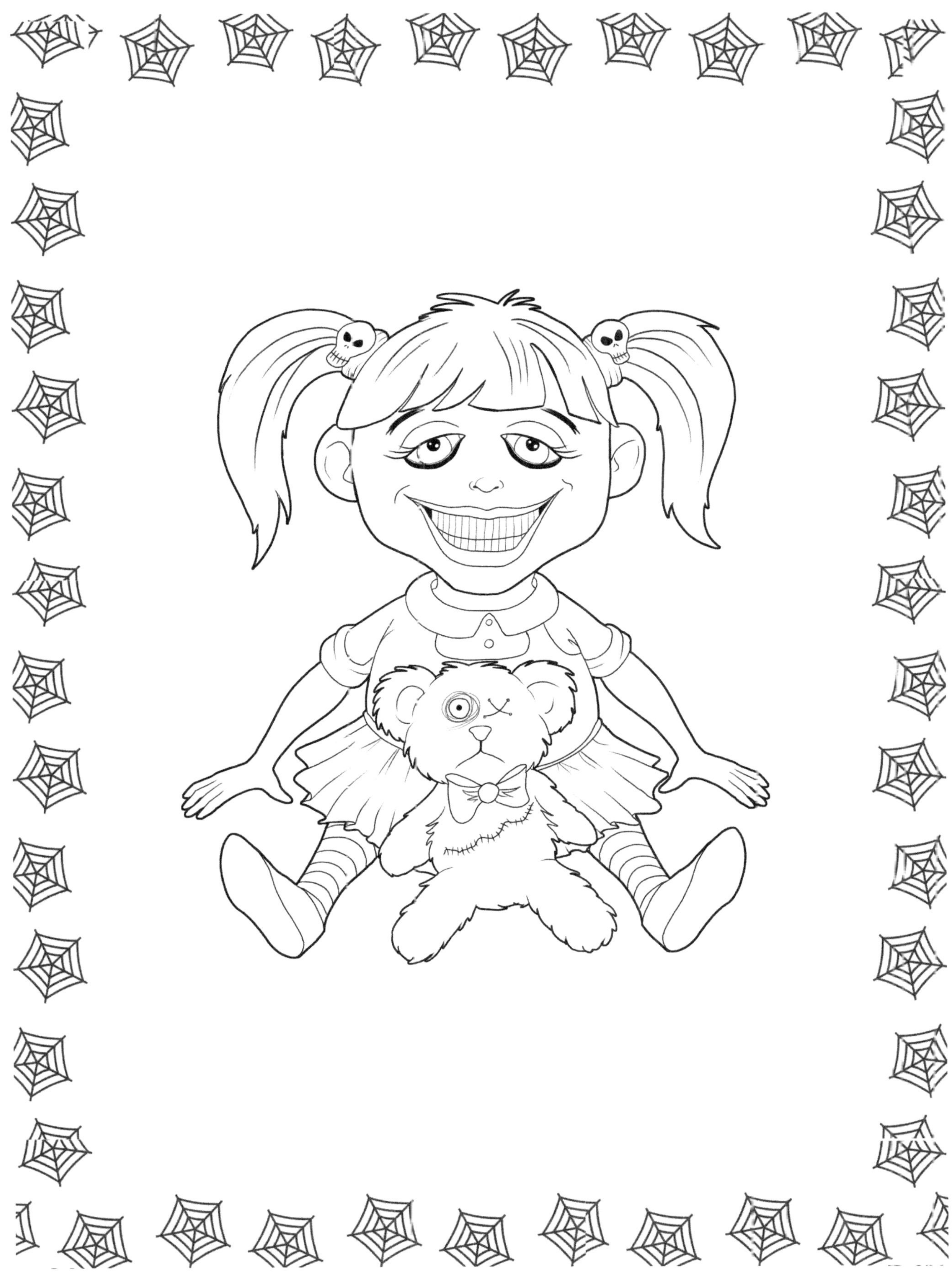

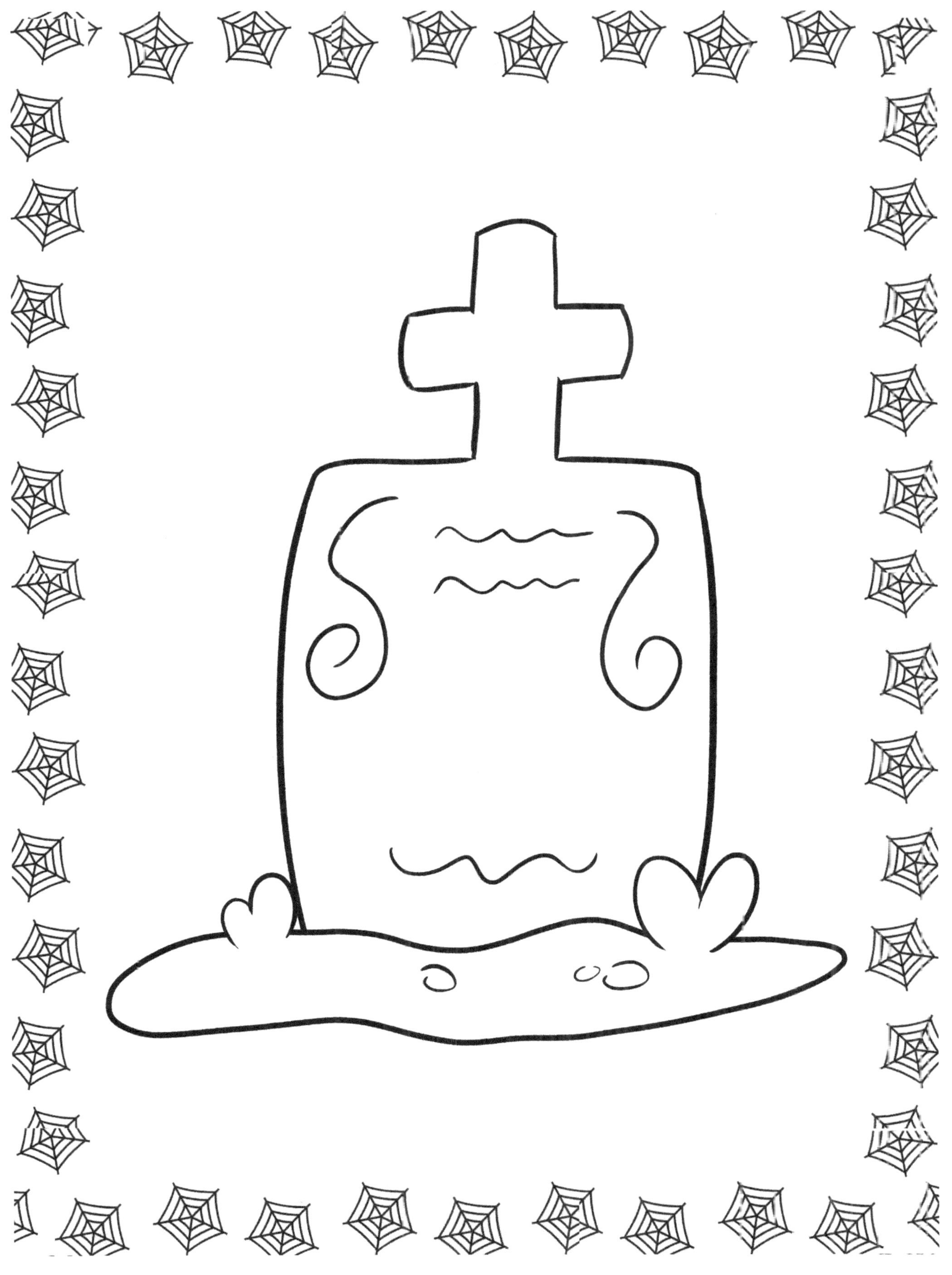

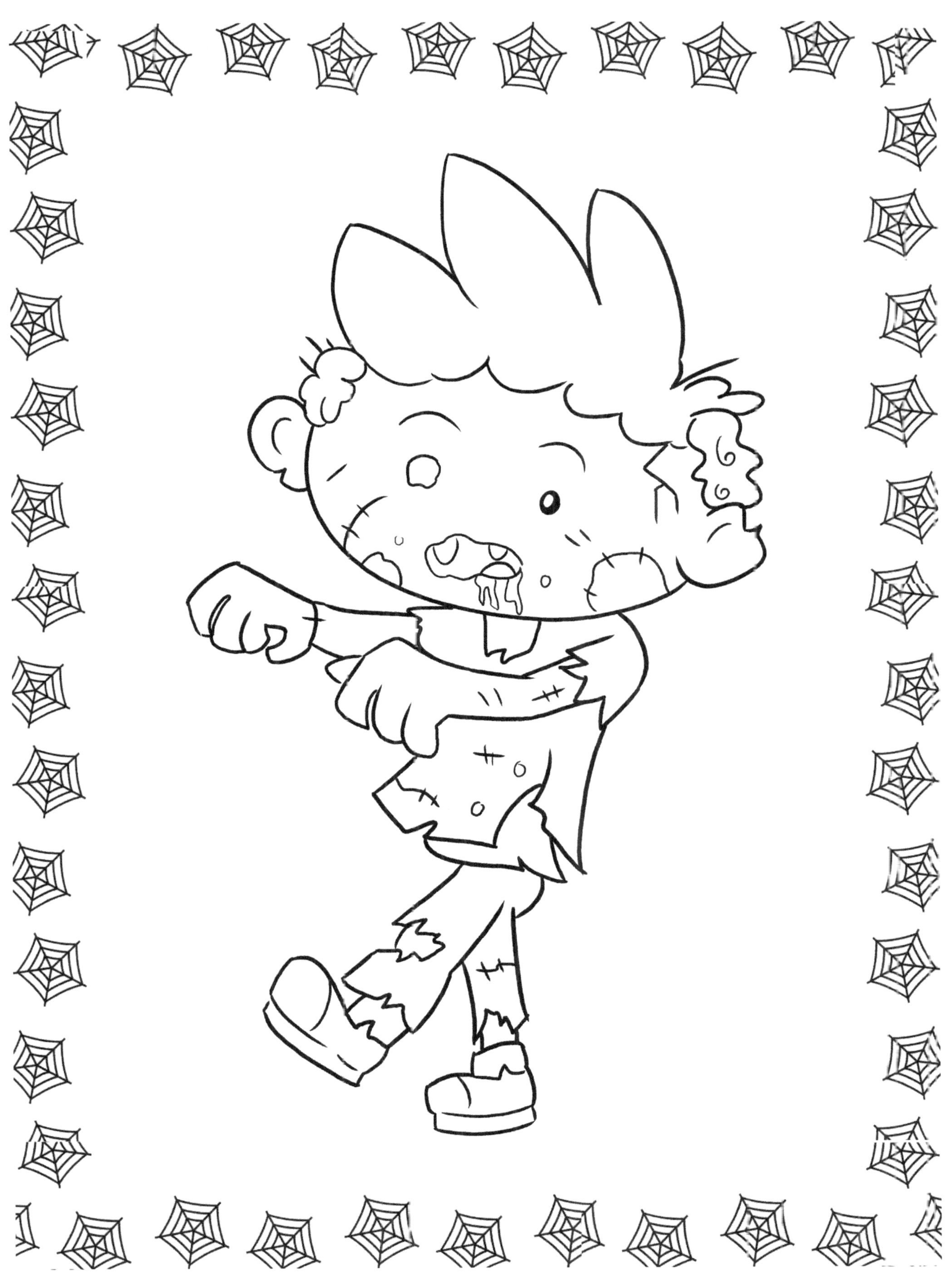

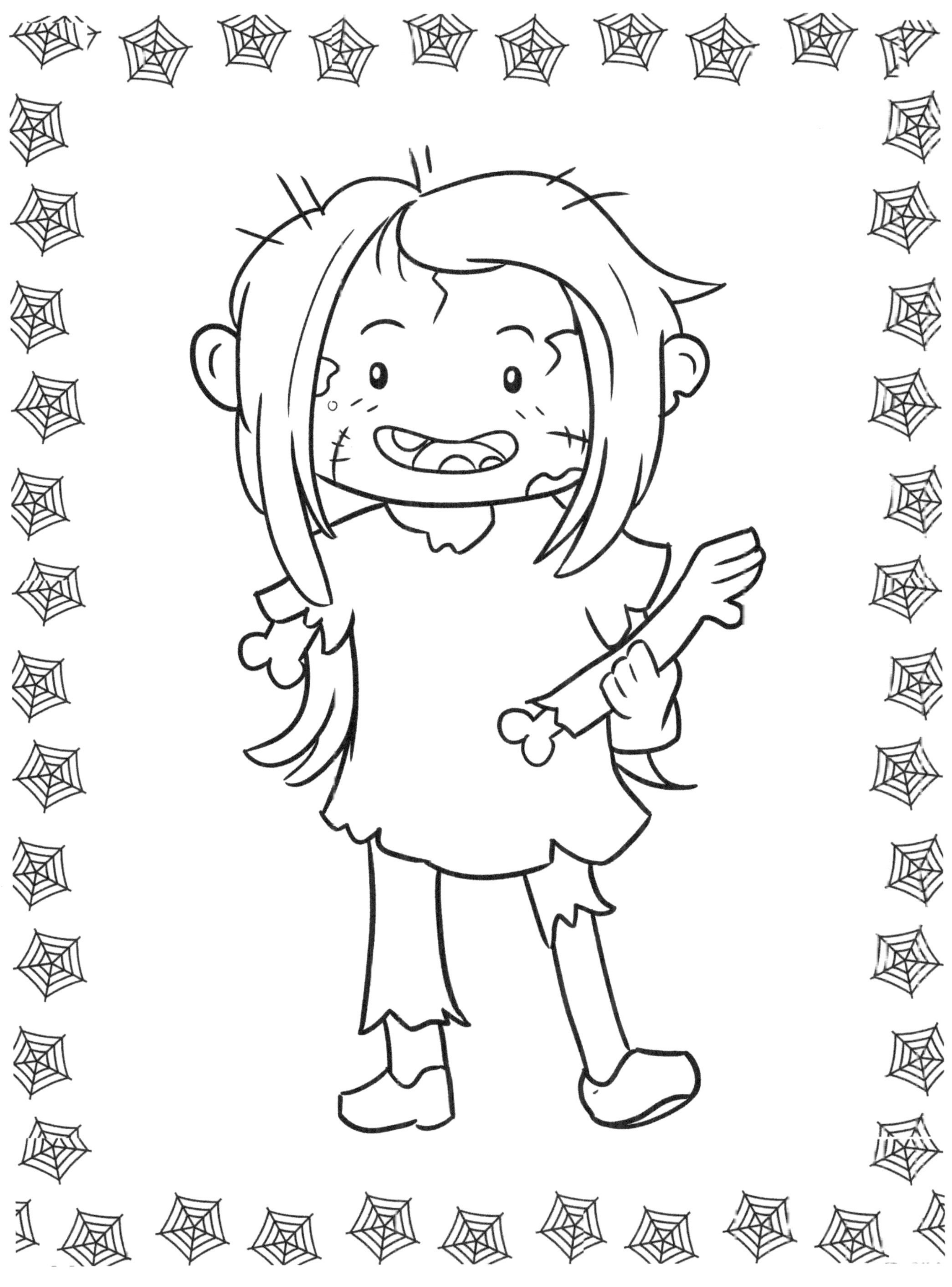

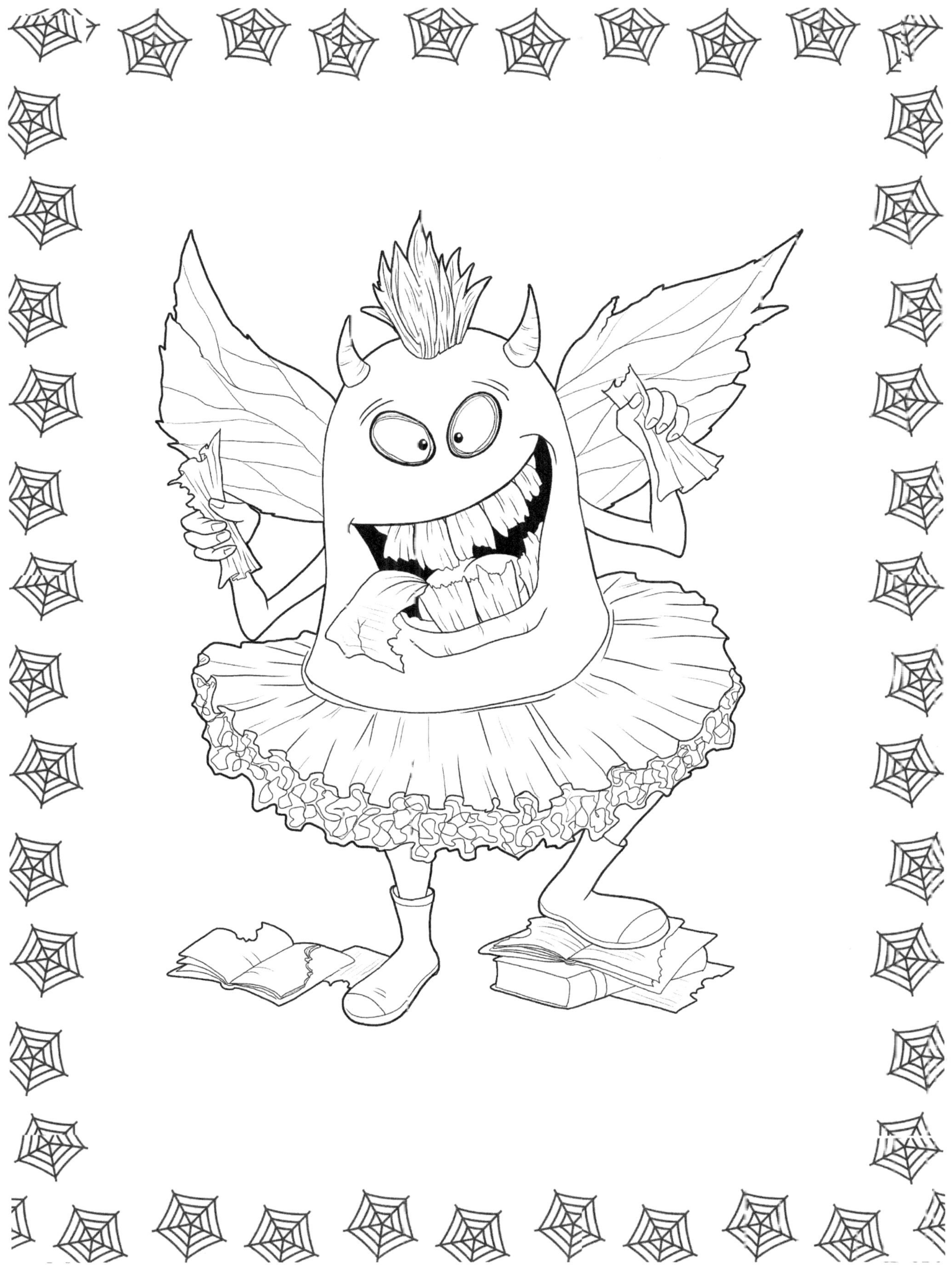

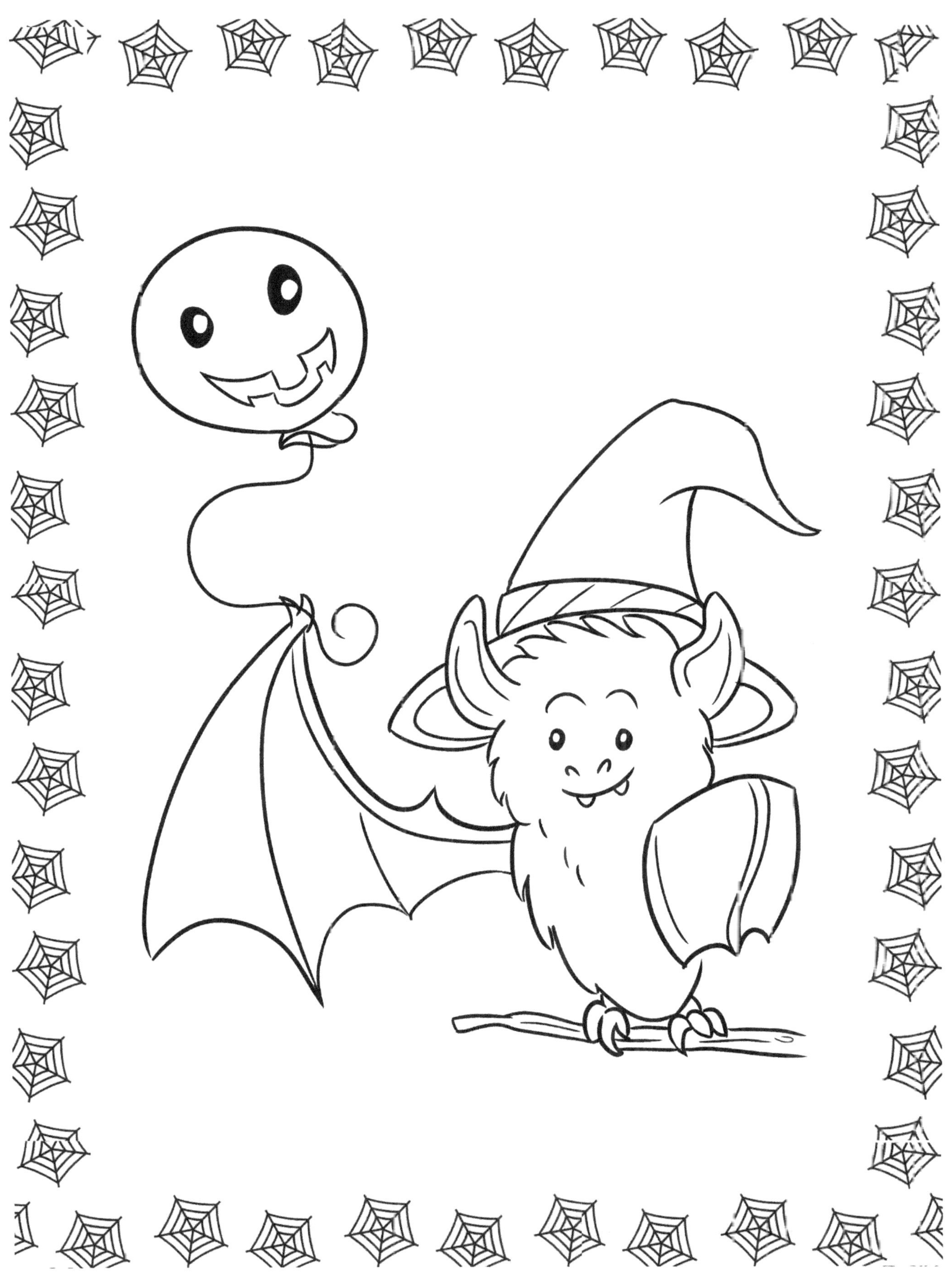

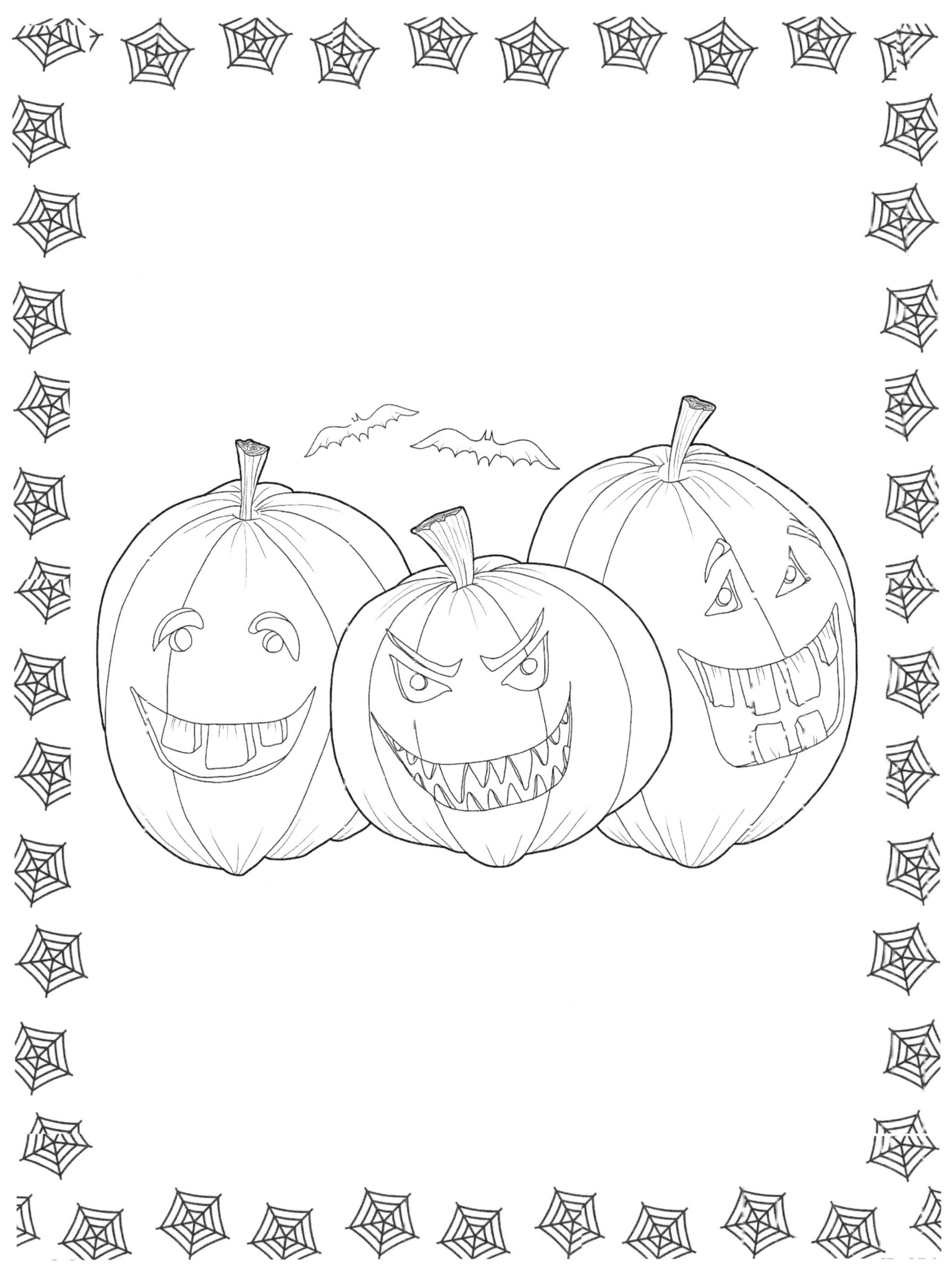

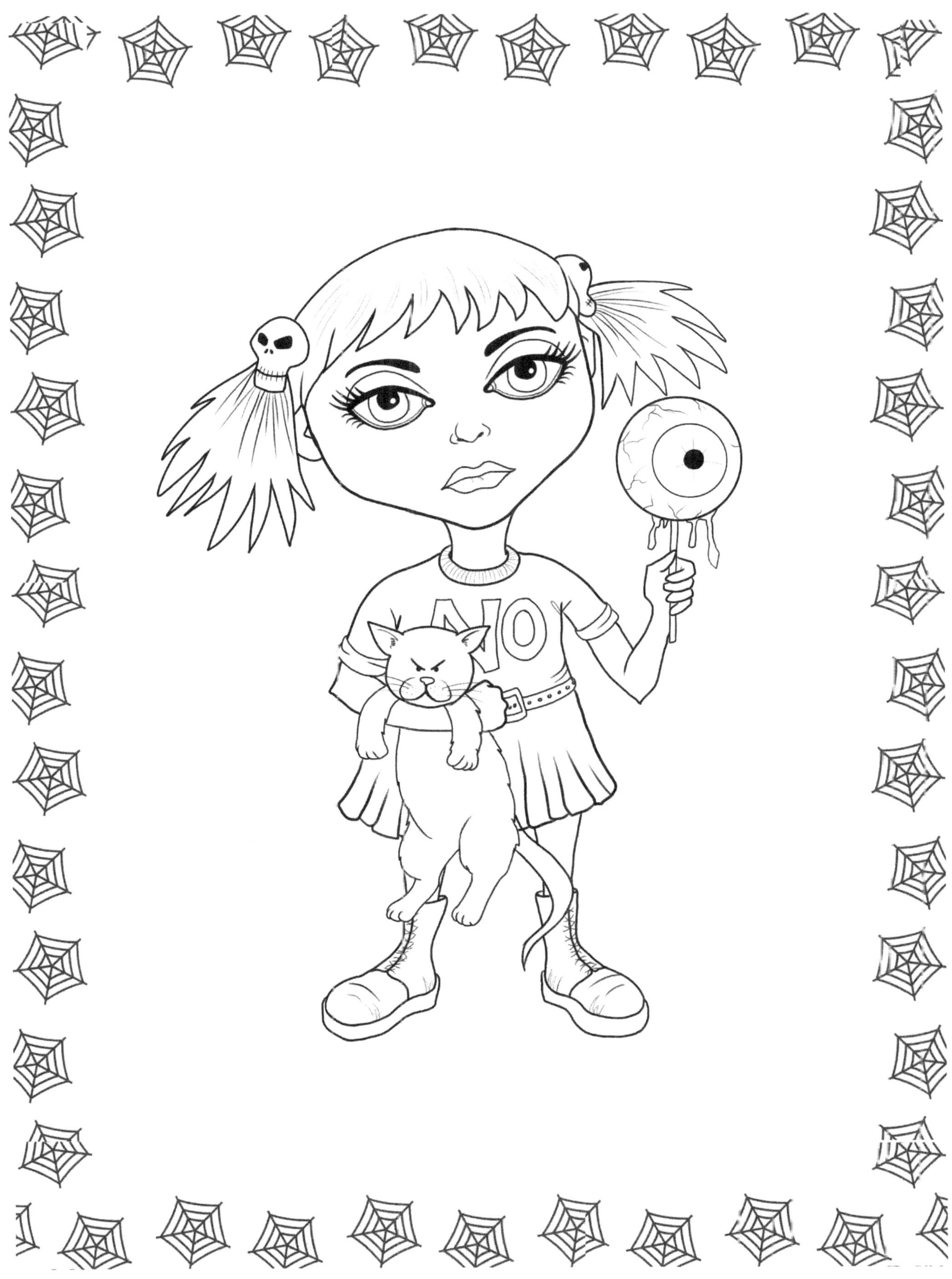

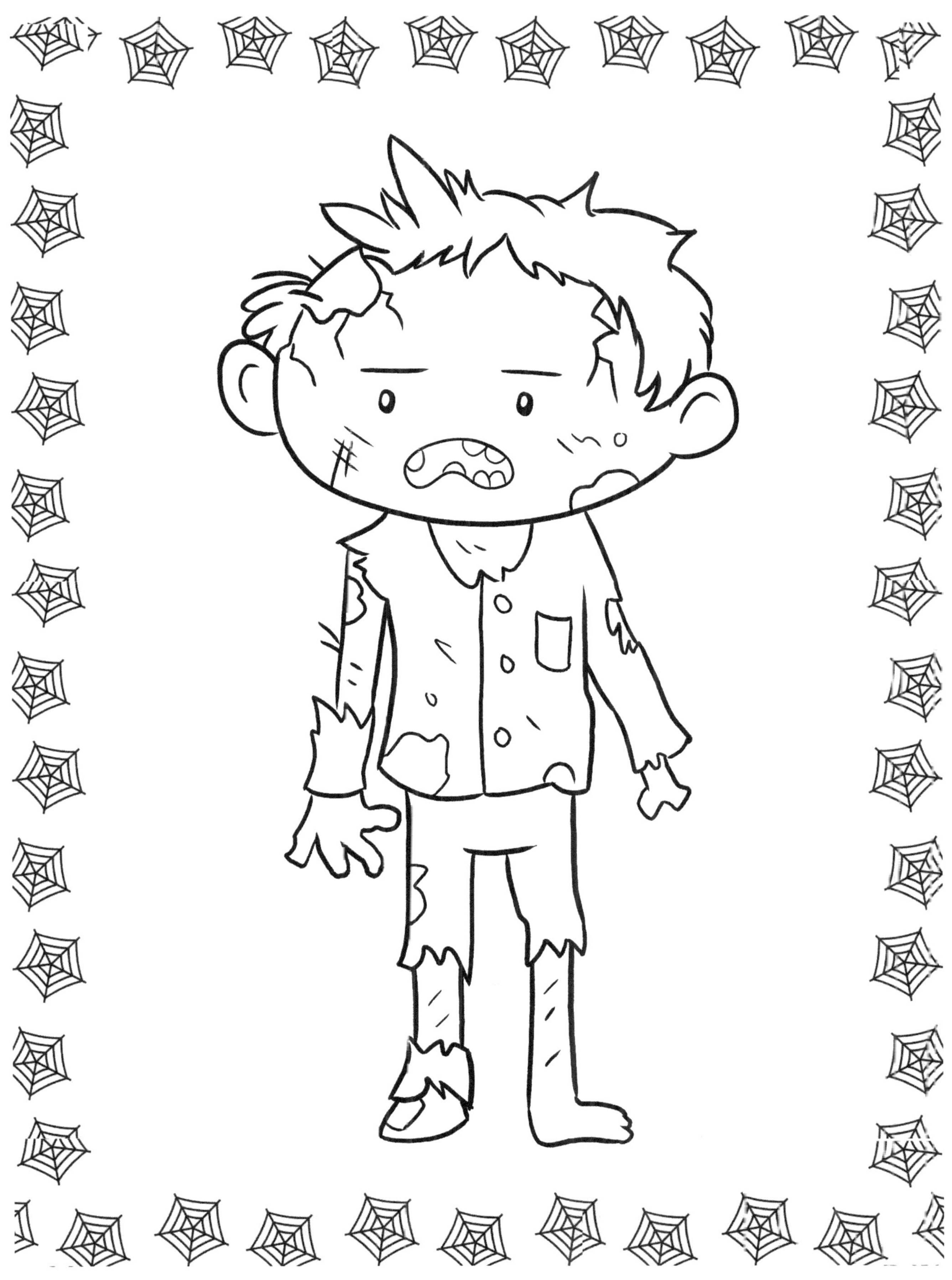

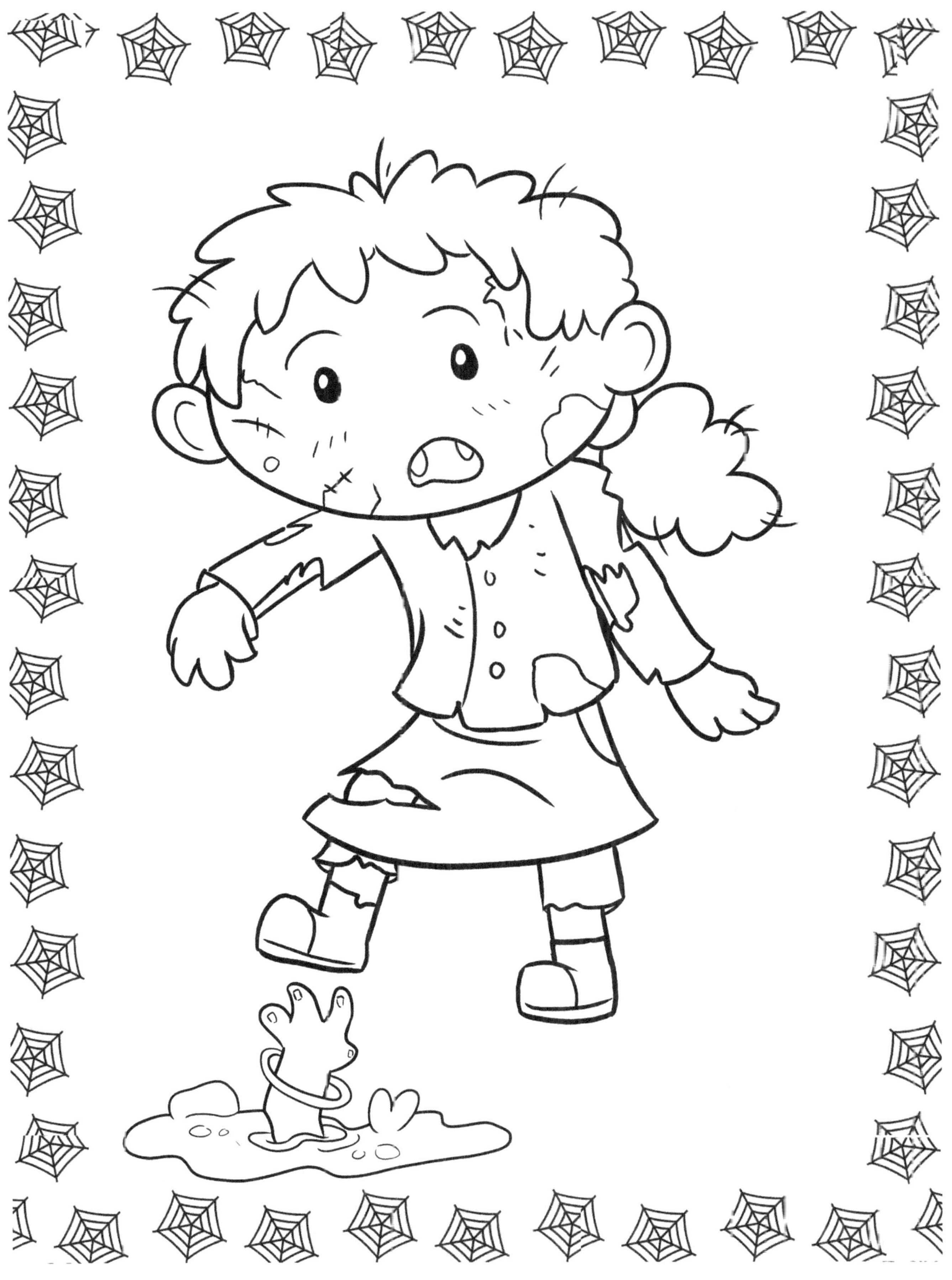

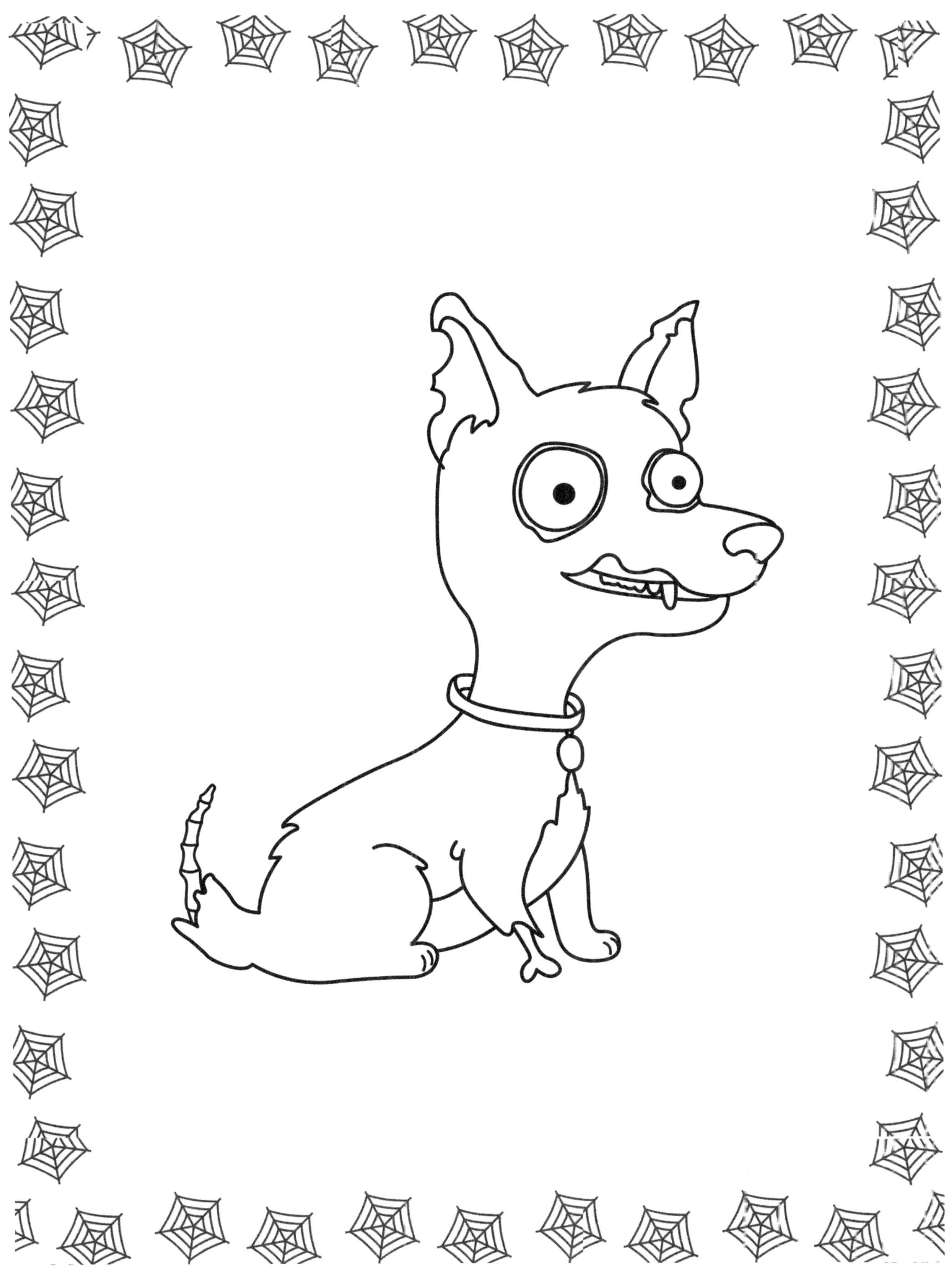

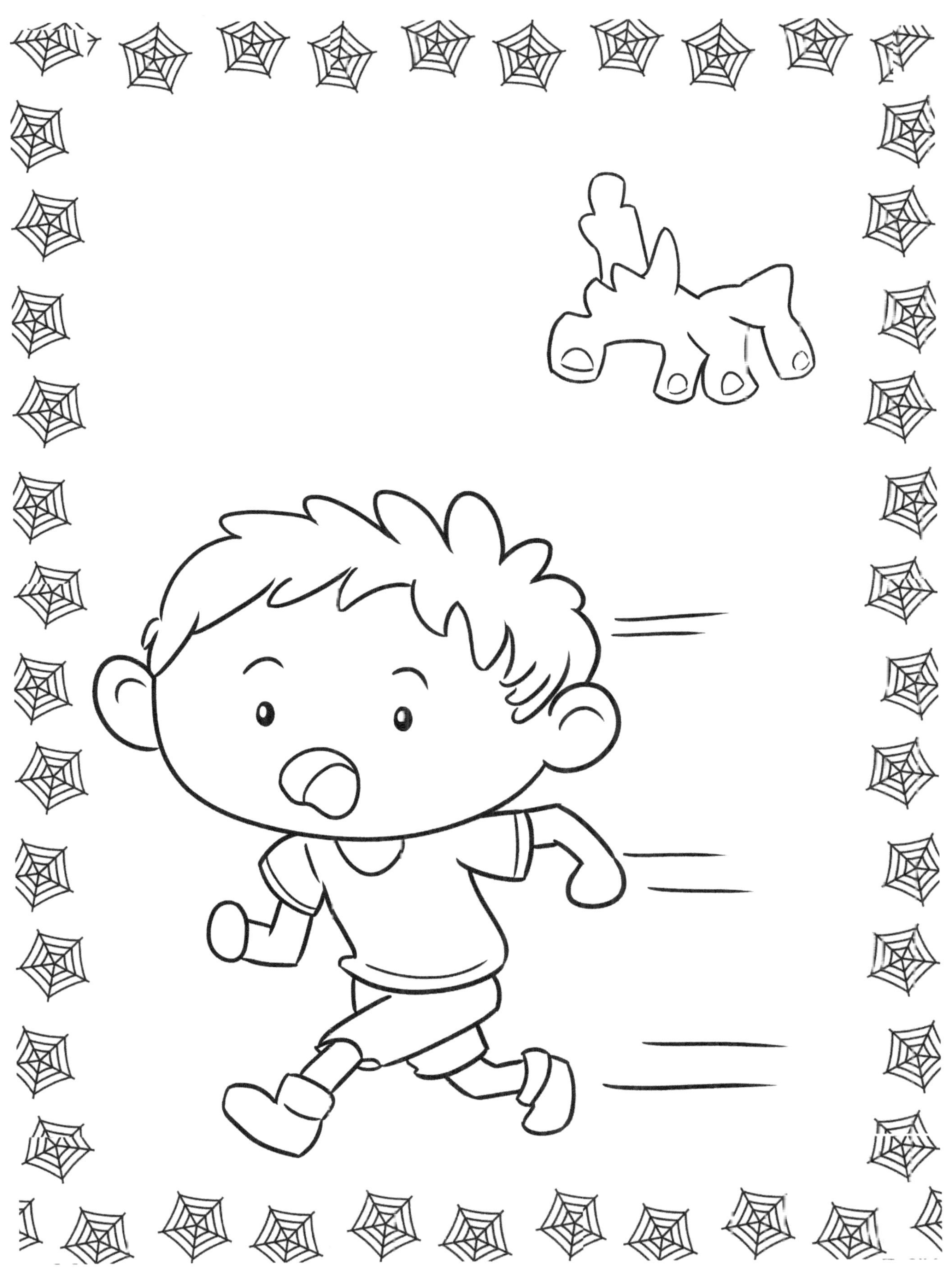

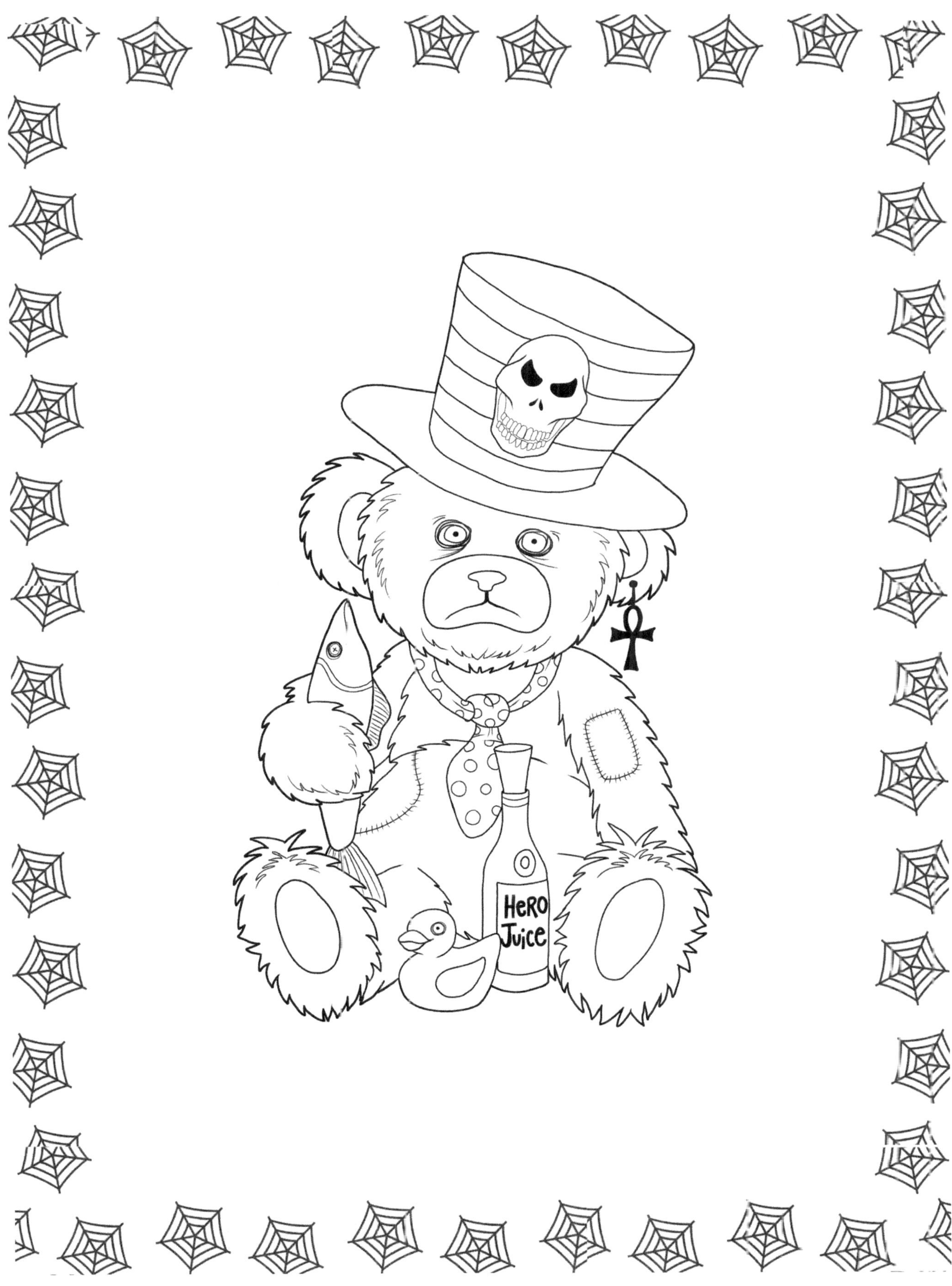

HeRO
Juice

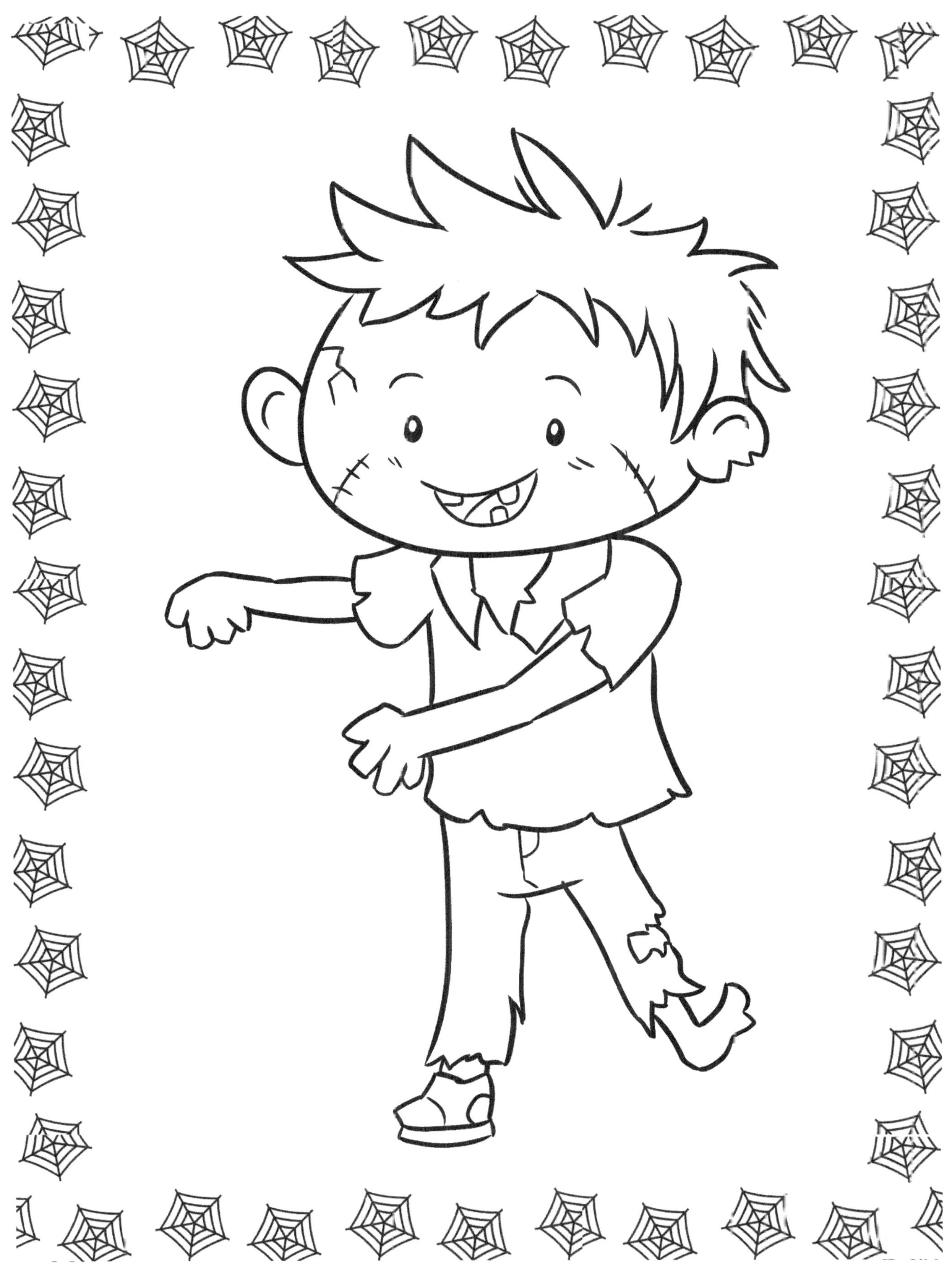

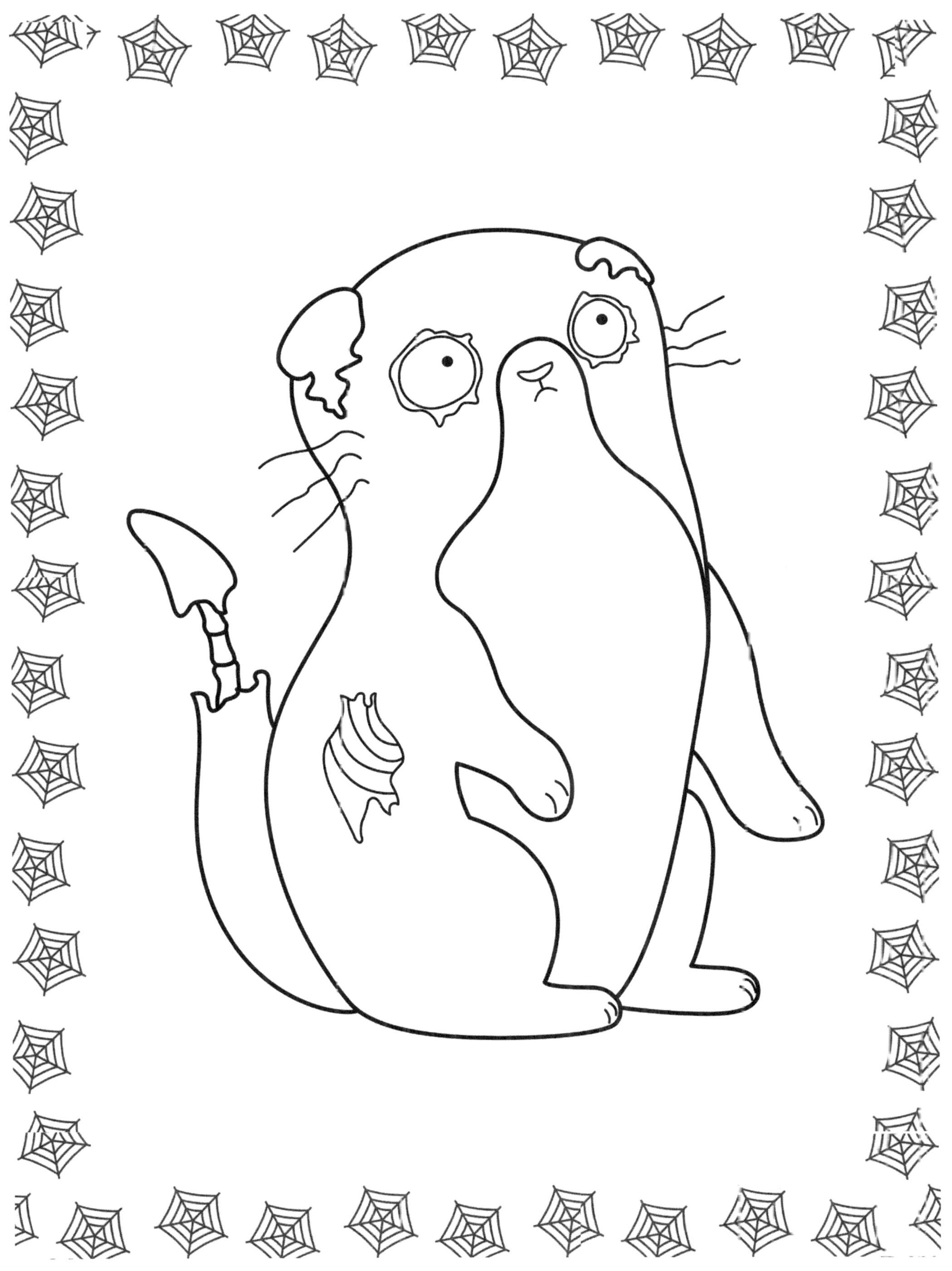

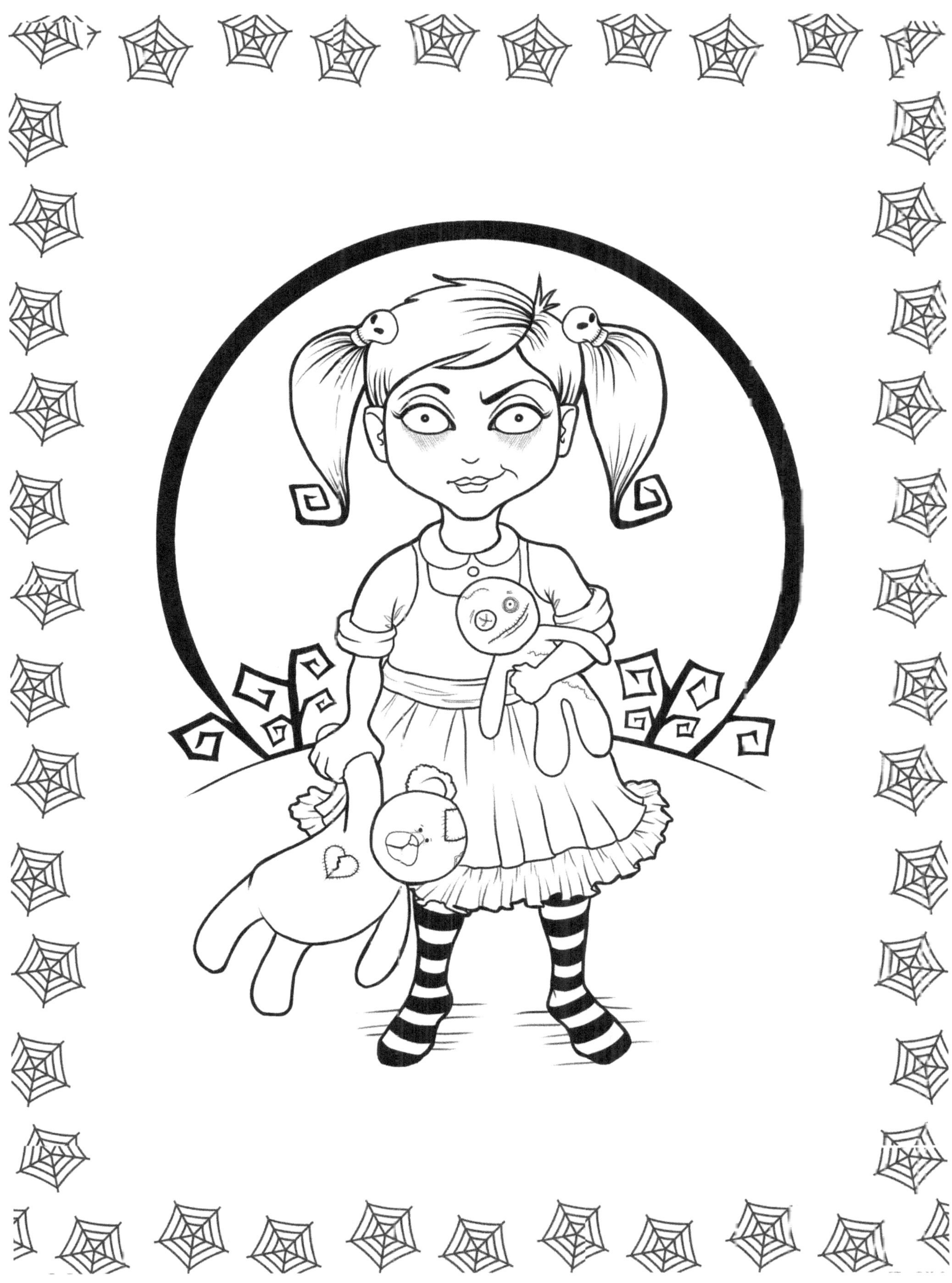

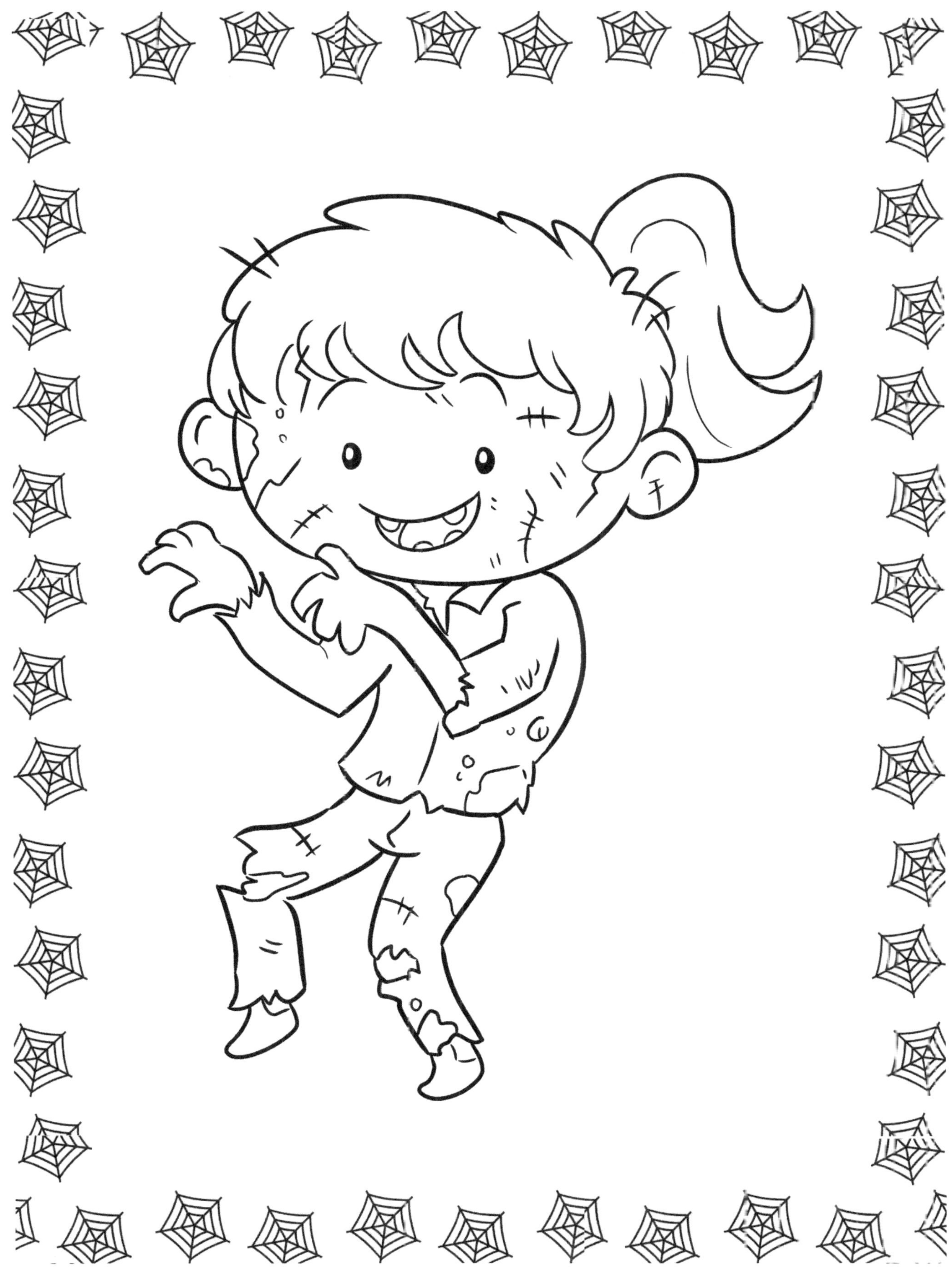

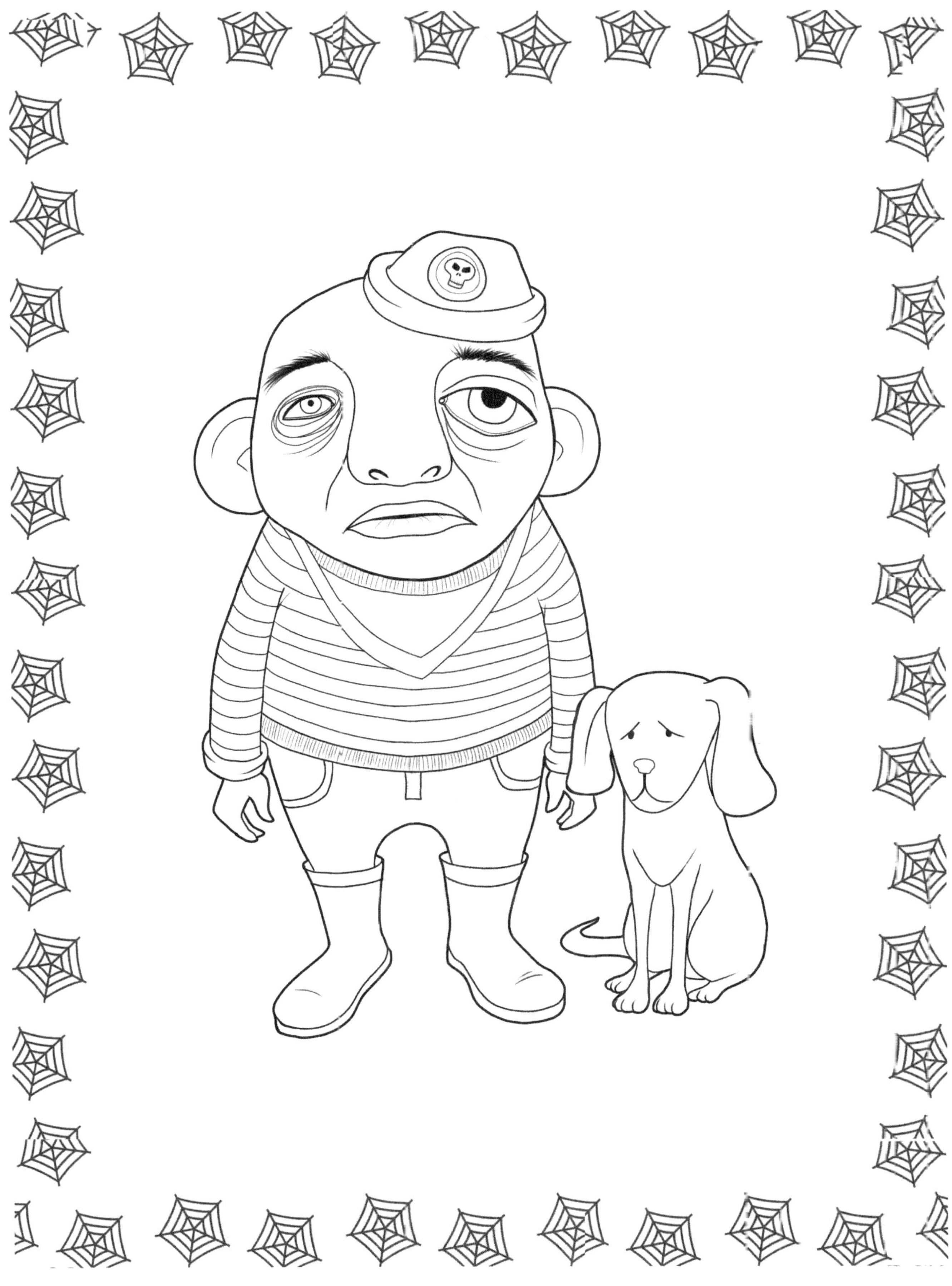

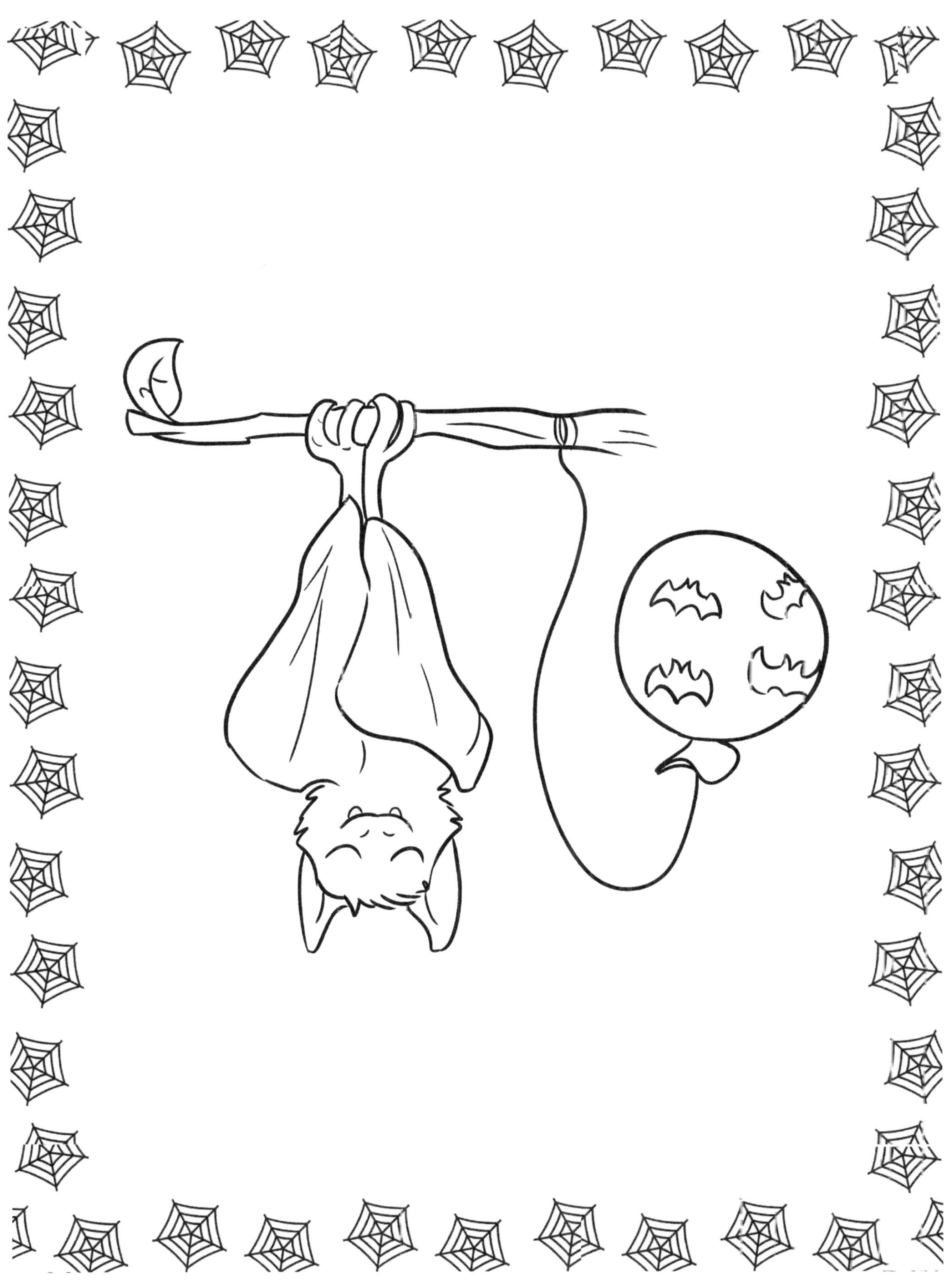

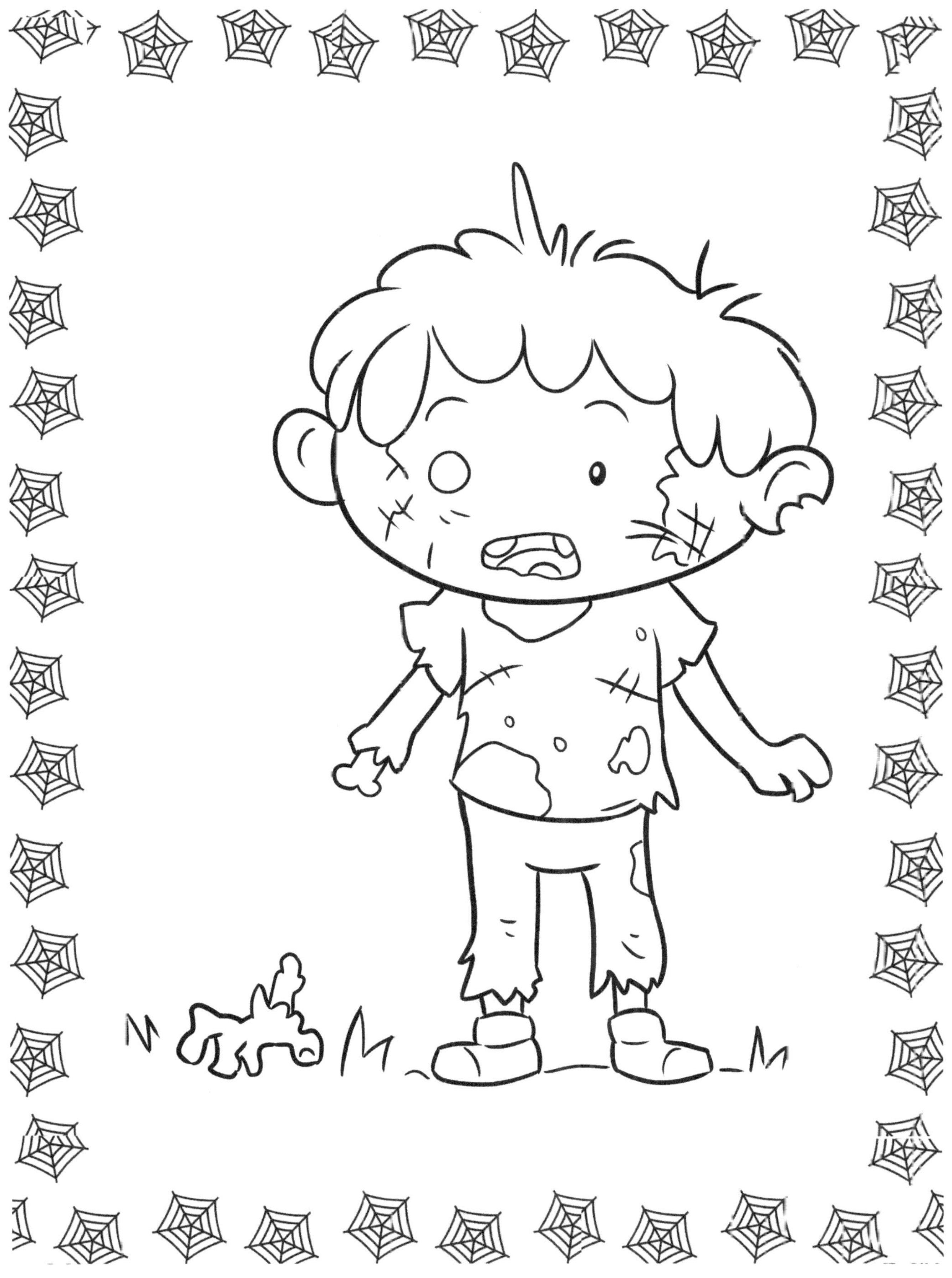

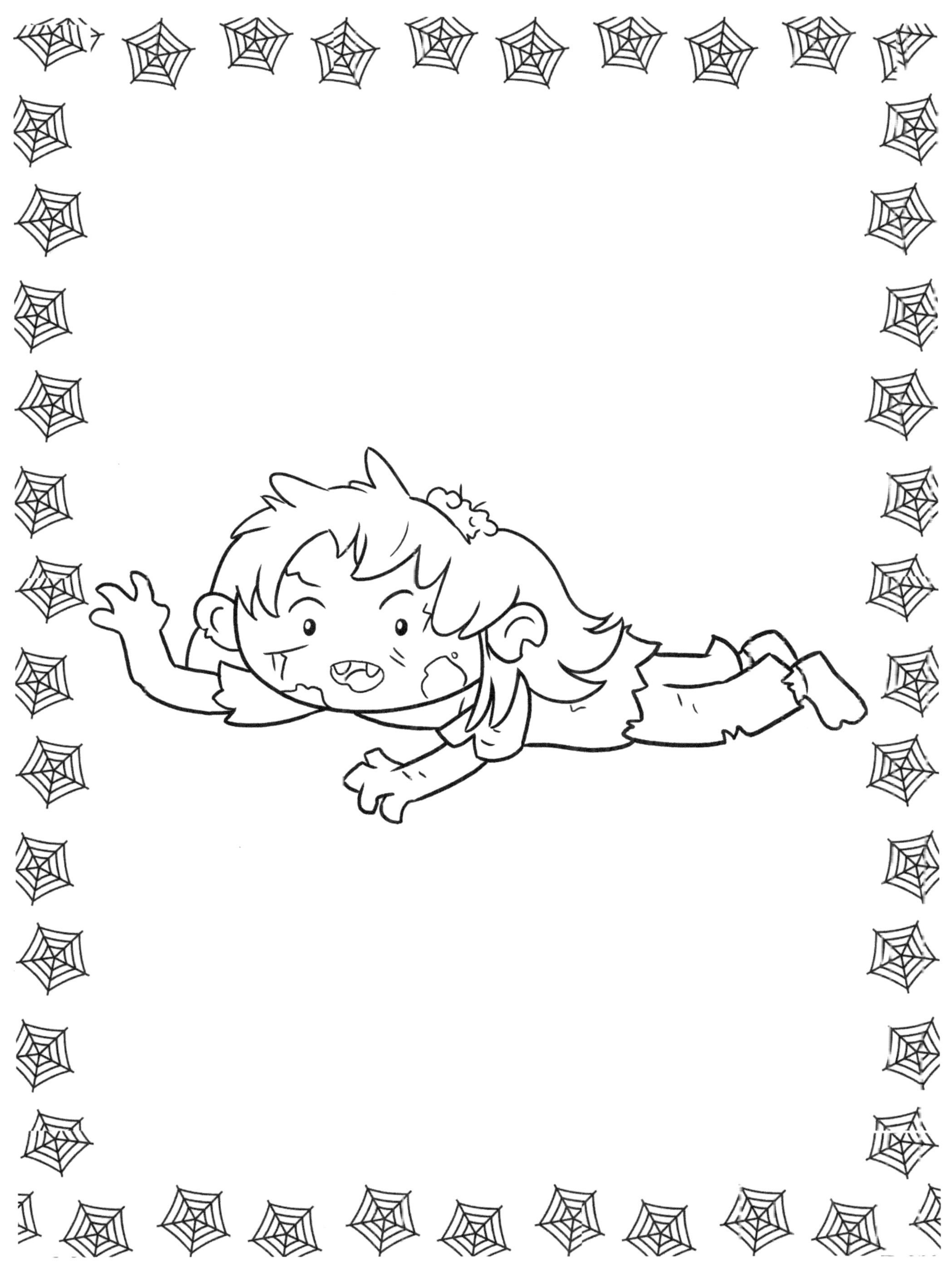

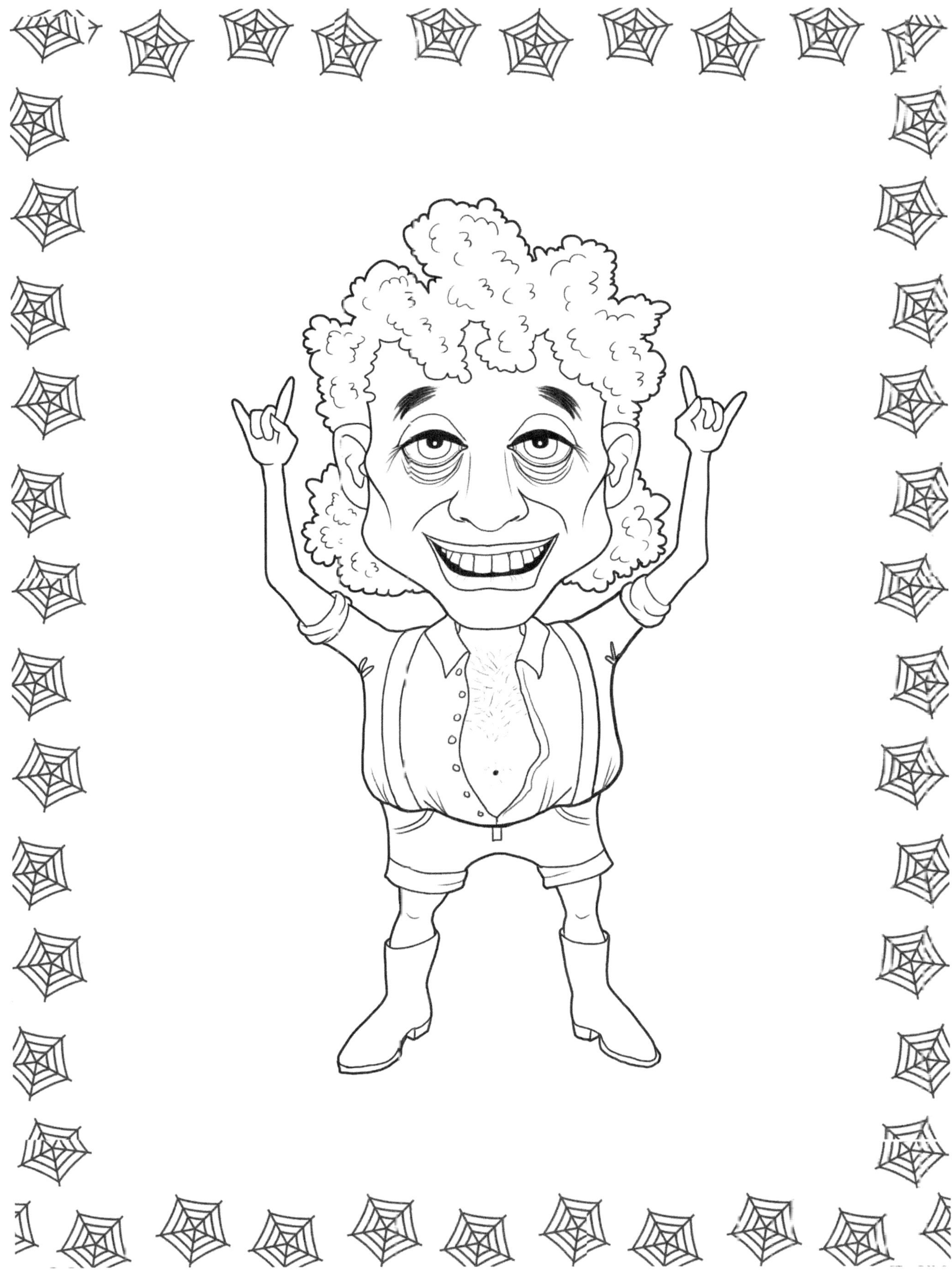

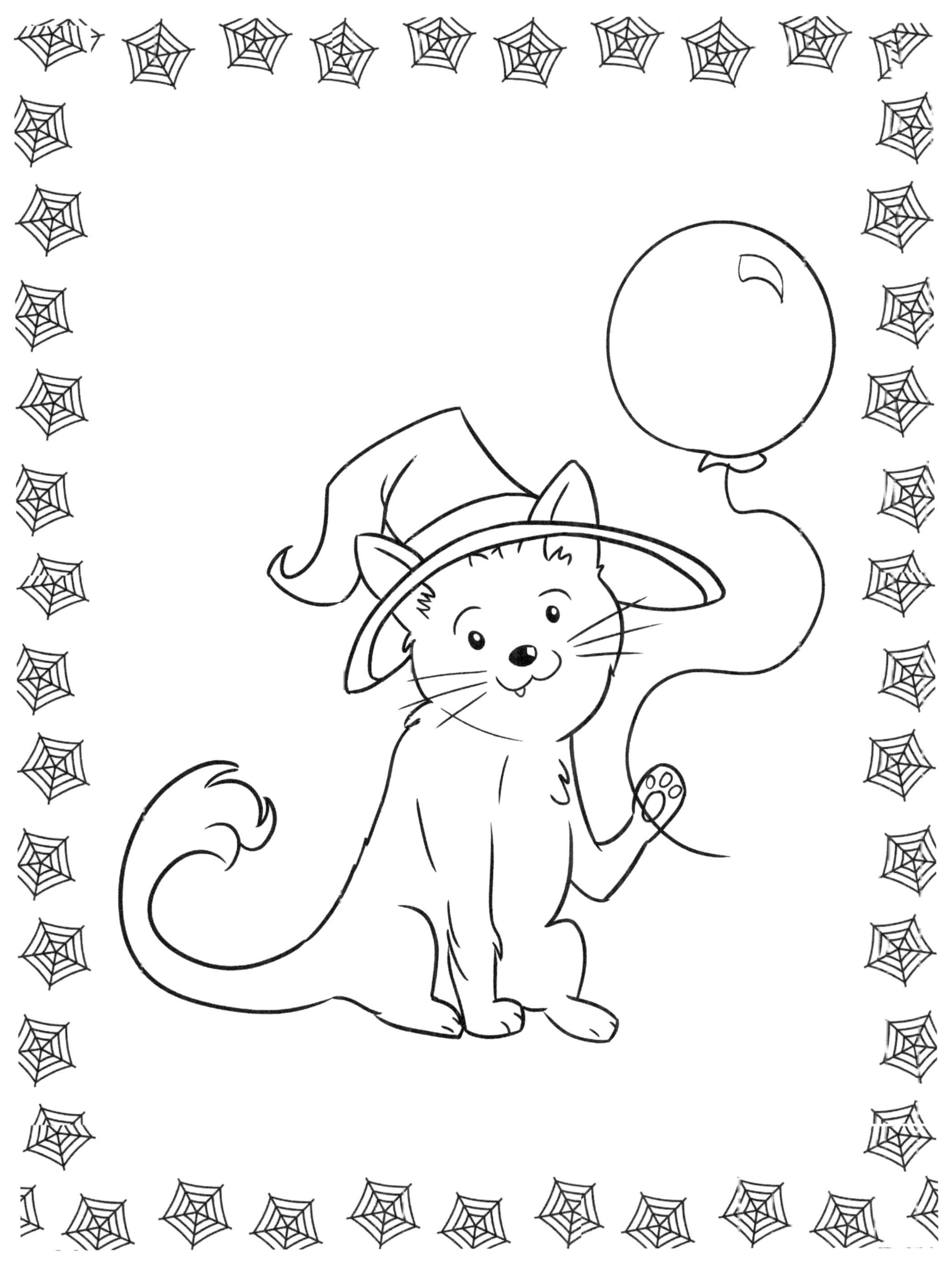

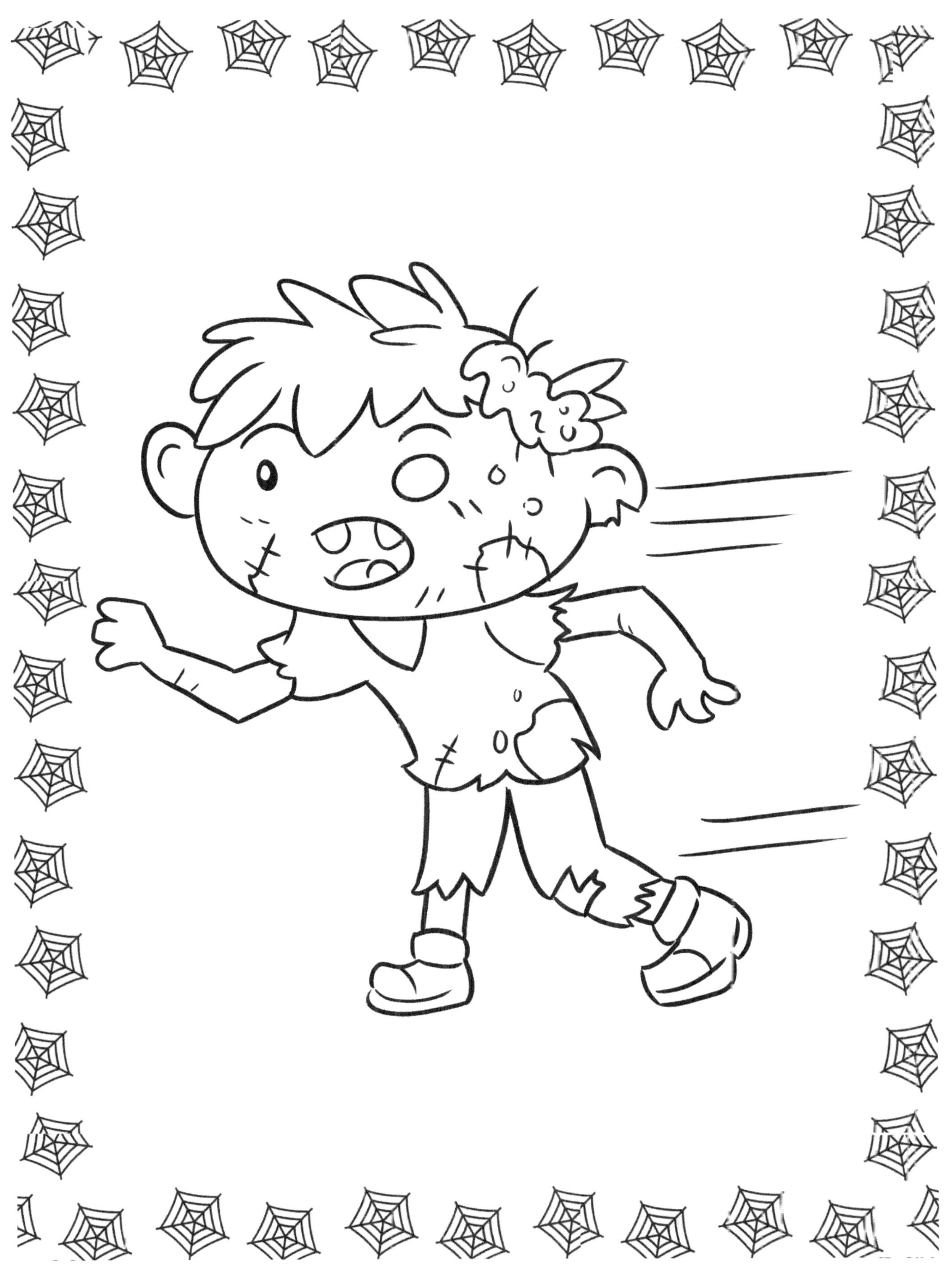

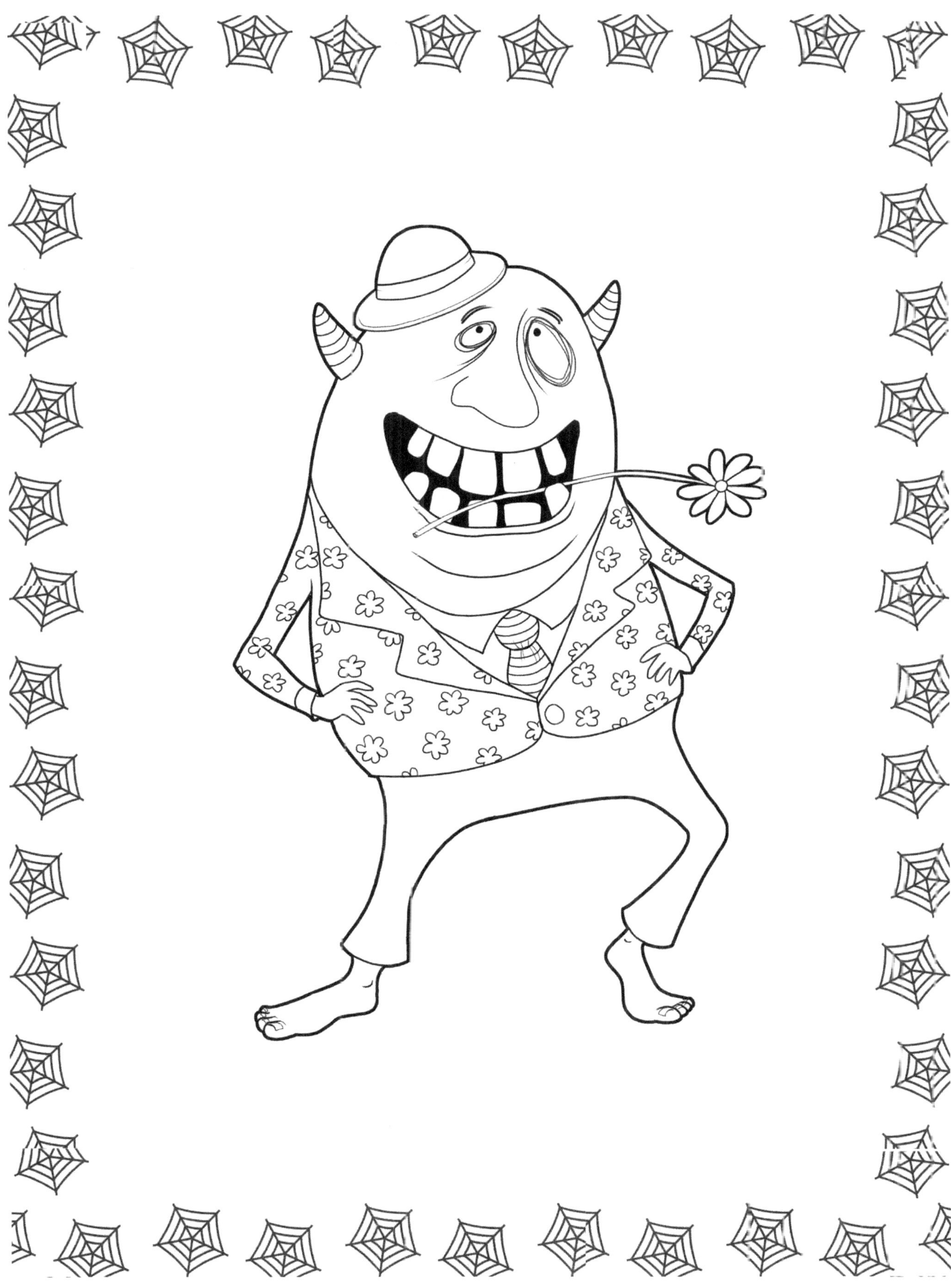

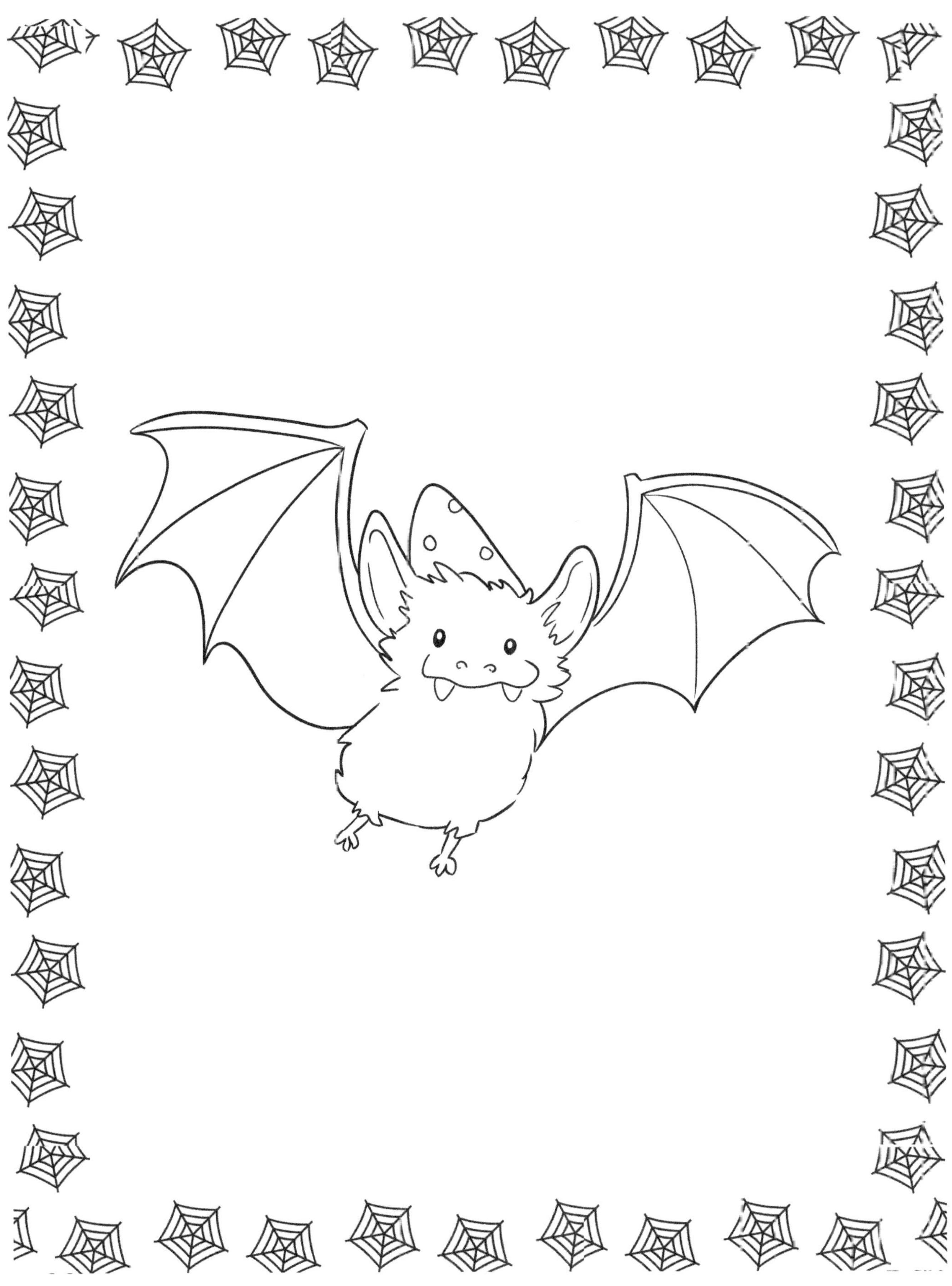

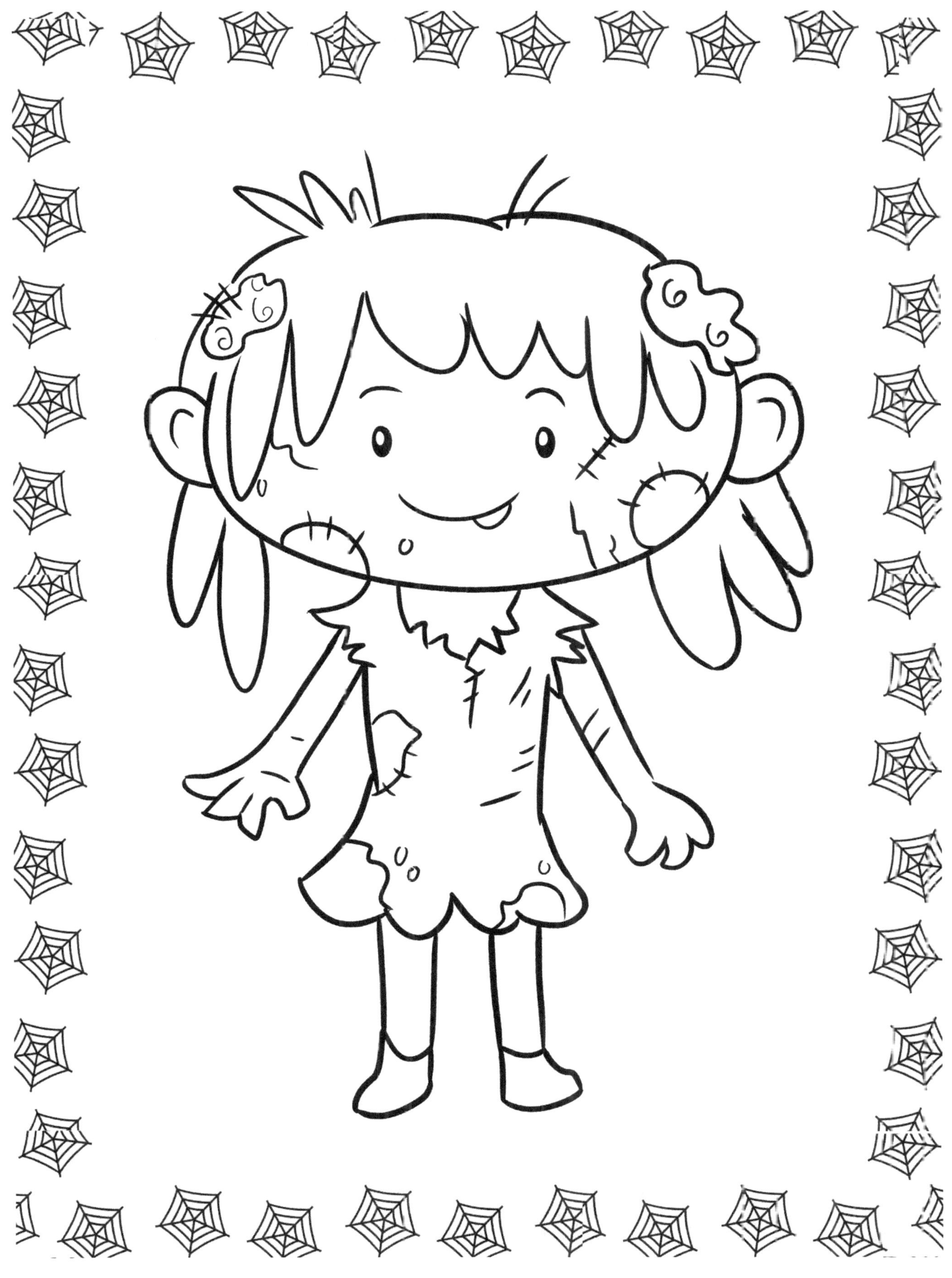

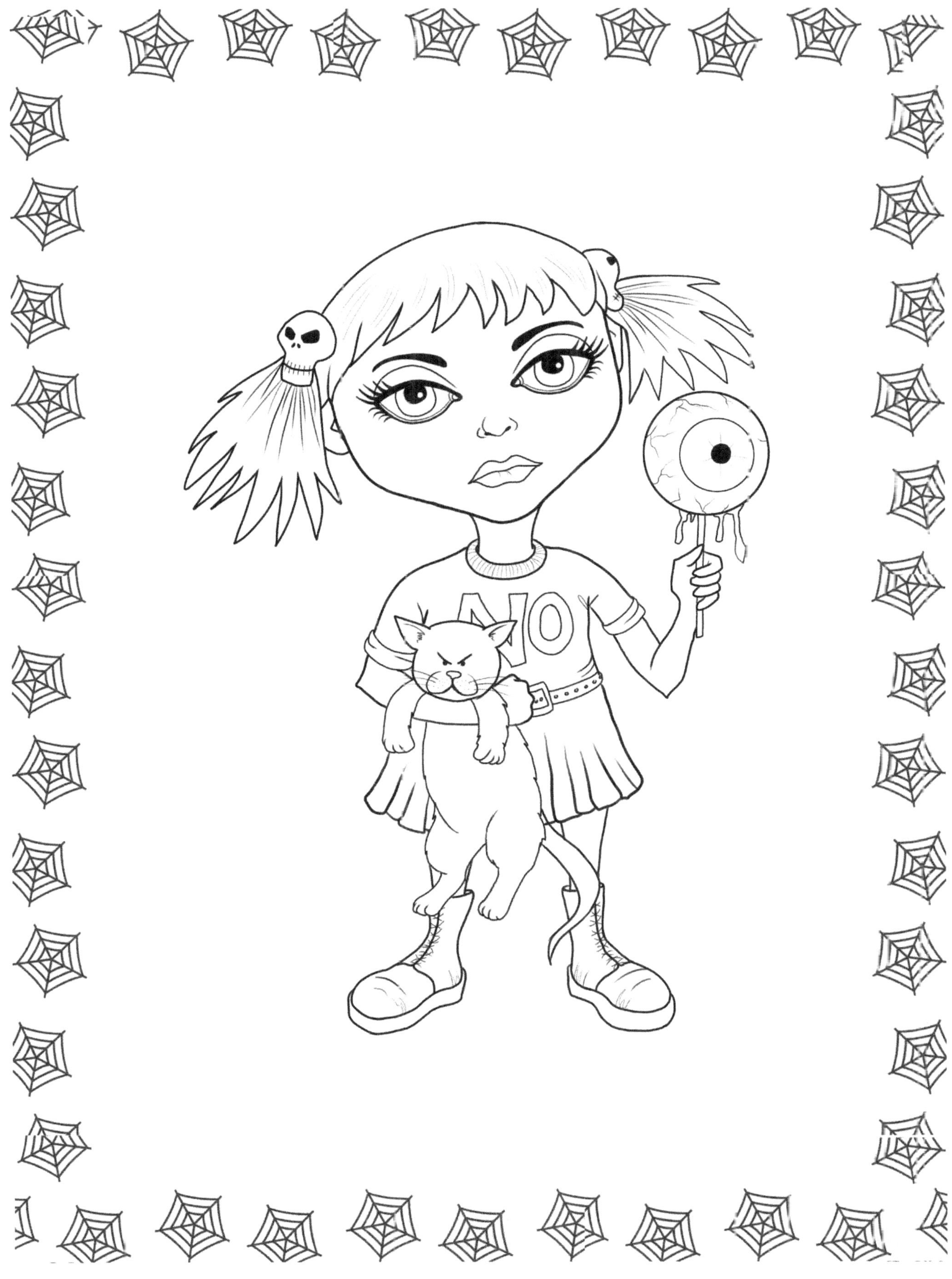
NO

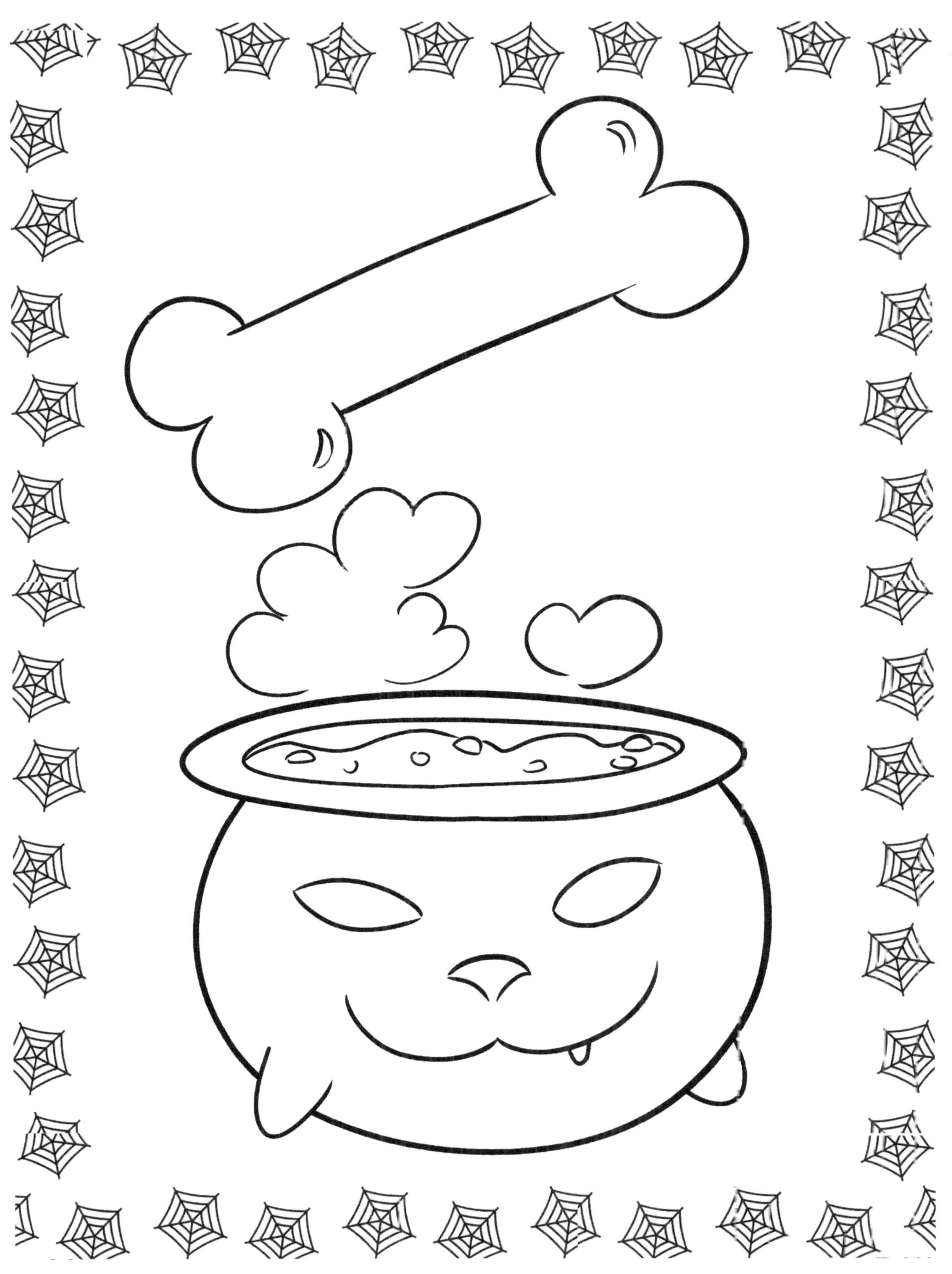

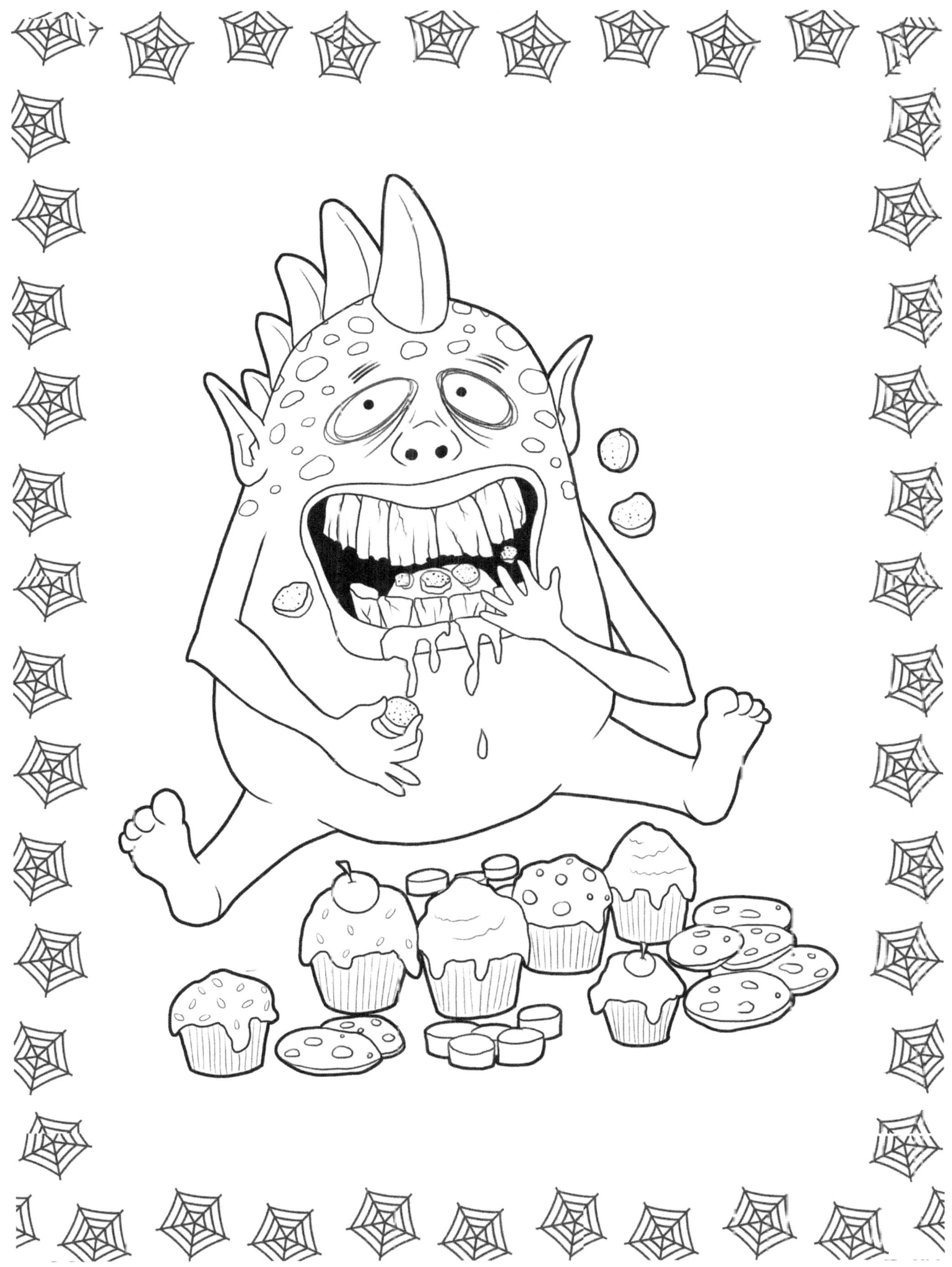

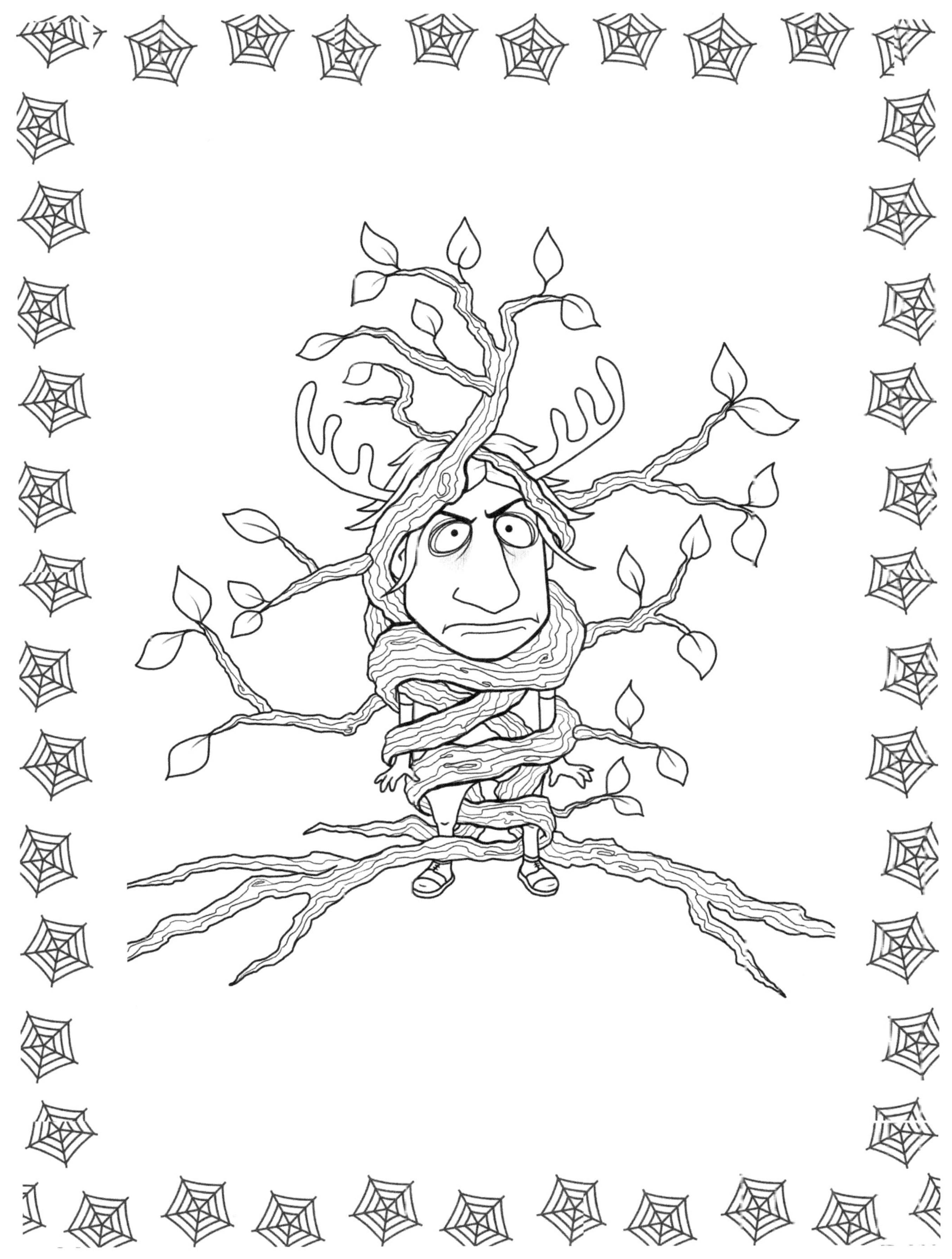

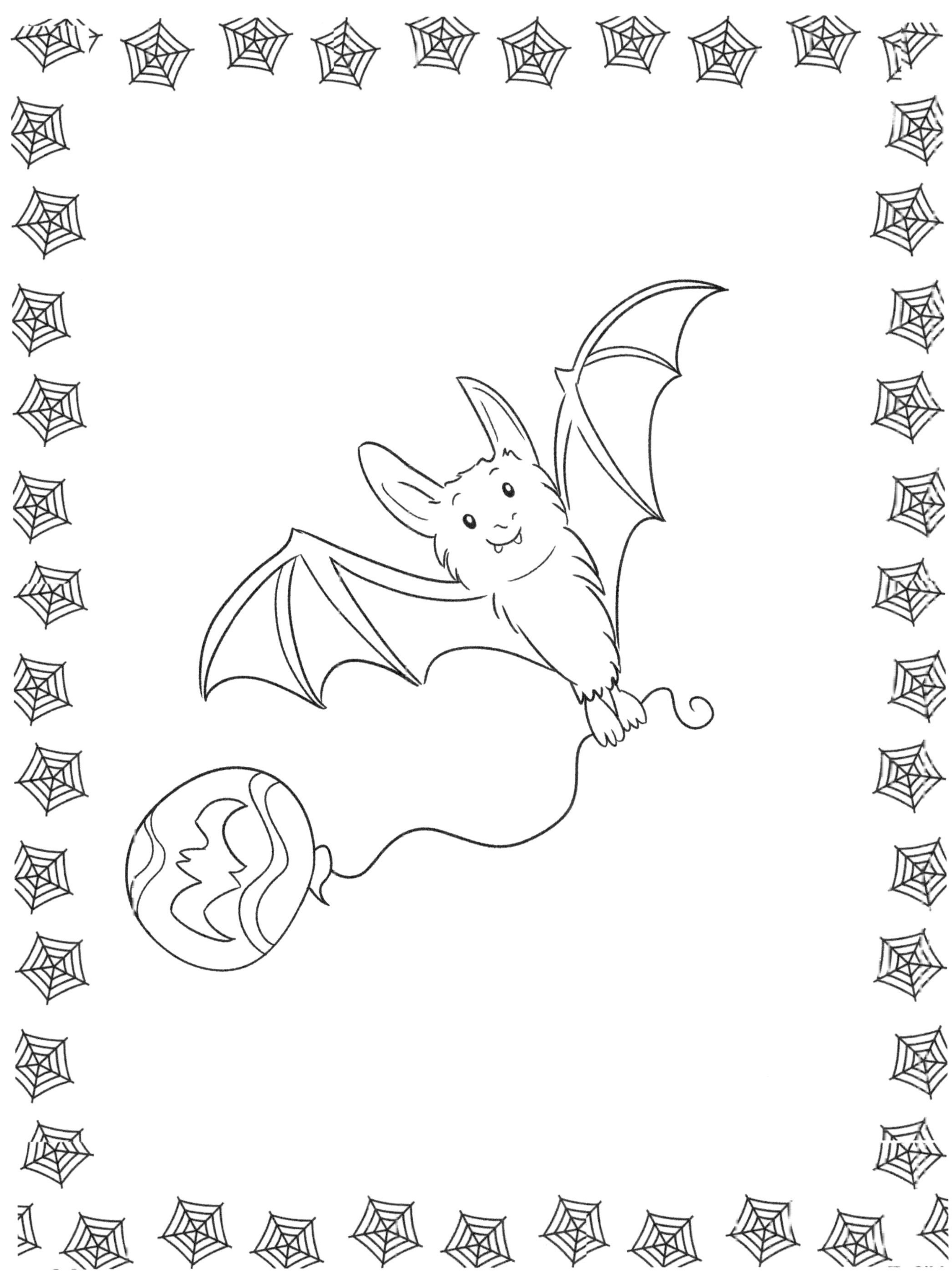

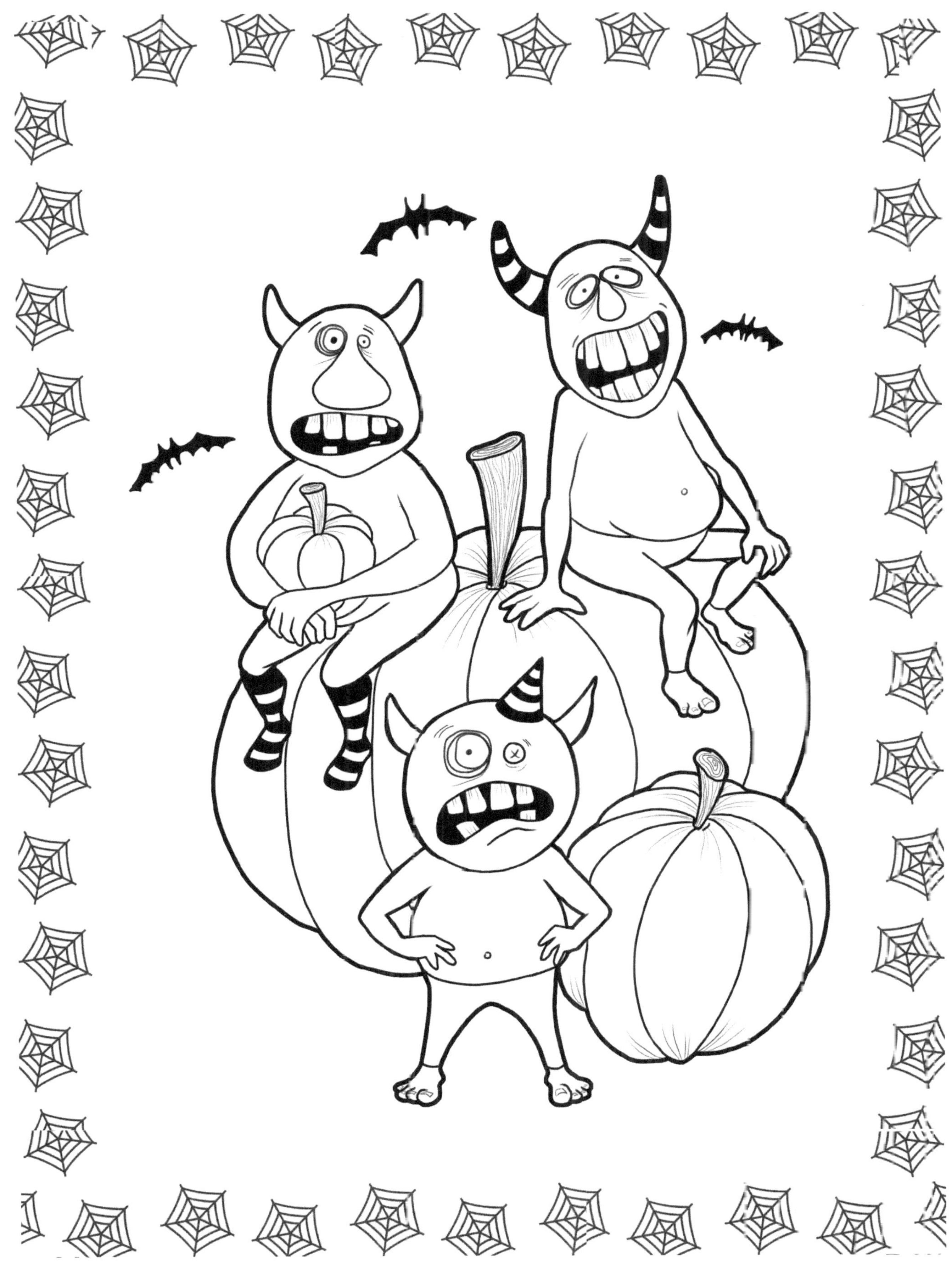

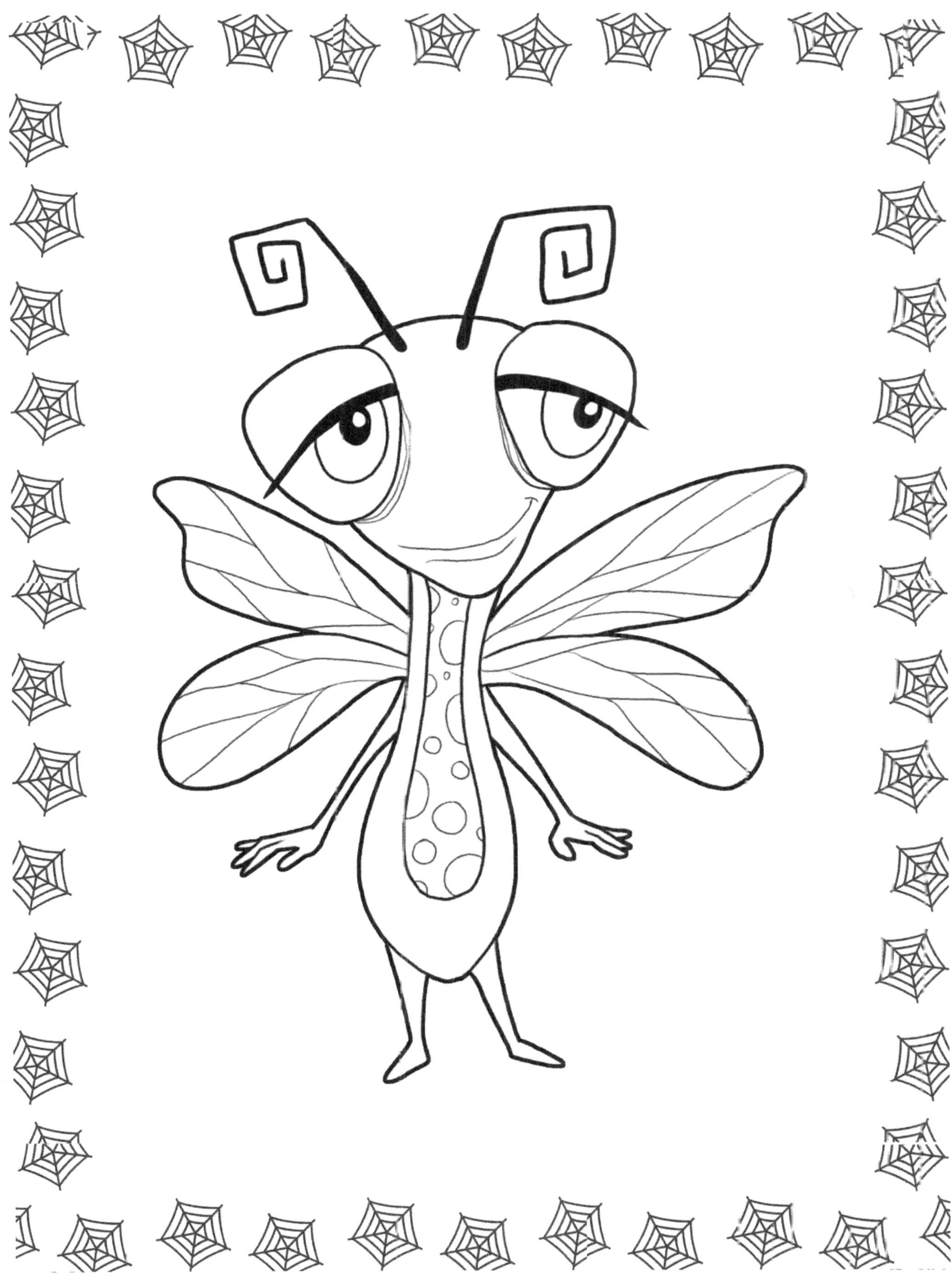

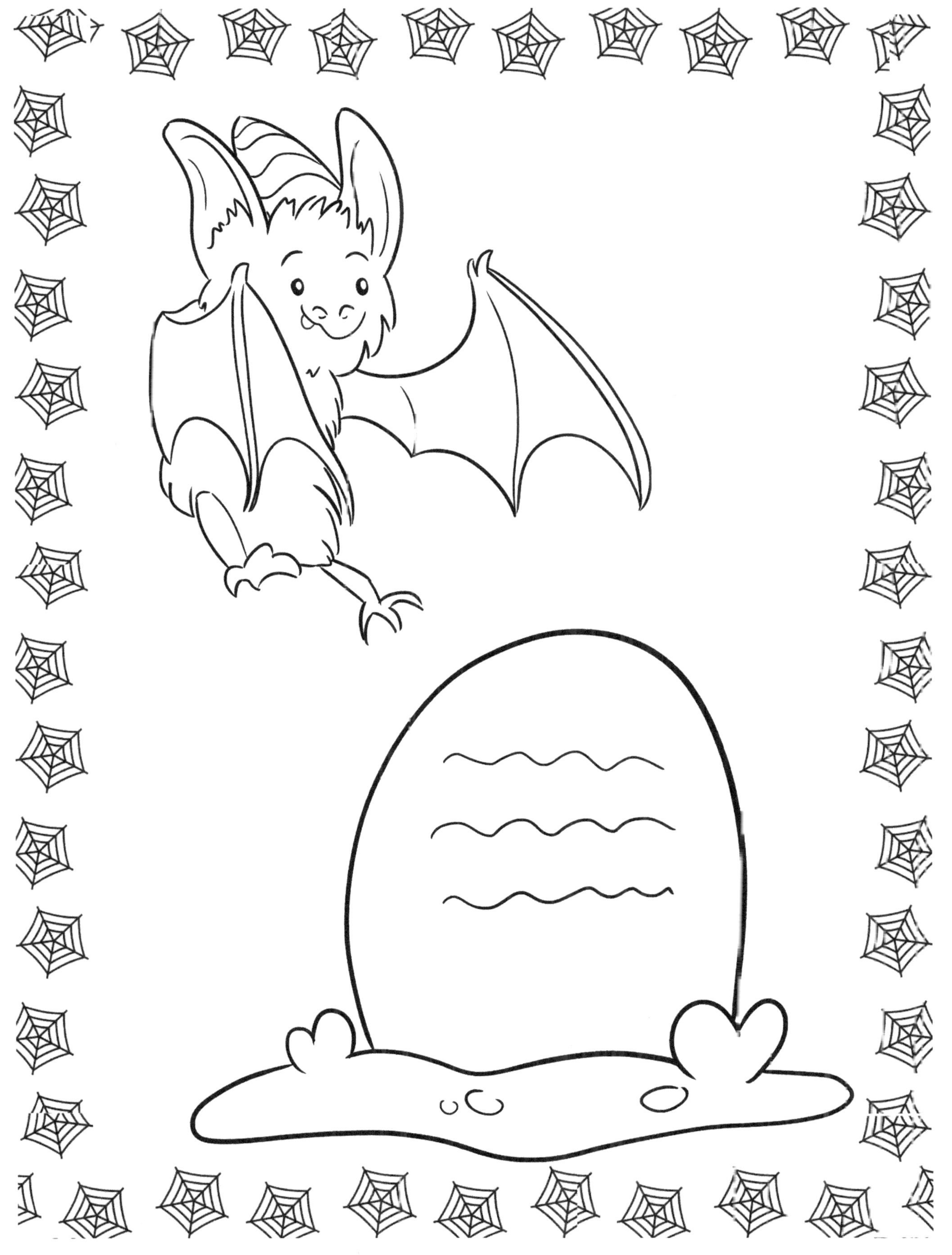

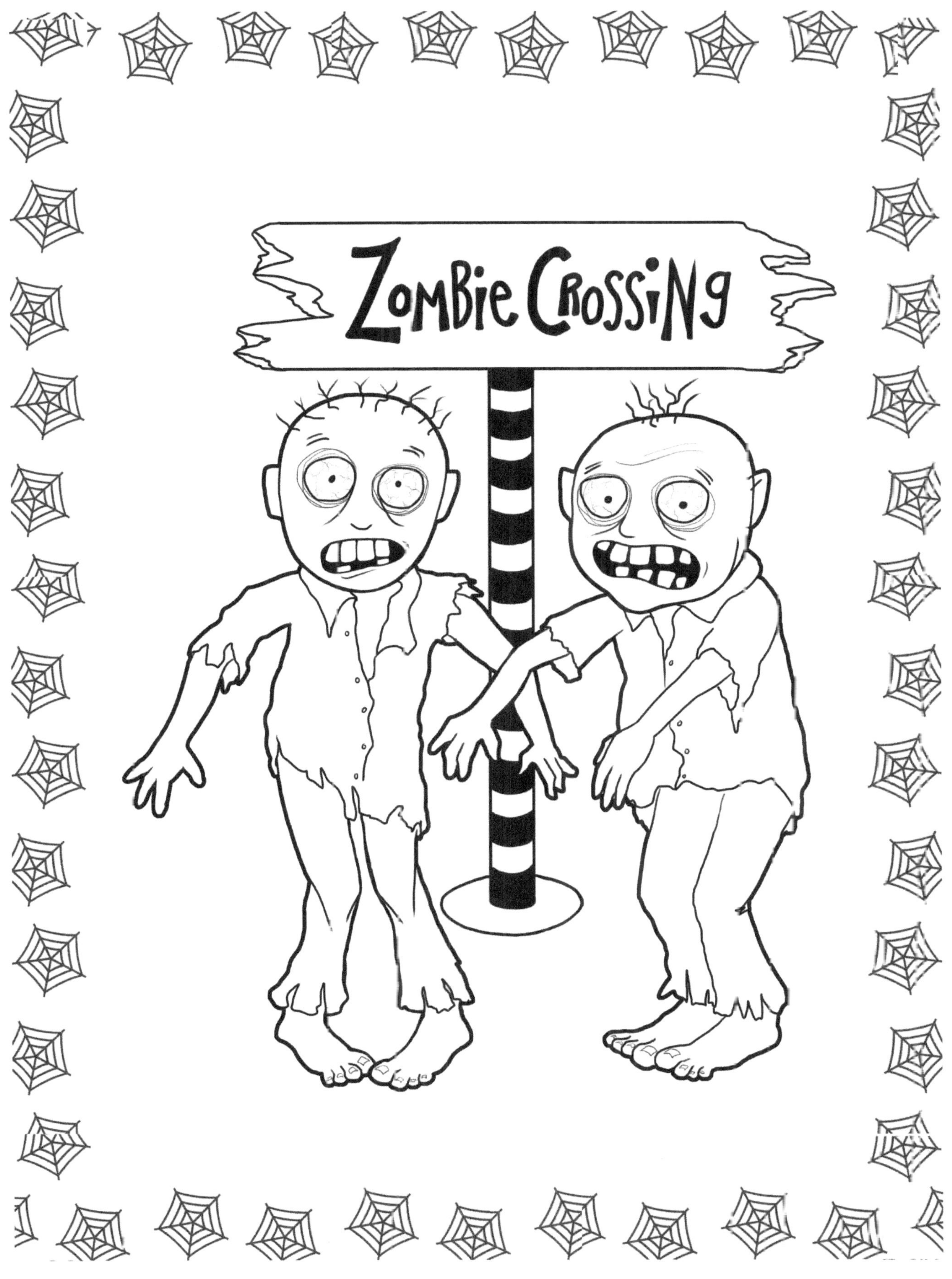

Zombie Crossing

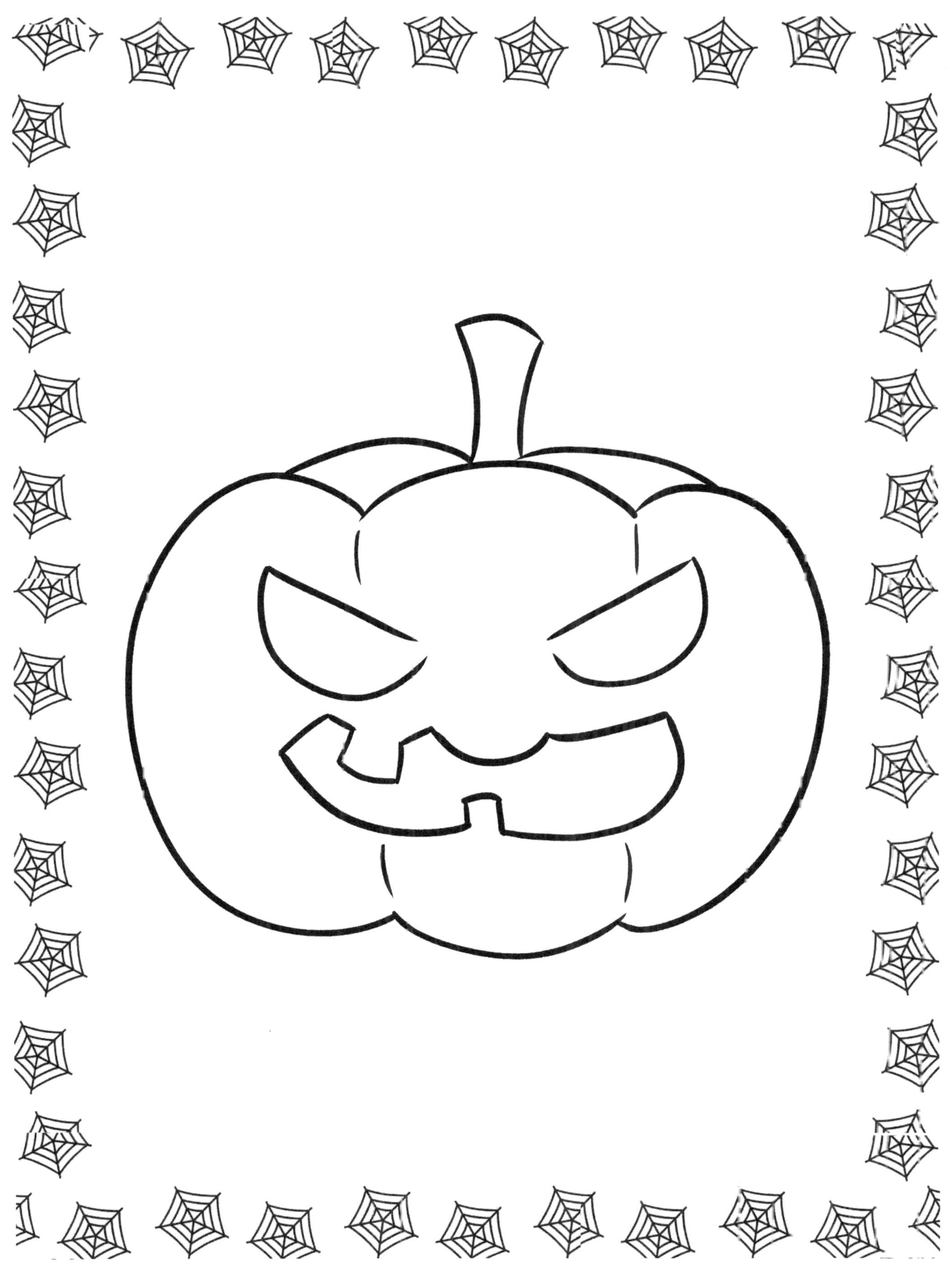

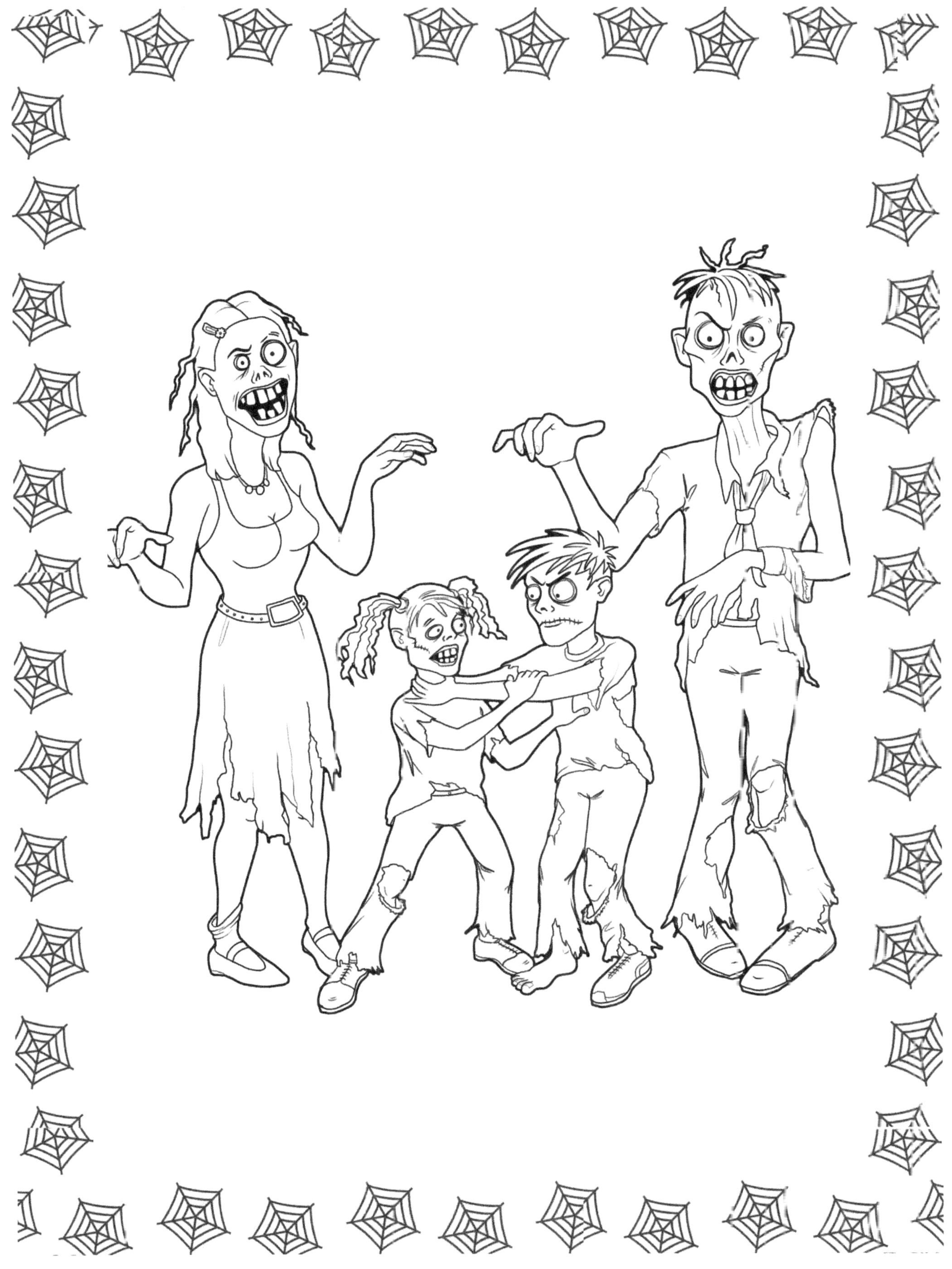

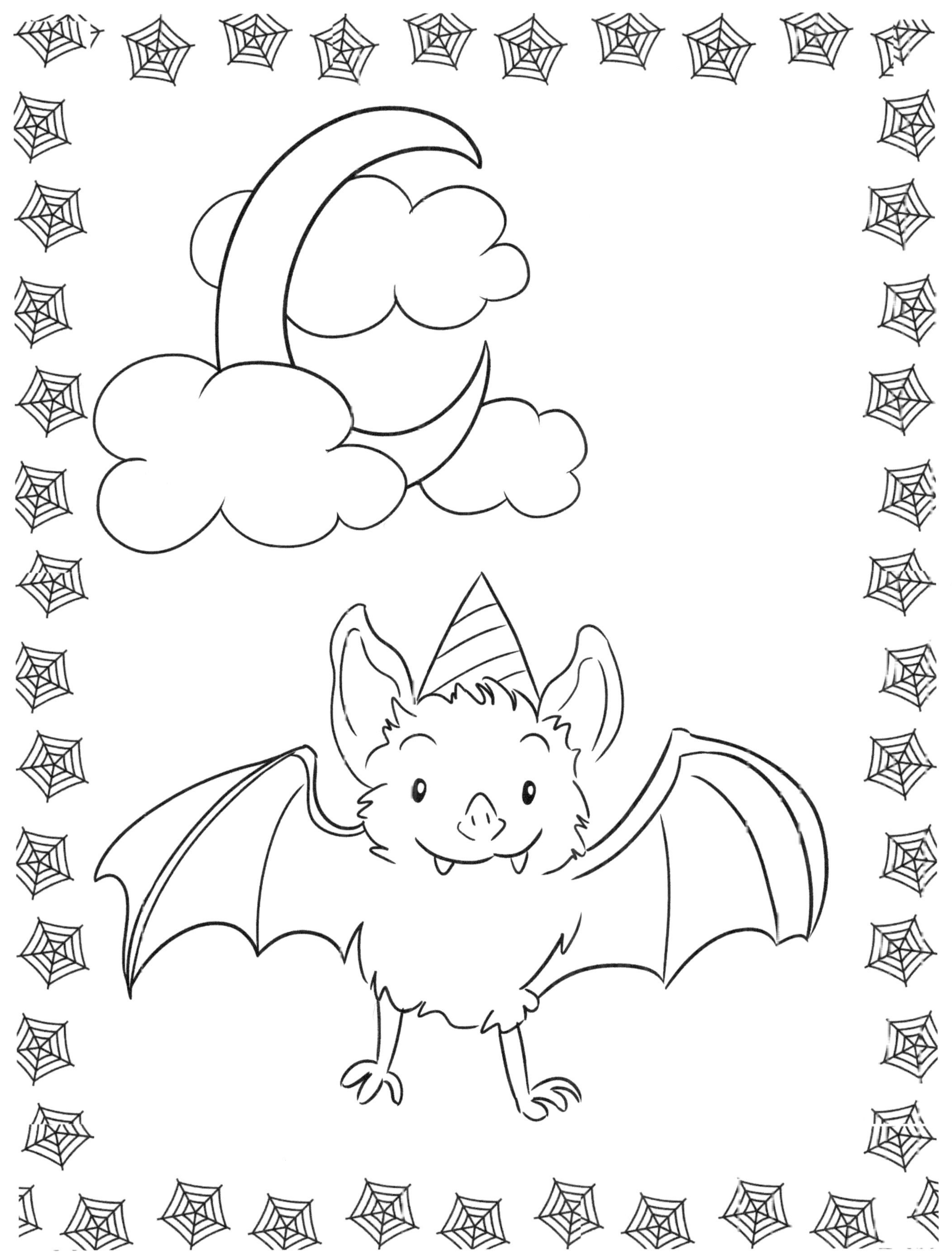

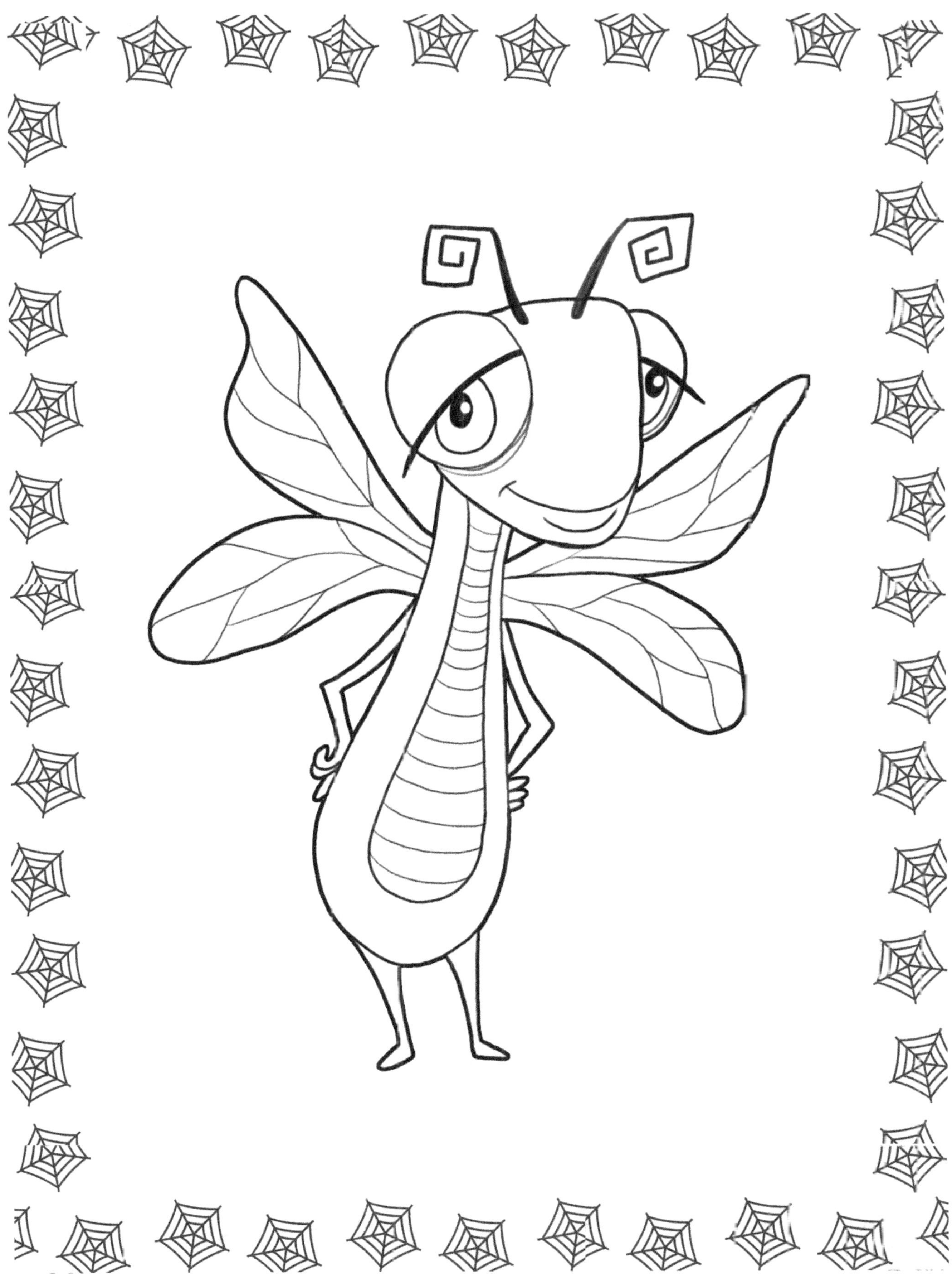

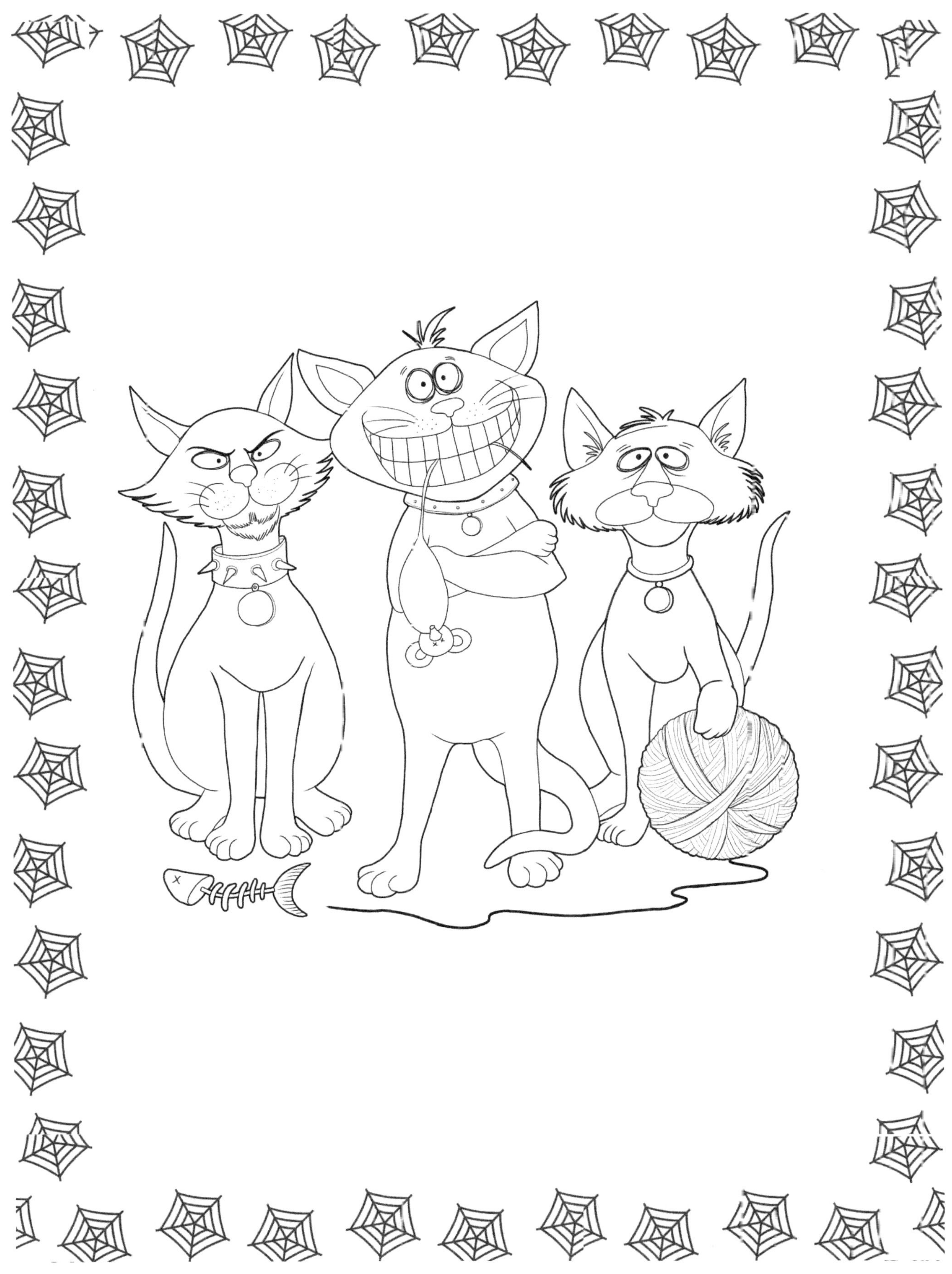

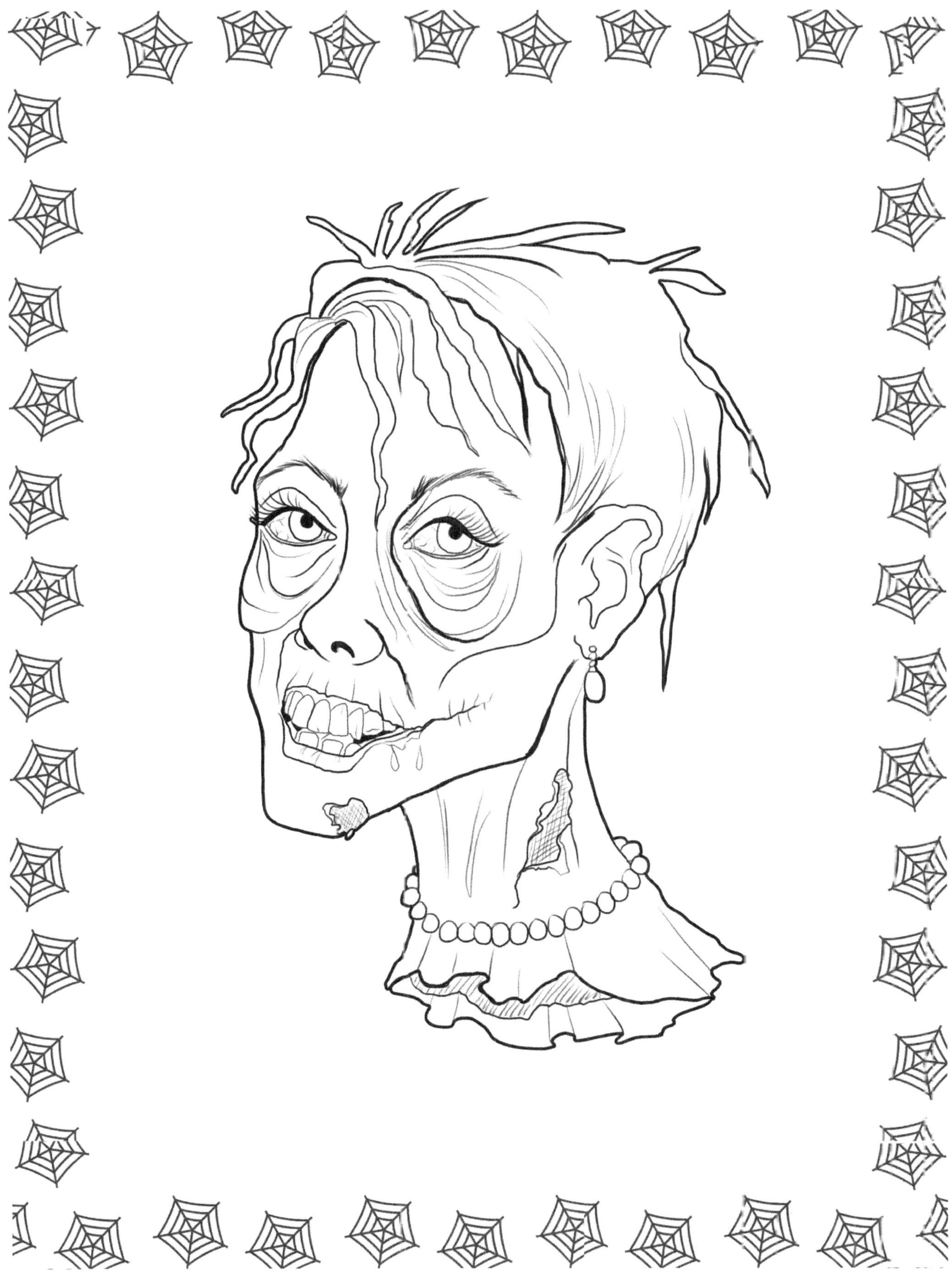

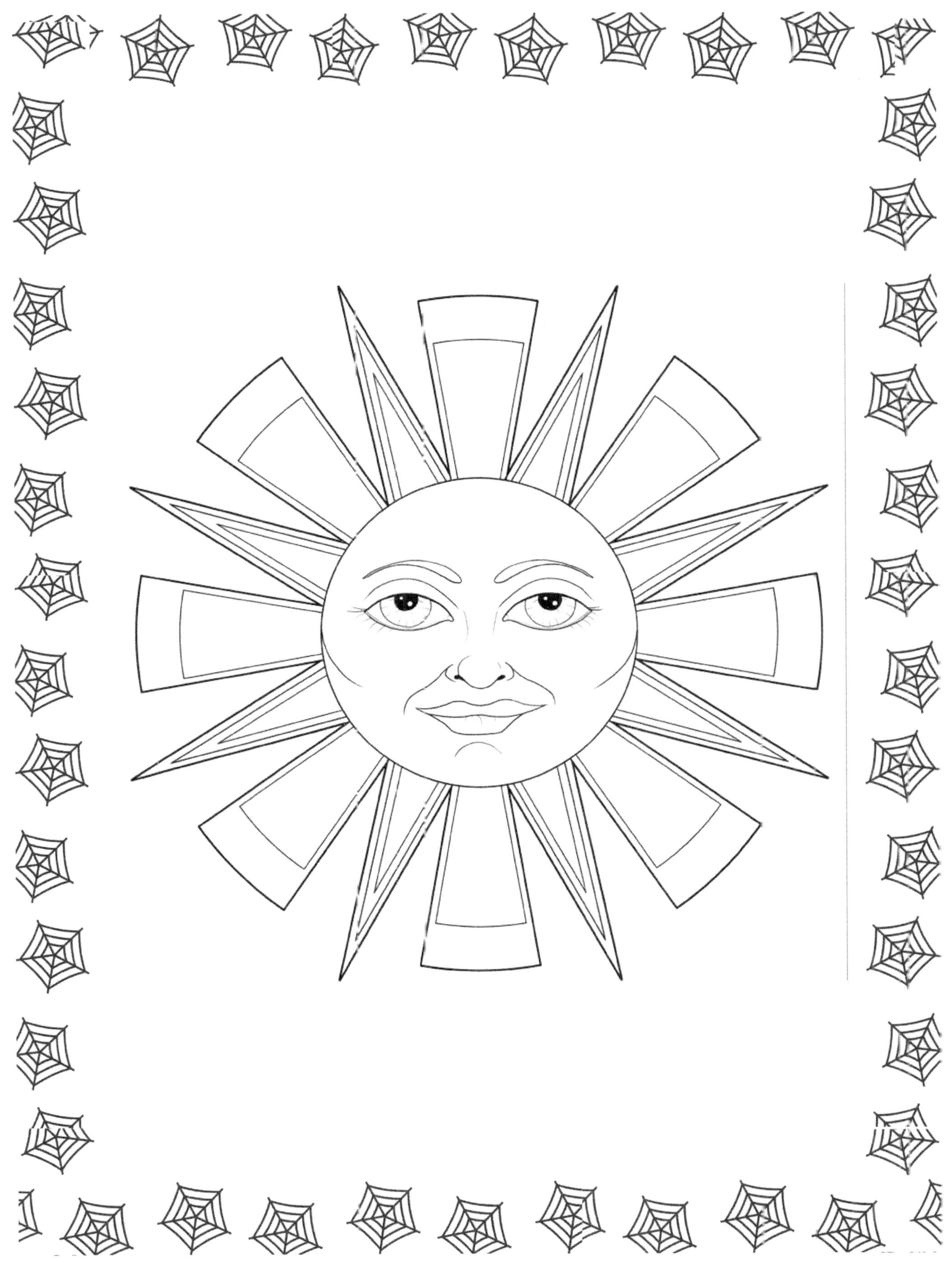

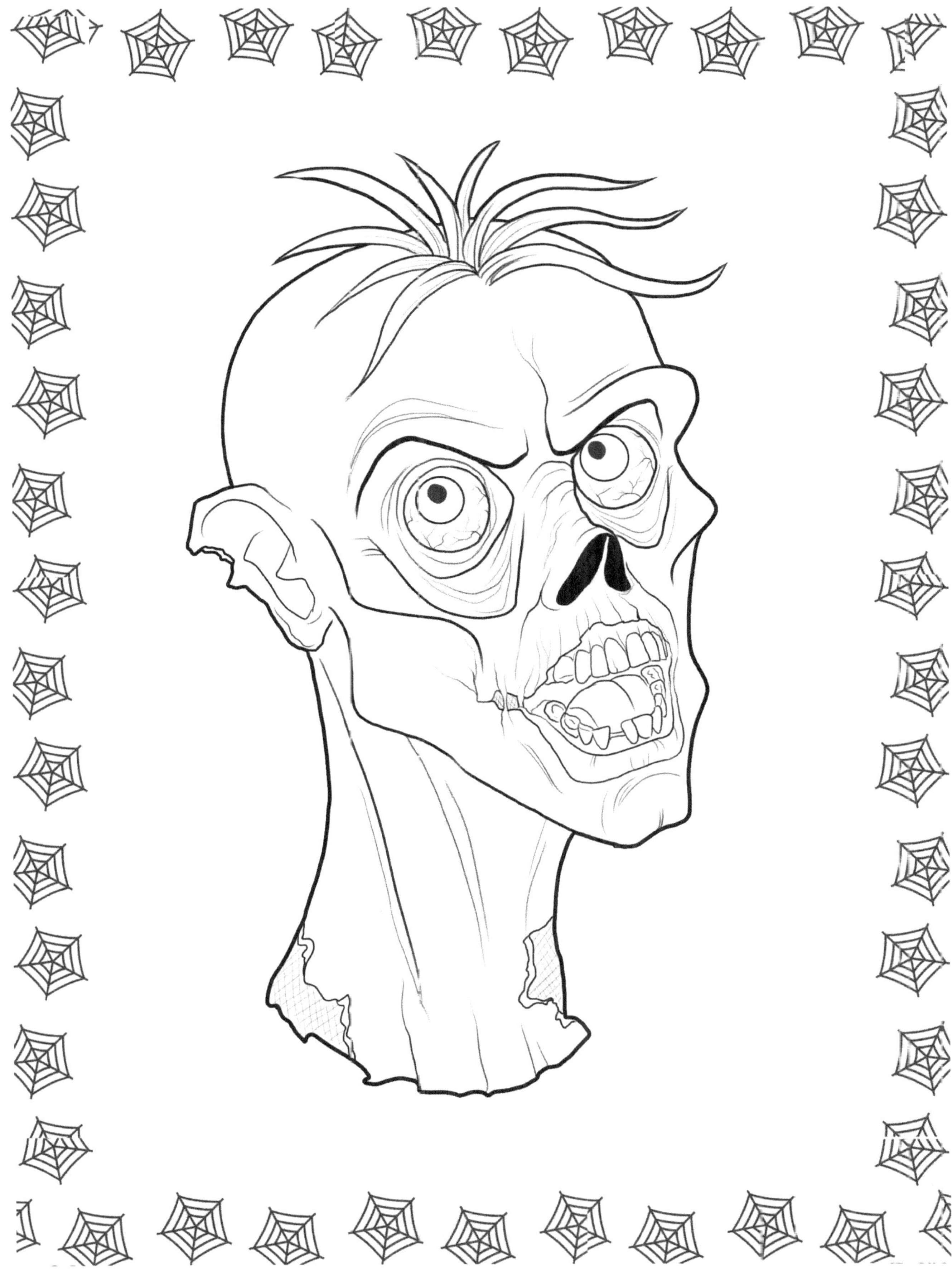

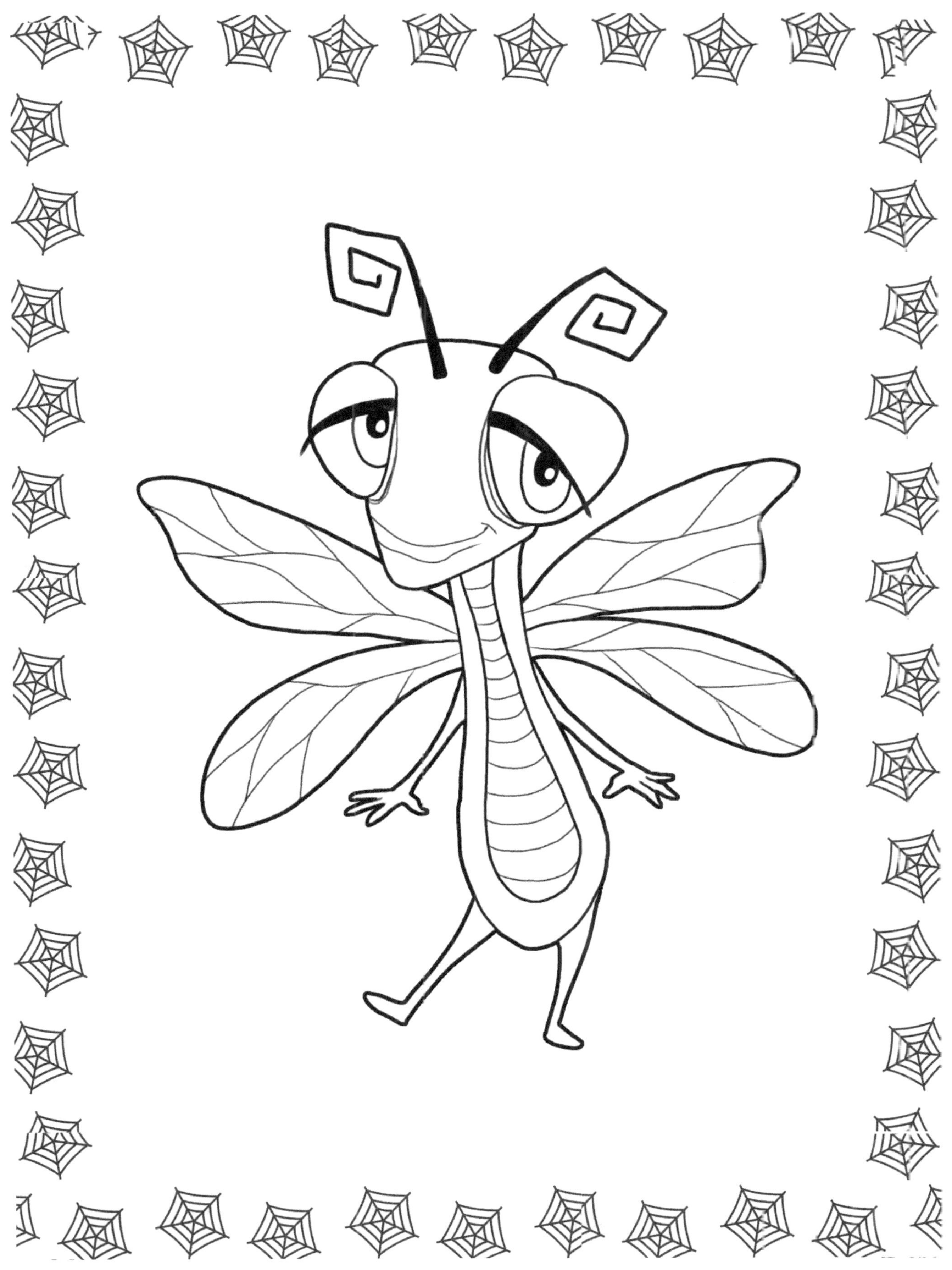

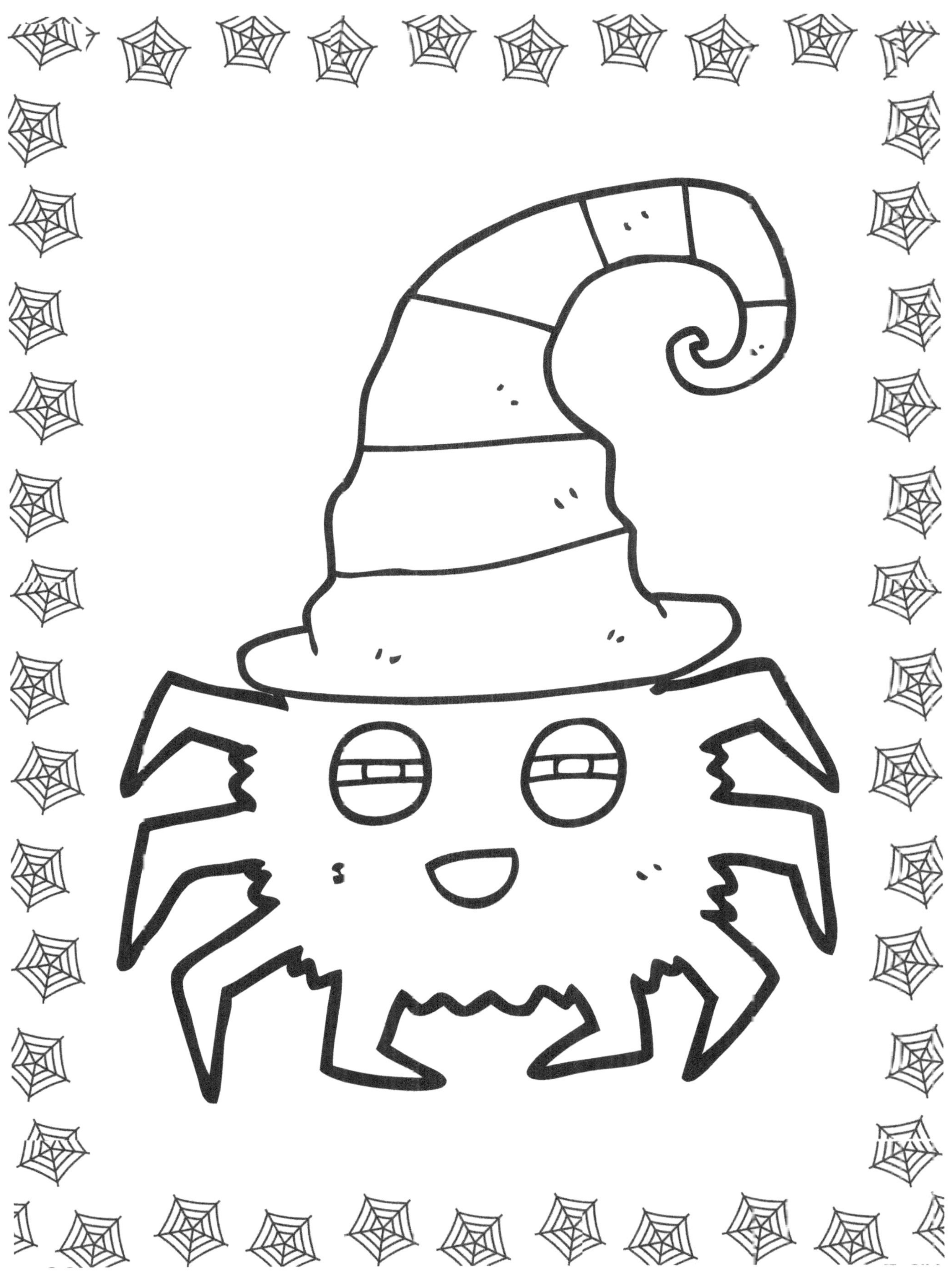

www.ingramcontent.com/pod-product-compliance
Lightning Source LLC
Chambersburg PA
CBHW081313250726
48662CB00008B/2553